review for
USMLE

**United States
Medical Licensing
Examination**

Step 2

National Medical Series

In the basic sciences

anatomy, 2nd edition
behavioral science, 2nd edition
biochemistry, 3rd edition
clinical epidemiology and
    biostatistics
genetics
hematology
histology and cell biology,
    2nd edition

human developmental anatomy
immunology, 2nd edition
introduction to clinical medicine
microbiology, 2nd edition
neuroanatomy
pathology, 3rd edition
pharmacology, 3rd edition
physiology, 2nd edition
radiographic anatomy

In the clinical sciences

medicine, 2nd edition
obstetrics and gynecology,
    3rd edition
pediatrics, 2nd edition
preventive medicine and
    public health, 2nd edition
psychiatry, 2nd edition
surgery, 2nd edition

In the exam series

review for USMLE Step 1,
    3rd edition
review for USMLE Step 2
geriatrics

The National Medical Series for Independent Study

review for USMLE

United States Medical Licensing Examination

Step 2

EDITOR

Edward F. Goljan, M.D.

Associate Professor of Pathology
Department of Pathology
Oklahoma State University College of Osteopathic Medicine
Tulsa, Oklahoma
Academic Coordinator
National Medical School Review
Newport Beach, California
714-476-6282

Williams & Wilkins

Philadelphia • Baltimore • Hong Kong • London • Munich • Sydney • Tokyo

A Waverly Company

**Williams
& Wilkins**

Test I:

The figure accompanying question 90 has been adapted with permission from Goldschlager N, Goldman M: *Principles of Clinical Electrocardiography,* 13th edition, Norwalk, CT, Appleton & Lange, 1989.

Test III:

The figures accompanying questions 25 and 65 have been adapted with permission from Goldschlager N, Goldman M: *Principles of Clinical Electrocardiography,* 13th edition, Norwalk, CT, Appleton & Lange, 1989.

Williams & Wilkins
Rose Tree Corporate Center, Building II
1400 North Providence Road, Suite 5025
Media, PA 19063-2043 USA

Accurate indications, adverse reactions, and dosage schedules for drugs are provided in this book, but it is possible they may change. The reader is urged to review the package information data of the manufacturers of the medications mentioned.

Printed in the United States of America

Library of Congress Cataloging in Publication Data

97 98
7 8 9 10

Dedication

To Kenneth Ibsen, Ph.D., for his tireless encouragement of thousands of medical students and the enrichment of their lives. You have made a difference!

Contents

National Medical School Review
4500 Campus Drive
Suite 201
Newport Beach, CA 92660
714-476-6282

Contributors

Grace Bingham, Ed.D.
President and Educational Consultant
Bingham Associates, Inc.
Toms River, New Jersey
Coordinator of Cognitive Skills
National Medical School Review
Newport Beach, California

Barbara Fadem, Ph.D.
Associate Professor of Psychiatry
Department of Psychiatry
University of Medicine and Dentistry of
   New Jersey
New Jersey Medical School
Newark, New Jersey
Director of Behavioral Science
National Medical School Review
Newport Beach, California

Edward F. Goljan, M.D.
Associate Professor of Pathology
Department of Pathology
Oklahoma State University College
   of Osteopathic Medicine
Clinical Associate Professor
Department of Obstetrics
   and Gynecology
University of Oklahoma College of Medicine
Tulsa, Oklahoma
Academic Coordinator
National Medical School Review
Newport Beach, California

Victor N. Gruber, M.D.
Founder and Executive Director
National Medical School Review
Newport Beach, California

Scot D. Hines, M.D.
Associate
Neuroscience Associates, PSC
Louisville, Kentucky
Director of Neurology
National Medical School Review
Newport Beach, California

Jasper McPhail, M.D., M.B.A.
Physician Manager
Metro Medical Associates
Dallas, Texas
Director of Surgery
National Medical School Review
Newport Beach, California

Eduardo Pino, M.D.
Assistant Professor of Pediatrics
Department of Pediatrics
Marshall University School of Medicine
Huntington, West Virginia
Director of Pediatrics
National Medical School Review
Newport Beach, California

Elmar Peter Sakala, M.D., M.A., M.P.H.
Associate Professor of Obstetrics and
   Gynecology
Department of Gynecology and Obstetrics
Director of Medical Student Education
Loma Linda University School of Medicine
Associate Professor of Nutrition
Department of Nutrition
Loma Linda University School of Public Health
Loma Linda, California
Director of Obstetrics and Gynecology
National Medical School Review
Newport Beach, California

Roderick Shaner, M.D.
Associate Professor of Clinical Psychiatry
Department of Psychiatry
University of Southern California School
   of Medicine
Los Angeles, California
Director of Psychiatry
National Medical School Review
Newport Beach, California

Anthony J. Trevor, Ph.D.
Professor of Pharmacology
Department of Pharmacology
University of California, San Francisco
School of Medicine
San Francisco, California
Director of Pharmacology
National Medical School Review
Newport Beach, California

Preface

Implementation of the single path to licensure for physicians who want to practice in the United States makes successful performance on USMLE Steps 1, 2, and 3 essential. In order to review for each examination as effectively as possible, students need to use the best study resources available.

This book is designed for medical students planning to take USMLE Step 2, an examination of the clinical sciences. The many areas of information assessed by the test require thorough review in order to ensure adequate preparation. In addition to study materials that review clinical content, students need material to help them gauge their ideas of content by practicing questions similar to those found on the actual examination.

Review for USMLE Step 2 contains a section to help students make the most of their studying (an examination preparation guide, which provides valuable suggestions for proper studying) and four practice examinations. The four composite question sets can be used in a number of different ways and at different times to meet particular purposes:

- As a diagnostic tool, or pretest, to check relative competency in the six clinical sciences before starting to review
- As a guide, or focus, for further study during the review process
- As a device for self-evaluation toward the end of the review to determine if clinical knowledge has reached a level that approximates, matches, or exceeds that expected for success on the USMLE Step 2

The questions in this book approximate both the topical distribution and complexity of those in Step 2. They are intended to be used as an integral part of a well-planned review process, rather than as an isolated resource.

Victor N. Gruber
Grace Bingham

Examination Preparation Guide

For most of you, USMLE Step 2 is not your first comprehensive national examination, nor will it be your last. With the introduction of USMLE Step 3 in 1994, the sequence of the single path to licensure will be complete. Demonstrating proficient performance is an ongoing reality in a physician's life, whether it is through standardized examinations, supervisory ratings, or through professional exchanges with colleagues.

During the past 10 years, medical schools have instituted a number of changes designed to make learning a more self-regulated process. The thrust of many of the innovations is toward increasing the independence and decision making of students who will be expected to continue their professional learning throughout their lives. The changes are consistent with recent findings from the fields of cognitive and educational psychology, which show that adults do better when they maintain responsibility for and feel in control of their own learning.

The topics presented in this examination preparation guide are directed toward assisting students in managing both the specific activities and the feelings associated with USMLE Step 2. You will be exercising your self-regulatory processes as you make decisions about what information to study, how to study it, how well to learn it, when to schedule it, and how you are feeling as you do so.

You may be a student who performed quite well in all your clinical courses; then again, you may be someone who passed everything but have a number of weak spots remaining. Perhaps your clinical training took place quite some time ago, and you are concerned because there are many topics you need to update. Regardless of which category best describes you, the realization that soon you will be facing USMLE Step 2—a national, standardized, comprehensive examination—may leave you wondering how best to prepare.

This part of the book is intended to guide your examination preparation to help you get the best return from your study investment by increasing your chances of successful performance. The ideas and suggestions discussed here have evolved from many years of experience working with hundreds of medical students in similar test preparation circumstances. In subsequent pages, you will read much more about each preparation component, but it might be best to start by looking at a few principles that have general applicability, regardless of your specific situation.

Develop a plan you can live with. Approach preparation for this examination with the belief that it is a manageable task, one that is within your capabilities to accomplish successfully. Be ready to acknowledge that it will require a commitment of time, effort, and appropriate study resources. Whether your motivation is high and you feel fired up or you are still trying to build steam, begin by engaging in some preliminary planning. You want to make the most effective use of whatever time you have available, regardless of whether it is months or just weeks before the exam. Be reasonable in your planning; you are more likely to stick to a plan that does not require drastic changes in your usual study habits. A few modifications to meet specific purposes will probably work best. Also keep in mind that it is better to plan regular periods of study, rather than establishing an all-or-nothing pattern (i.e., loading up study activities at one stretch, followed by long periods of neglect).

Study in an active, fully engaged manner. It may seem odd to make such a statement to students who have been learning and studying all of their lives. Yet, experience has shown that for some students, studying has been largely a routine process, one engaged in but never really analyzed. Many students cannot identify what particular study strategies are most useful to them.

To study actively means to **approach studying as if on a search,** seeking to find and extract meaning from any domain of information rather than being led by the study material. Viewed in this way, studying becomes a series of deliberate acts, each of which accomplishes a specific goal. As you proceed with your review, always be aware of **what** you are doing, and **why** you are doing it. You are the one controlling the study process.

Avoid the common pitfalls. Students take many different study routes when preparing for a Board examination. After receiving their test results, some are quite satisfied, feeling that their scores are consistent with the time and effort they expended reviewing. Others, although they may have passed, are a bit puzzled because they believe their scores do not reflect what they really know. A small number of students are not successful and experience feelings of anger and bewilderment about what went wrong for them. It is helpful to consider some ineffective behaviors that have caused problems for students preparing for Board examinations.

Studying what is already known. Students often spend an inordinate amount of time reviewing topics that are already part of their repertoire, hoping that if they have them mastered, it will compensate for their lack of knowledge in other areas. Obviously, decisions about which topics require mastery, and which can be learned with less proficiency, should be made carefully. Most students have a pretty good idea about which topics in each clinical science absolutely must be learned. To bypass any of them now, even if they have been troublesome in the past, would be risky. For any Board examination, your review will need to be comprehensive but priorities will still have to be set based on your particular needs.

Studying for a declarative test. Students sometimes use study materials too literally. That is, they learn information almost exactly as it is presented in a particular resource, as if they were memorizing a script and would be expected to "declare" their knowledge in the same form. Board questions will not require you to repeat what you know, but will require you to use your knowledge as a base for making decisions about diagnosis, treatment, and prognosis; forming judgments; and drawing conclusions or inferences. To do this with comfort on the examination, **practice these activities as part of the review**.

Misjudging the examination. Students occasionally fall victim to their misjudgments about the examination. For example, those who were unsuccessful will sometimes say they "had no idea" the examination would be as "detailed" as it was, or as "comprehensive," or that some of the questions would have "such long stems," and so on. Other students report that their estimates of how much they thought they could accomplish within their study sessions were way off the mark. Obviously, few of us are able to plan every facet of this type of review with unerring accuracy. It is expected that as you proceed, you will have to modify or fine tune some features of your study plan. To do so, however, you need to be self-observant and attend to any feedback that tells you something needs to be changed while there is still time to do it.

Losing focus (scattering). Even students who have laid out a reasonable review plan sometimes fall victim to "scattering." For example, Tim completed all of the activities he had planned for the first 3 weeks of his review. He was feeling rather good about his efforts until he started talking to Jane, and discovered that she had taken an entirely different approach in her plan. Doubts begin to surface: Perhaps he should try Jane's plan? She is using a different book; maybe it is better? There are many variations of this example, but the outcome is usually the same—valuable time and effort are lost as students change their study plan midstream. They lose their focus as well as their sense of accomplishment. Developing a sensible plan that suits your needs minimizes the temptation to scatter your efforts.

Avoiding question practice. Many students still perceive testing solely as an evaluative activity, something you do only when you have reached complete mastery. As a result, some get to the end of their review without having practiced the very behaviors expected on the examination. They tell themselves they will get to the questions "later," when they "really know it," but in many cases time runs out. Self-testing should be part of the entire review process, an ongoing activity serving a number of purposes.

Not managing feelings. Students preparing for a comprehensive examination experience a wide range of emotions, from an "upbeat" sense of control to frustration, despondency, or anger. Some students still carry the burden of anxiety from previous unsuccessful Board examination experiences. It is not hard to understand why students experience such stress when one considers the importance of these tests in their lives. It is possible, however, to reduce stress and minimize negative self-evaluation through the use of effective learning strategies, practice testing, and positive self-reinforcement.

USMLE Step 2: What to Expect

Since their introduction, much has been said about the "new" USMLE Steps 1 and 2 examinations for licensure. Questions still arise about whether they differ substantially from the former National Board of Medical Examinations Parts I and II examinations, or whether the changes are mainly structural [e.g., elimination of K-type (multiple comparison) questions, inclusion of extended-matching questions]. There is no doubt that most of the questions in Step 2 describe a vignette giving pertinent information and then require the examinee to provide a diagnosis, choose a treatment option, select the next step in management, and so forth. However, questions requiring recall of specific mechanisms or details of disease processes are still represented. Step 2 is a sophisticated, carefully constructed examination designed to elicit a wide range of clinical knowledge and skills.

Following is a brief summary of what can be found in much more detail in the materials distributed to students when they register for the Step 2 examination (i.e., "Bulletin of Information," "Step 2—General Instructions, Content Outline, and Sample Items"). **Both booklets should be read in their entirety before taking the examination.**

Description. The purpose of USMLE Step 2 is to assess medical knowledge and the understanding of clinical sciences that are essential to providing patient care under supervision, including emphasis on health and disease prevention. There are three categories used for organizing clinical science material: physician task, population group, and disease process. Of the four subdivisions in the physician task category, understanding mechanisms of disease and establishing a diagnosis receive substantial attention in question construction, as can be seen by the percentages in the "General Instructions" booklet.

Format. USMLE Step 2 is a 2-day multiple-choice examination consisting of four 3-hour test books with approximately 200 questions in each book. Each book includes items from the wide range of topics included in the examination: internal medicine, obstetrics and gynecology, pediatrics, preventive medicine and public health, psychiatry, surgery, and any other areas considered essential to the provision of care under supervision.

Question types. There are two types of questions on USMLE Step 2: **A-types,** which have one best answer, including those questions that are negatively phrased, and **B-types,** which are matching sets. Each type is grouped together, with the highest proportion of questions being A-types. The B-types each start with a list of four to twenty-six options, which are used for all items in the set. The "General Instructions" booklet describes strategies for answering each type of question.

Scoring. Each question is worth one point if answered correctly, and passing is based on the total score. Raw scores are converted to a standard score scale with a mean of 200 and a standard deviation of 20. The minimum passing score for Step 2 is 167. A two-digit score is also reported, in which a score of 75 is equivalent to the minimum passing score on the three-digit scale. The percentage of items that correspond to these passing scores generally falls between 55% and 65%. Scores are reported to examinees with a pass/fail designation, a score on the three-digit scale, and a corresponding score on the two-digit scale. Graphic performance profiles summarizing areas of strength and weakness are also included.

Components of Successful Preparation

Whether you are planning to review independently or to participate in a structured review program, the preparation components that lead to successful performance will be the same. In a review program they are built into the design of the course. Students preparing on their own will need to include these components intentionally as part of their overall study plan.

Strengthening Knowledge of the Clinical Sciences

There is no question that the foremost agenda item of any review is to retrieve knowledge and strengthen recall of a vast amount of clinical material. For some students, this may simply mean reactivating what was previously learned and learned well. Other students, in addition to reviewing, may need to clarify topics that are still confusing, or to acquire "new" information about topics insufficiently learned the first time. Obviously, the scope and stability of prior knowledge will influence the amount of time and effort required for the review, as well as the type and extent of study resources to be used.

Each student represents a unique profile when it comes to making study decisions. Those who know themselves and use both self-observations and data from past performances will be in a better position to know which topics in each clinical area are already under their control, which need a bit more emphasis, and which require concentrated, intensive effort.

Diagnostic information. There are two sources of information you can use to help yourself get started. First, find your **performance scores from your clinical courses**. Take a sheet of paper and arrange them in descending order beginning with your best score. If you have taken a **recent composite clinical diagnostic test,** arrange these scores in the same manner and place them next to the other data. (If you have not taken a recent clinical test, there are directions for doing so using one of the tests in this book in the section "Using These Practice Exams.")

Now look at the two sets of scores and make some observations. Think of your hierarchy of six clinical areas as three bands with two sciences in each band, "top," "middle," and "relatively weak." Are there any consistencies? For example, do you show the same two sciences in the top band even if their positions are not exactly the same? Make similar comparisons about the other two bands. Are there any unusual patterns for which you cannot account (e.g., a science that you have always considered your strength falls near the bottom in your diagnostic test)? The goal of this level of comparison is either to confirm your self-perceptions of strength and relative weakness in each clinical area, or to uncover an area that warrants more attention than you had intended to give it.

A third source of information is available to students who have already taken Step 2 and were not successful. Obviously, data from a recent examination should be analyzed and given careful attention, particularly the graphic material that shows areas of strength and weakness.

Where to begin. Having identified your clinical science profile of strengths and needs, which one should you start studying first? There are different points of view, most of them based on student reports of what worked for them. One strategy that has been used successfully by many students is to study two sciences concurrently, a strong one teamed with a weaker one (described more fully in the section "Effective Time Management"). Another strategy is to start with the sciences in the middle range since they are the ones that stand the highest chance of being raised to a proficient level. When you start to review sciences that fall in the weak range, select and study the essentials first, then fill in with other topics. Be careful of spending so much time on a troublesome area that you do not move on to others that are just as important and more available to understanding.

Effective Time Management

It seems that no matter how much time students set aside to prepare for a comprehensive examination, most reach the end feeling that they need more time to feel *really* ready. The amount of time needed to prepare adequately will vary according to factors such as the strength of prior knowledge, motivation, and the pressure of other life events. Unless you are planning to devote all of your time to studying, it is wise to start 3 months before the exam, or earlier, if possible. This is based on an estimate of 4 to 5 hours of study each day (25–30 hours per week) or about half the number of hours per week of a student in a full-time, 6-week review course.

Develop a study schedule by allocating segments of time to each clinical area, either by hours, days, or weeks. For example, if you are scheduling by weeks, you may decide that for you, 1 week for reviewing psychiatry will be sufficient, but internal medicine will need at least 2 weeks. Continue estimating across the remaining clinical sciences, taking into consideration the results of your previous performances. If possible, leave the last 2 weeks unscheduled for returning to topics that need more study, for comprehensive self-testing, and for focused follow-up study. As you implement your schedule, modify your estimates as needed for particular topics.

Blocks of study time. Assuming you plan to study 4 to 5 hours each night, you might consider dividing those hours into two study blocks. This allows you to study two clinical areas each evening, if you wish: one that is weaker and therefore requires more time, and another that is relatively strong, and can be allocated a little less time. The advantage of studying two sciences concurrently is that you will move through your strong science with more ease and feel a sense of accomplishment, even if the weaker science is not yet firmly under control. If you find that pattern too confusing, you can devote all of your study hours to one science until that one is completed, then start reviewing another.

Setting goals for each study period. Begin each study session by identifying a few goals you think can be accomplished within that period. They need not be elaborately stated; simply trying to articulate what you think is important makes it more likely that you will be studying actively. Try to target three or four essentials (i.e., concepts, procedures, treatments) that you wish to make a firmer part of your knowledge base. By the time you have completed the study period, your awareness of the material will have been heightened and your recall strengthened. A number of recent studies confirm the benefits of setting study goals.

Additional suggestions. A number of other time management suggestions follow. If any apply to you, decide if it would be in your best interest to modify the behavior that interferes with your effective use of time.

1. **Plan what you would like to accomplish** by writing lists of tasks. Prioritize them from those that must be done to those that are not absolutely essential.
2. **Develop schedules,** even though you may find you cannot follow them exactly as planned. It is better to adjust an already existing schedule than to operate without any structure.
3. **Use record-keeping devices** to help you stay organized; appointment books and large desk calendars that show a whole month can be used to jot notes for long-range study planning.
4. **Set realistic deadlines.** It is self-defeating to set arbitrary completion targets if you know there is little or no chance of meeting them.
5. **Make use of your best time of the day** (i.e., when you feel most energetic) and schedule tasks that require the most concentration during those periods.

6. **Avoid starting too many tasks** and not being able to finish any of them. Bring some tasks to closure so that you can feel a sense of achievement.
7. **Keep fighting procrastination.** The temptation to put tasks off until later will always be there. Avoid using chores or telephone calls as a convenient excuse to avoid studying. Family and friends want to be supportive; they will understand.

Using Appropriate Study Materials

Finding just the right study materials for managing a productive review of clinical sciences can sometimes prove frustrating. Although a number of study resources are available on the market, each differs in purpose, format, depth, and comprehensiveness of coverage. If still available, **your own notes, outlines, charts, or handouts are excellent resources** because they are organized in ways that have personal meaning for you. They probably contain cues that will jog your memory. In making your selections from published materials, four types are useful to consider.

Review books. Summarized or compacted information resources are available for each of the six large domains of clinical information (i.e., internal medicine, obstetrics and gynecology, pediatrics, preventive medicine and public health, psychiatry, and surgery). These books should provide just enough narrative (without being excessively wordy) for you to reactivate each topic. Some series include study questions at the end of each topic, and a comprehensive examination at the end of the book.

Textbooks. It is unlikely that you will have time to reread the texts that were excellent resources during your initial mastery of clinical material. However, you should identify and have available a preferred text for each of the clinical areas to use as a supplementary reference if you find that some topics in your concise review materials are not as detailed as you might wish.

Question books. A number of Board examination question books are currently available. Although they vary in many ways, two criteria should be met by all of them. First, the questions should approximate the format and level of complexity of the USMLE Step 2 examination questions. Second, answers should be sufficiently explanatory. Question books can be classified into three types. (Suggestions for their use are provided in the section "Monitoring Study Progress.")

1. Books consisting of **questions organized by topic,** representing all major topics in each of the six clinical sciences.
2. Books of **randomly arranged questions** representing all pertinent topics in each clinical science. These are typically used after review of all topics in a science has been completed.
3. **Mixed composite sets of questions** representing the full range of topics in all clinical areas and approximating the format of the USMLE Step 2 examination. (This book is an example.)

Computerized question sets. There are now a few of these question banks available from various publishing companies. Some offer explanations for incorrect responses, whereas others simply indicate which option is correct. Most are organized so that you can call up a batch of questions by topic within a science, by mixed topics, or by randomly arranged questions in all of the clinical sciences covered on the Step 2 examination.

Using Productive Study Strategies

The goal of most students when reviewing for any examination is to study the largest number of topics in the shortest period of time. The question to ask yourself as you review material should be, "Is this information already a part of my knowledge base and do I just need to **retrieve and consolidate** it or is it something about which I need to **extend** my knowledge?" In other words, what will it take for you to make that information sufficiently firm so that you can recall it dependably at examination time?

Preview. One strategy is to take any topic or subtopic and preview its organization in whatever study resource you are using before doing any reading. **Notice particularly how the topic and its subtopics are interconnected** and whether the main thoughts are linked to one another in a meaningful way. Pay attention to your reactions of familiarity or unfamiliarity with the material; they are your first cues about how smoothly you will proceed as you try to study. If you are participating in a structured review course, previewing before lectures is a useful technique that helps you get more out of the lecture.

Proceed briskly. Process most of what you read at a pace that is brisk but allows you to extract meaning and make sense of what you see. **Move through the ideas as if you were a camera with a zoom lens;** if you encounter a concept, procedure, or explanation that does not make sense with what you have just been reading, slow your pace, "zoom in," and focus a bit more closely. Varying your processing rate is one way to implement an active study approach.

Recap. Although studying at a brisk pace is recommended, you will need to restrain yourself from moving through topics so rapidly that you end up reviewing superficially. One way to avoid this is to pause after each subtopic or other meaningful block of information and **summarize** or **restate** the most important ideas you have just reviewed. Allow yourself a few minutes to relate what you just studied to other topics; that is, to **think about** the material and to **think with it**. A particularly valuable study activity is to imagine how you would explain a given procedure to another person.

Reformat. Reformatted materials, such as **charts, outlines, index cards,** and **diagrams,** can be quite useful because the arrangement is personalized by you and, therefore, more easily remembered. It is best to reformat information early in your review—not too close to the examination deadline.

Take notes. Students often ask whether they have time to construct their own notes and what kinds of notes they should be keeping. There is not time to construct your own notes if you typically take elaborate, detailed notes. Assuming that you are using well-organized, condensed review materials, there should be less need to summarize what is already a summarized version. There will be times, however, when you want to restate something in a way that makes it more meaningful to you. Do not let the task of taking notes become so lengthy and time-consuming that little time remains to learn and remember what is in those notes.

One note-taking device is the personal "study laundry list." As you study each clinical science, record specific items you want to review again by noting the page number and the name of the subtopic, mechanism, or procedure. You may also add a brief explanation or note particular points that are problematic for you. These reduced notes are handy during the last few days before the exam, when you want to make sure you still recall what you studied in the earlier weeks of the review.

Synthesize. If you have confidence in the study materials you have chosen, you will probably need to do little synthesizing from multiple sources. **Try using one reliable review source** as you "road map" each of the clinical areas and supplement with other materials only if you really need to do so. It is inefficient to try to cover the same topics in many sources. However, if you are using a set of your own notes on a particular topic, you may still want to check another resource. If you do, read your notes first, then look for differences in the other source and highlight them.

Recall. One of the questions most frequently asked by students trying to review vast amounts of information is, "What can I do to help myself remember all the material?" Some of the strategies that follow are useful for improving memory skills.

1. **Categorical clustering.** Use materials that are well-organized and meaningful; they are more likely to be remembered. Each science has subdivisions or categories into which information can be organized. These subdivisions recur and can be recognized readily

as you become familiar with a particular science, and they form your cognitive framework for that science. When studying, think in terms of clusters of categories rather than trying to recall isolated items or lists.

2. **Visual imaging.** This is a valuable skill for physicians. It is one you have probably used throughout your medical training, and it is one that can be used in your review. For example, revisualize an anatomic structure and draw it from memory; sketch the grainy surface of a particular cell; recall the vivid stain of a laboratory test; picture ECG tracings and the meaning of each pattern; or revisualize the sequence of a surgical procedure. It is also helpful in storing such visual images to tie in an oral statement about what you see. In addition, as you review, try to place yourself mentally in the situation where you first acquired your knowledge of the subject. Try to bring it back, along with any perceptual cues that may be associated with the information (e.g., form, shape, color, texture).

3. **Rehearsal.** There will be relatively few occasions when you will need to repeat information verbatim. Therefore, rehearsing only by **rote repetition has limited usefulness**. More often, the expectation will be that you understand and can apply information in a variety of forms. There are other ways to consolidate material in long-term memory that are more strategic because they emphasize relationships or the logic or structure of the material.
   a. **Analogies** involve associating what you are learning to a concept or idea that is already familiar to you.
   b. **Paraphrasing** is a good way to find out if you have really made sense of a concept or are just repeating words.
   c. **Inferences** are like bridges from your partial knowledge to what you are trying to remember. What you already know can help you form reasonable guesses or estimates about what you are trying to recall.

4. **Cumulative distributed practice.** When you need to remember lists or strings of items, learn a few blocks of information at one session and take a break. At the next session, review those blocks first, then add a few more. Follow the same procedure until the list is firmly in your memory. Distributed practice produces stronger consolidation.

5. **Mnemonics** are mental cues used to associate a wide range of information. Medical students usually have heard a few from other students or have constructed some themselves. Among the most common types of mnemonic devices are:
   a. **First letter mnemonics** use the first letter of each item to be remembered. For example, "kinds of tumors leaping promptly to bone" refers to kidney, ovary, testis, lung, prostate, thyroid, and bowel. Any mnemonic device, no matter how silly or bizarre, is useful if it has particular meaning to you.
   b. **Acronyms** are words that have some relationship to the material to be remembered. The first letter triggers recall. For example, BITE-M for the muscles of mastication (i.e., buccinator, internal pterygoid, temporalis, external pterygoid, masseter).
   c. **Method of loci** may be the oldest mnemonic device around. In preliterate societies, orators used it to help themselves remember their speeches. Think of a very familiar location, one that you can "see" mentally, such as your bedroom. Place what you want to remember in various spots around the room. When you want to recall, revisualize the locations and bring back the ideas, concepts, or items you placed there.

6. **Study with peers.** Many students find it very helpful to meet periodically with others to study. If you opt to join a study group, try to keep the size of the group small (from two to five people), so that everyone has an opportunity to participate rather than to simply be a passive listener. Members of the group will benefit more from this kind of study if each one has given the material some attention before the group meeting. This preliminary review increases the chance that the session will be spent reinforcing learning by integrating ideas, clarifying confusing concepts, and drawing relationships, all of which

make recall more dependable. Group question and answer sessions, using Board-type questions, are effective for practice in applying test-taking strategies. Here, too, the most efficient use of time is made if students attempt the questions on their own first, then meet to discuss their choices with the group.

Applying Effective Test-taking Skills

General test-taking skills. What follows in this section and others are principles that increase the likelihood that what you learned and can recall from your review will translate into correct responses on multiple-choice examinations. This first set is applicable to most test-taking situations.

1. **Read carefully for comprehension, not speed,** and respond to questions in **sequence.** Mark every item on your answer sheet as you go along, even if you are not completely sure of your choice. Note in your book the questions to which you want to return if there is time.

2. **Keep a positive attitude.** Suppose the first question you see as you open the test book is a particularly difficult one, and you can feel yourself becoming anxious. After giving it a try, go right to the second question, which in all likelihood will feel more accessible. The point is to get into a positive frame of mind and have a good attitude concerning the examination.

3. **Be alert to key terms** in the question stems such as negatives (i.e., except, not, least) and words such as "primarily," "frequently," "most often," "most likely," and so on, or notice transition words that signal a change in meaning such as "but," "although," "however."

4. **To change or not to change a response** still puzzles students. The prevailing viewpoint is to change if you have thought of additional information; otherwise, let your original response stand.

5. **Pace yourself.** You will have approximately 60 seconds per question. Avoid dwelling on any one question or rushing to finish. Set up check points in your test booklet of where you want to be at the end of the first hour and second hour. You will know before you get close to the end whether you need to adjust your pace.

Analyzing questions. When you first read a question and look at the options, the answer may not be immediately apparent. Do not be tempted just to pick an answer and move on. It is at this point that you can be systematic and apply fairly straightforward reasoning skills of logic and deduction to narrow five options to two or three possibilities.

1. **Search for key information.** As you read the question stem, highlight key information (e.g., age, symptoms, lab results, chronic or acute condition, distinctive facts in the history). **Notice particularly the request of the question** in phrases such as, "the most likely diagnosis is," "the most appropriate initial step in management is," "which initial diagnostic evaluation is most appropriate?" Take a quick look at the last line of the stem before reading the specific information in the remainder of the stem, especially if it is lengthy.

2. **Analyze options.** As you reach each option, your objective is to **try to eliminate** those that are inconsistent with the information you highlighted in the stem. For example, if a question concerns a 65-year-old woman, you would eliminate a treatment that you know applies only to children.

3. **Cue each option.** As you consider each option, mark down your initial reaction. In an A-type question (i.e., single best answer) there are four "false" options and one that is true. For negative A-type questions, the reverse applies. As you read each option, cue

those you are sure of with a symbol such as "F," "N," or a minus sign. Cue true responses with a "T," "Y," or a plus sign. Cue those options you are uncertain about with the symbol you are using and a question mark. In arriving at your decision, focus your attention only on those options cued with question marks.

4. **Analyze structural clues in words.** Pay attention to the meaning of prefixes, suffixes, and root words. They can sometimes help you decide whether to eliminate an option.

Approaching questions stragically. The following examples show how you might approach questions found in USMLE Step 2.

Example
A 25-year-old woman has a blood pressure of 145/95 after multiple readings on two separate visits. There is no family history of hypertension. Physical examination is unremarkable. Which of the following is the most likely cause of this woman's hypertension?
(A) Essential hypertension
(B) Turner's syndrome
(C) Fibromuscular hyperplasia of the renal artery
(D) Pheochromocytoma
(E) Oral contraceptives

Analysis: The fact that there is nothing remarkable in the physical examination allows you to eliminate B, C, and D, which are conditions that would show other symptoms. That leaves options A and E. The age of the patient and the absence of a family history of hypertension make option A unlikely. The patient may be using oral contraceptives, which are the most common medical cause of hypertension in a woman. Therefore, the best choice is E.

Comment: It is quite possible that when you read this question the answer was immediately apparent. However, practicing analysis of what seems to be a rather easy question makes it more likely that you will apply it to more difficult questions when necessary.

Example
A 19-year-old man with a history of chronic lung disease, pancreatic insufficiency, and infertility most likely has which one of the following disorders?
(A) a_1-Antitrypsin deficiency
(B) Cystic fibrosis
(C) Kartagener's syndrome
(D) IgA deficiency
(E) Klinefelter's syndrome

Analysis: This looks like a differential diagnosis question, which means that some of the disorders will have one or more of the three symptoms but only one will have all three. Infertility is a symptom of Klinefelter's syndrome, but chronic lung disease and pancreatic insufficiency are not, so E is eliminated. Kartagener's syndrome has to do with ciliary motility, which would indicate chronic respiratory disease, but probably not the other two symptoms. Your hunch is to eliminate C. Of the three remaining options, you know the most about cystic fibrosis. You know that it is definitely associated with chronic lung disease and pancreatic insufficiency, but you're not sure about infertility. However, you choose B.

Comment: Your sequence of deductive reasoning might not have followed exactly the pattern above, but the important point is to weigh evidence carefully before arriving at a differential diagnosis. Even after applying analysis, you might not feel completely certain, but you will have increased the probability of accuracy.

Relying on test question cues. The ability to use the characteristics or the formats of the test itself to increase your score is sometimes referred to as "test wiseness." It is possible to make use of idiosyncrasies in the way the questions are constructed to decide on the correct choice. This technique should be used only if you are unable to answer the question based on direct knowledge or reasoning. The following are examples of the principles of test wiseness, but you may have little opportunity to use them on USMLE Step 2 because the experts who construct the questions eliminate these cues.

1. **Length of an option.** If an option is much longer or much shorter than the others, it is more likely to be correct.
2. **Grammatical consistency.** Options that are not grammatically aligned with the stem are probably false. There is grammatical alignment between the stem and the correct answer.
3. **Specific determiners.** Words such as "all," "always," "never," and so on overqualify an option and are likely to be false.
4. **Overuse of the same words or expressions.** Some test makers have a tendency to repeat words or phrases in the options. If you are unsure of an answer, select from the options with the repeated words or phrases. Another variation of this principle is to select an option in which a key word from the stem is repeated.
5. **Numeric mid-range.** When all options can be listed in numeric order (e.g., percentages), the correct choice will most often be one of the two middle values.

Guessing. The following might be termed "last resort" strategies but you should be aware of them.

1. If you have eliminated one or two options, but have no idea about the remaining ones, choose the first in the list.
2. If you have a number of questions left to do and time is running out, **do not leave blanks.** Choose A, B, or C, and fill in the same letter for all remaining questions.
3. If you are unable to eliminate any options, choose A, B, or C.

Monitoring Study Progress

Preparation for an examination such as USMLE Step 2 spans a number of weeks or months. It requires that you be able to track your own progress and accurately **assess the state of your knowledge.** Perhaps more than at any other time in your medical training, you will be the one imposing structure on yourself and making decisions about how to proceed. Although the need to self-monitor seems obvious, many students do not make it an intentional part of their review. The importance of self-monitoring cannot be overemphasized.

The main objective of self-monitoring is to make accurate decisions regarding which areas in each science are firmly under your control, which topics are fairly well mastered but still need reinforcement, and which topics are still shaky and require more intense study. There are several valuable sources of study-monitoring information.

Self-observations are thoughts, impressions, or reactions that you gather about yourself as you move through various phases of the review. For example, if you are part of a review course and are attending lectures, think about whether the content is making sense, whether new material fits in with what you already know, and how well your follow-up study of the new material is going.

While studying on your own, you might feel productive and focused, or you may feel distracted and find it difficult to get started on your study agenda. The study resources you are using may be just right for what you are trying to review, or the material may seem too sketchy and superficial.

If you do some of your studying with peers, other opportunities arise for self-observations. You may find that you can recall material and talk confidently during discussions, or your knowledge may seem shallow compared with that of others in the group. You may be able to elaborate on or clarify topics, or you may seem to lack pertinent details. You may be able to respond promptly and accurately to most questions, or you may find it difficult to recall material you thought you learned.

The examples above are just a small sample of what you might observe about your own study behavior. Self-observations should not be ignored; they may be signalling that all is well or that there is a need to modify some aspect of your study routine. Using self-observations in combination with quantitative data from self-testing will help you make more accurate study decisions.

Self-testing. The value of engaging in self-testing has been noted in other sections. These types of monitoring activities are data based; that is, they provide numeric scores for charting your progress. The following are suggestions for implementing a self-monitoring sequence along with some simple record keeping.

1. **Diagnostic tests.** If you do not have recent information about your performance in the various clinical sciences, it would be best to engage in some form of diagnostic testing to establish some baselines. One possibility is to use one of the tests in this book for that purpose. Steps 1 through 6 in "Using These Practice Exams" can be applied to any other diagnostic test(s) you may wish to use.

   a. After completing steps 1 through 6, record the results of your diagnostic test.

   b. After you have completed your initial study of all areas, you may want to retake the diagnostic examination as a "post-test" and compare results.

   c. If the diagnostic test you used was lengthy, your post-test check can be a sampling of every other question to see how much improvement you made following your first pass at the material.

   d. If your performance has not yet reached the level you are aiming for, continue to analyze errors and focus on follow-up study.

2. **Monitoring progress using published question sources.** These books or computerized banks of Board-type questions are similar to those found on the target exam. Not surprisingly, there are differences among them in the scope and depth of coverage, question difficulty, extent and clarity of answers, and whether they include questions that measure higher-order learning outcomes (e.g., application of knowledge, analysis, synthesis, evaluation). These practice questions serve two main functions: (1) to determine in what areas and to what degree further study is needed, and (2) to make further study more focused, productive, and dependable. After taking a diagnostic test or a pretest, begin your study of a topic and periodically test yourself to get feedback on what additional follow-up study is needed. Try to do some self-testing throughout your review, not just at the end. The sequence outlined below is a desirable one.

   a. As each major topic is completed in a clinical science, sample a batch of 25 to 50 Board-type questions that test the essential information.

   b. After all topics in a science have been reviewed, take a comprehensive test of mixed topics within that science.

   c. Follow the same procedure for all other clinical sciences included in the review. d. After all clinical sciences have been studied, take a comprehensive composite test with randomly arranged questions that cover the content addressed by the examination. This should simulate the format of USMLE Step 2.

3. **Suggested procedures when using Board-type questions**

   a. It is strongly suggested that you do not do questions one at a time and then read the correct answer. The purpose of self-monitoring is not to study particular questions, but to have questions indicate something to you about your progress.

   b. **Use a separate sheet of paper as an answer sheet** instead of answering questions in the book. This will give you space to make notes as you do error analysis. It also keeps questions clean for future retakes, if needed.

c. **Adhere to the same time limits as expected on the target examination** (no more than 60 seconds per question). When you have finished the whole set, score your responses. If an answer is correct, do not mark it in any way. If it is incorrect, put a bracket around it. **Do not record the correct answer next to it, and do not read the correct answer at this time.** Compute an accuracy percentage by dividing the number correct by the total number of questions.

d. **Keep a record of your scores,** and note whether your accuracy level is approaching the 55% to 65% expected for passing the Board examination or whether it is far above it or far below it. The nature of your follow-up study will vary according to your results. If your score is quite low, it would be better to review the entire topic again rather than to analyze individual errors.

e. If you can afford the time, **give the incorrect questions another try**. If you are correct on the second attempt, your information was close but not on target. Follow-up study for this question may be minimal. However, if you are still incorrect on the second try, more sustained study is needed.

4. **Error analysis** is an important dimension of data-based assessment because you move beyond the score to analyzing more specific aspects of your study and test-taking behavior. The objective is to use your errors to help you diagnose what needs to be changed or fine-tuned.

a. Were there patterns of errors (e.g., were more rheumatology and renal questions missed than any others in the area of medicine, or were questions related to DNA principles consistently missed regardless of the clinical area with which they were associated)?

b. Was there a pattern in the question type missed (e.g., negatively phrased A-type questions)?

c. Did you misread or misunderstand the point of the question?

d. Was your answer close but you had trouble recalling specific details?

e. Were errors made, although you "knew the facts," because you were unable to make a decision between two management plans, make a prediction about disease progression, form a judgment about appropriate intervention, engage in differential diagnosis? In other words, were you unable to transform your information to meet the request of the question? Did you note that one type of question request was missed more than any other?

5. **Follow-up study.** After completing error analysis and noting your observations, you can develop a follow-up study agenda. You will need to decide what kinds of focused study activities will be most appropriate.

a. If you found patterns of error, you now have a heightened awareness of what topics you need to reinforce. Did the resources you used explain these topics adequately? When you take a comprehensive clinical test at a later time, note if you are able to answer questions related to those topics with accuracy.

b. If a particular kind of question format was a problem, check the appropriate strategy for dealing with such questions, then select a different set of questions about the same topic but practice only the format you missed. Note if the same pattern shows up when you do questions on a different topic.

c. If you misread or misunderstood the point of questions, remember to highlight key information in the question stem and to focus on comprehension rather than speed.

d. If you found yourself forgetting details, reading the correct answers and attending to the specifics that you forgot may be sufficient. Or, you may want to make a list and construct a mnemonic device to help you recall.

    e. If most of your errors are related to the request of the question, you need to strengthen your ability to identify the information that the question assumes you know (e.g., mechanism of a particular disease, initial management, emergency management, chronic care). Try practicing the question analysis procedures with a peer in which you make your thinking overt. Feedback about why your analysis of a question is faulty can be helpful.

    f. If no particular patterns are found and your errors are scattered, simply reading the correct answers may be sufficient to lock in the information.

Managing Your Feelings

If preparing successfully for USMLE Step 2 were strictly a cognitive activity, there would be no need to deal with the affective dimension. However, there is general agreement that emotional and cognitive processes are so closely linked that feelings, attitudes, and beliefs can either enhance or sabotage intellectual functioning. The pressure of trying to complete vast amounts of work in a limited amount of time and the need to demonstrate proficiency to receive favorable evaluations makes students susceptible to stress.

    Test anxiety is a phenomenon that has affected almost all of us at one time or another, usually in relation to a specific course or a particular examination. There have been hundreds of studies of test anxiety but the findings that are of most interest to students preparing for an exam like USMLE Step 2 are:

1. Practicing and using learning strategies facilitate performance.
2. The more frequent a student's contact with tests of a specific type given for a specific purpose, the less likely he or she is to be subjected to extreme anxiety.
3. The best defense against test anxiety is a combination of strong review of subject matter, practicing tests similar to the target test, and positive self-reinforcement throughout the process.

    Positive self-reinforcement. Most of us at some time or other have tried to talk ourselves into a change of mood or tried to convince ourselves we could do a particular task. As you begin preparing for this examination, part of your self-monitoring should include an awareness of your moods and general state of being. Using positive self-reinforcement means being sensitive to when you are about to give yourself a negative self-evaluation and intercepting it with a positive one. You need to make it an intentional activity. Making positive self-statements and following through increases the chances that **you are the one in control**.

    If you find yourself starting to think about "What if I don't . . .," stop immediately and practice positive self-talk (e.g., I'm the same bright student I have always been; I will make it if I continue to study," or "I'll remember this material because my self-testing shows I'm making progress," or "Get back to the topic; if I still want to worry, I'll worry at 10:30. It is only 9:30 and I want to continue studying.")

    It is also important to give yourself positive reinforcement for your efforts. Take note of when you have worked well and give yourself a positive message, or schedule some type of pleasurable activity. In fact, make it a practice to allow for an enjoyable, self-renewing activity each day.

Using These Practice Exams

The least effective use one can make of the four practice exams in this book is to "study" the questions and answers literally by reading them one at a time and then checking the correct answer. Although the questions have been carefully chosen to be representative of the domains of information found in Step 2, simply "knowing" the answers to these particular 800 questions does not ensure a passing grade on the exam. The questions in this book are intended to be an integral part of a well-planned review, rather than an isolated resource. If used appropriately, the four question sets can provide self-assessment information beyond only a numeric score. They can be used (1) as a diagnostic tool (pretest), (2) to guide and focus further study, and (3) for comprehensive self-evaluation.

As a diagnostic tool. It is possible to use each set of 200 questions as a screening device to gather diagnostic information about relative performance across the six large clinical areas. In each 200-question test, the sampling of each subject is not large but, for those who have been away from clinical study for a while or who have no other recent clinical performance data, using a practice exam in this manner provides a form of feedback before starting to review. It also allows students to respond to Board-type questions similar to those on the examination so they can experience the structure and complexity of the questions and acquire a sense of what they "feel" like.

1. Select any one of the first three tests in this book. It does not matter which one you choose, since they are all approximately equal in terms of topics represented and question difficulty.
2. Allow yourself the same amount of time as would be allowed on the real Boards (approximately 60 seconds per question).
3. Use a separate sheet of paper for your answers (instead of writing in the book). This will make it easier for you to score, analyze, and interpret results.
4. Score your responses (but do not read the correct answer to the question or record the correct response next to your incorrect one). Compute an accuracy level by counting the number of correct responses and dividing by the total number of questions. This will give you the percent correct. Note your score, but be careful not to overreact to this initial score, whether it is a high one or a low one. Remember that this type of sampling provides a rough indication of how familiar or remote clinical material seems to you prior to review. Not reading the correct answer to these questions may seem a bit strange at first, but by not doing so now, you will be able to use these questions again later in your review as a "post-test" to check progress.
5. It is most important to know your distribution of errors across the clinical areas. To find out, categorize each error ("surgery," "internal medicine," "pediatrics"). If in doubt about how to categorize a particular question, check the reference listed in the answer, and use that to make your decision.
6. Arrange the clinical areas in a hierarchy from relatively strong (few errors) to relatively weak (many errors). Did you do well in those sciences you thought you would do well in, and vice versa, or were there some surprises (unexpected highs or lows)?

To guide further study. In keeping with the review approach proposed in this book, you will begin by first reviewing material in each clinical science. After completing all of them, you will reach a point where you think your knowledge is close to what is needed to hit the passing level on the exam (but not complete "mastery"). At this point, try another set of 200 questions from this book to find out if your estimate of content control is correct. It would be useful to discover how close you are after having completed just your "first pass" at the material. The results of your test, if analyzed carefully, should make it possible for you to use your last few weeks (or even days) in more focused, targeted study rather than random review. Obviously, in carrying out a study schedule, it would be wise to plan to finish a "first pass" while enough time remains for you to do the necessary follow-up study.

1. Follow the first five steps described previously.
2. Analyze errors using the guidelines described in the section "Monitoring Study Progress."

3. Focus your follow-up study on the content areas or specific subtopics noted to still be weak. Pay attention to whether a particular pattern of errors has emerged (for example, on questions requiring a judgment on management, or on questions requiring an up-to-date knowledge of genetic principles).

For self-evaluation. As the reality of the last week before the exam hits students, some begin to experience feelings of approach/avoidance; they "want to know" and yet they "don't want to know" how close their review efforts have brought them to the numbers needed to pass. Students who have engaged in self-testing throughout their review are less likely to avoid the last level of evaluation. They have been getting performance data all along and adjusting their study agenda.

There are a few different ways to handle the last round of self-testing. Some students feel less anxious if they do all final testing in the first few days of the last week and reserve the rest of the time for follow-up study. Other students prefer to start the week with a composite test, continue with further study, and then take another test two or three days before the exam.

1. If you have used one set of questions previously as a "pretest," it would now be informative to start with those questions as a post-test. Follow the steps described earlier and compare performance (both total score and across each clinical science).
2. The three remaining tests can be used separately as three individual question sets, or they can be combined into one 600-question test.
3. Another possibility is to use the three remaining tests and do every other question. This provides a 300-question test sample early in the week, with 300 questions remaining for a subsequent test.
4. If none of the tests has been used for prior testing, you might take every other question from all four tests (400 questions) and follow-up later with the remaining 400 questions.

Score interpretation. Keeping in mind that the percentage of items needed to pass the USMLE Step 2 is between 55% and 65%, how should you interpret accuracy levels from your self-testing? Although any practice test sample suggested here is smaller than the approximately 800 questions that comprise the Board exam, it can nevertheless give you some useful feedback. On your tests, percentages between 55% and 60% are encouraging. Percentages between 60% and 75% show you are moving beyond the bare minimum needed for passing. Scores of 75% and above are indicators of substantial strength.

Grace Bingham, Ed.D.

Test I

QUESTIONS

DIRECTIONS: Each of the numbered items or incomplete statements in this section is followed by answers or by completions of the statement. Select the ONE lettered answer or completion that is BEST in each case.

1. A 19-year-old obese black woman with right upper quadrant pain has calculi present in the gallbladder on ultrasound examination. Physical examination shows mild splenomegaly. Laboratory studies show a mild normocytic anemia, with an elevated reticulocyte count. Many of her red blood cells are reported to have no central areas of pallor. The mechanism most likely responsible for her anemia and subsequent gallbladder disease is

(A) absent iron stores
(B) inflammation
(C) extravascular hemolysis
(D) bile salt deficiency
(E) a hemoglobinopathy

2. A 51-year-old patient presents to the emergency room in convulsive status epilepticus. The first means of medical management should be

(A) inserting a tongue blade
(B) administering an intravenous (IV) bolus of 50% dextrose
(C) ensuring that the airway is open and the patient is oxygenating
(D) injecting 5 mg of IV diazepam followed by a loading dose of phenytoin
(E) inducing pentobarbital coma

3. Which assumption about the menstrual cycle is used in Nägele's rule for establishing the estimated due date?

(A) The predominant hormone in the luteal phase is progesterone
(B) The normal length is 28 days
(C) The follicular phase may be of variable duration
(D) The midcycle surge of luteinizing hormone (LH) is absent with anovulation
(E) The predominant hormone in the follicular phase is estrogen

4. Pathologic fractures are most commonly the result of

(A) chronic osteomyelitis
(B) trauma from motor vehicle accidents
(C) secondary infection from an open wound
(D) primary bone disease or metastasis

5. A former arsonist now feels remorseful and spends time planting trees and volunteering as a firefighter. This reaction most strongly suggests the psychodynamic defense of

(A) undoing
(B) denial
(C) sublimation
(D) dissociation
(E) intellectualization

6. The diagram shows the findings of test X for colon carcinoma in a normal population and in patients with colon cancer.

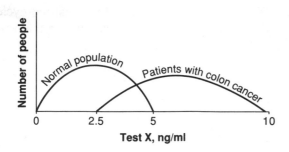

Test X, ng/ml

Which statement about establishing reference intervals (normal range) for this test and interpreting them is true?

(A) If the reference interval is 0–2.5 ng/ml, the test has 100% specificity

(B) If the reference interval is 0–2.5 ng/ml, a patient with a test result of 4 ng/ml must have colon cancer

(C) If the reference interval is 0–5 ng/ml, the test has 100% sensitivity

(D) If the reference interval is 0–5 ng/ml, a test result of 4 ng/ml may represent a true-negative (TN) or a false-negative (FN)

(E) If the reference interval is 0–5 ng/ml, the number of FNs and false-positives (FPs) increases

7. Which gestational age gives the most accurate estimation of weeks of pregnancy by uterine size?

(A) Less than 12 weeks

(B) Between 12 and 20 weeks

(C) Between 21 and 30 weeks

(D) Between 31 and 40 weeks

(E) Over 40 weeks

8. A 65-year-old man with a 40 pack-year history of smoking associated with productive cough presents with a 15-pound weight loss over the last 3 months and recent onset of streaks of blood in the sputum. Physical examination reveals a thin, afebrile man with clubbing of the fingers, an increased anteroposterior diameter, scattered coarse rhonchi and wheezes over both lung fields, and distant heart sounds. A chest x-ray exhibits left hilar adenopathy, dilated tubular markings, and flattened diaphragms. A sputum cytology using Papanicolaou's stain test shows numerous cells with deeply eosinophilic staining cytoplasm and irregular, hyperchromatic nuclei intermixed with inflammatory cells. The most likely diagnosis in this patient is

(A) tuberculosis

(B) small cell carcinoma of the lung

(C) a pulmonary embolism with infarction

(D) bronchiectasis

(E) a squamous cell carcinoma of the lung

9. An 8-year-old child presents with low-grade fever, arthritis, colicky abdominal pain, and a purpuric rash limited to the lower extremities. Laboratory studies reveal a guaiac-positive stool, a urinalysis with red blood cell (RBC) casts and mild proteinuria, and a normal platelet count. The most likely diagnosis is

(A) systemic lupus erythematosus (SLE)

(B) Rocky Mountain spotted fever

(C) idiopathic thrombocytopenic purpura (ITP)

(D) Henoch-Schönlein's vasculitis

(E) poststreptococcal glomerulonephritis

10. A 35-year-old man with nausea and vomiting, vertigo, nystagmus, tinnitus, and nerve deafness in the right ear most likely has

(A) mastoiditis
(B) a cerebellar tumor
(C) vertebral-basilar arterial insufficiency
(D) a glioblastoma multiforme
(E) acoustic neuroma

11. Which physical finding is more typical of a multiparous than a nulliparous cervix?

(A) Increased bluish hue
(B) Purulent discharge
(C) Retracted squamocolumnar junction
(D) Transverse-appearing external os
(E) Absence of scarring

12. Boerhaave's syndrome would most likely be associated with

(A) gastroesophageal reflux
(B) bulimia
(C) tension pneumothorax
(D) gastric ulcer disease
(E) a tear in the esophagus or stomach

13. An executive who states that losing his job has been helpful in that it gives him more time to spend with his family is using the psychodynamic defense of

(A) derealization
(B) compensation
(C) displacement
(D) rationalization
(E) projection

14. The number of live births per 1000 women in the population between 15 and 44 years of age describes

(A) fertility rate
(B) reproductive rate
(C) birth rate
(D) perinatal rate
(E) obstetric rate

15. This scenario concerns the 1993 case–fatality rate for rabies in Anytown, USA, which has a population of 100,000. The number of deaths in 1993 from all causes including rabies was 2000. At the beginning of 1993, 12 patients with rabies diagnosed the previous year were under treatment. In 1993, 100 new cases of rabies were diagnosed. There were 7 deaths from this cohort of newly diagnosed patients. Five patients died in 1993, and two died in 1994. The rabies case–fatality rate during 1993 for Anytown, USA, was

(A) 5/7
(B) 5/100
(C) 100/2000
(D) 100 minus 7/2000
(E) 9/100

16. A 35-year-old nonsmoking woman has progressive dyspnea, fatigue on exertion (with occasional syncopal episodes), and retrosternal chest pain. Her history is negative for thromboembolic disease or rheumatic heart disease. Physical examination reveals a normotensive patient with increased jugular venous pressure, a left parasternal heave, accentuation of P_2, and a decreased carotid pulse. No heart murmurs are present and breath sounds are normal. Pertinent laboratory studies include hypoxemia, normal Pa_{CO_2}, and polycythemia. Dilatation of the right and left main-stem pulmonary arteries and clear lung fields are noted on chest x-ray. The electrocardiogram reveals right axis deviation and right ventricular hypertrophy. The most likely diagnosis in this patient is

(A) mitral stenosis with right heart failure
(B) chronic obstructive lung disease with right heart failure
(C) pickwickian syndrome
(D) primary pulmonary hypertension
(E) polycythemia rubra vera

17. A 44-year-old man presents with the acute onset of dysarthria, a right Horner's syndrome, hiccoughs, right ataxia, sensory loss to pinprick over the right face and left body, and intact cognition. The initial unenhanced computed tomography (CT) scan of the brain is normal. The best means of acute medical management would be

(A) heparinization and observation
(B) right carotid endarterectomy
(C) left carotid endarterectomy
(D) outpatient follow-up
(E) surgical decompression of the cerebellum

18. The definition of maternal mortality rate is the number of maternal deaths

(A) per 1000 births
(B) per 1000 live births
(C) per 10,000 births
(D) per 10,000 live births
(E) per 100,000 live births

19. What is the most common cause of epistaxis in the pediatric population?

(A) Allergic rhinitis
(B) Nose-picking
(C) von Willebrand's disease
(D) Idiopathic thrombocytopenic purpura (ITP)
(E) Nasal angiofibroma

20. A 53-year-old woman with hyperthyroidism and a multinodular thyroid gland on physical examination most likely has

(A) Hashimoto's thyroiditis
(B) Graves' disease
(C) a papillary carcinoma
(D) Plummer's disease
(E) a follicular adenoma

21. The correct formula for calculating the perinatal mortality rate is

(A) fetal deaths + neonatal deaths per 1000 births
(B) stillbirths + neonatal deaths per 1000 births
(C) stillbirths + neonatal deaths per 1000 live births
(D) abortions + stillbirths per 1000 births
(E) abortions + stillbirths + neonatal deaths per 1000 live births

22. A 23-year-old man presents with bizarre delusions, a blunted affect, and tangential thought processes. Which characteristic indicates an unfavorable prognosis?

(A) An extensive premorbid history of social withdrawal
(B) A family history of schizophrenia
(C) A sudden onset of symptomatology
(D) Magnetic resonance imaging (MRI) that shows no gross changes in brain morphology
(E) Catatonic symptomatology

23. Which statement about incidence of a disease is correct?

(A) Incidence is the existence of a disease at a particular moment in time
(B) The numerator and denominator need not be related
(C) The duration of the time period must be stated
(D) The numerator is greater than the denominator
(E) The numerator includes the total population at risk

24. A 65-year-old man with urinary retention secondary to benign prostatic hyperplasia develops high fever, shaking chills, hypotension, and sinus tachycardia with a full pulse. His skin is warm and dry. A complete blood count reveals an absolute neutropenia. The hemodynamic findings in this patient are most likely the result of

(A) endotoxemia with complement system activation
(B) reflex vasodilation secondary to a reduced cardiac output
(C) high-output failure secondary to peripheral vasoconstriction
(D) reflex vagal stimulation with reduction in cardiac output
(E) endothelial damage secondary to bacterial invasion of the cells

25. Based on general bony architecture, the most common female pelvic shape is

(A) gynecoid
(B) android
(C) anthropoid
(D) platypelloid
(E) obstetroid

26. Which nutrient normally in high concentration in cow's milk could lead to an increased renal solute load in an infant if the milk is not appropriately diluted with water?

(A) Linoleic acid
(B) Linolenic acid
(C) Calcium
(D) Protein
(E) B-complex vitamins

27. An absence of ganglion cells in the myenteric plexus of the rectum would most likely be associated with

(A) bleeding
(B) excessive mucus in the stool
(C) constipation
(D) fecal soiling
(E) meconium staining of amniotic fluid

28. Which disorder is associated with peculiar calmness?

(A) Conversion disorder
(B) Simple phobia
(C) Obsessive-compulsive disorder
(D) Hypochondriasis
(E) Melancholic depression

29. A 23-year-old woman who is 39 weeks pregnant with her second child is having regular uterine contractions every 3 minutes. Which criterion is best for assessing if a parturient has entered the active phase of labor?

(A) The cervix is effaced over 90%
(B) The contraction duration is over 30 seconds
(C) The presenting part is low in the pelvis
(D) The cervical dilation is at least 4 cm
(E) The membranes are ruptured

30. Which statement about prevalence of a disease is true?

(A) It measures the risk of acquiring a disease
(B) It may be quantitatively lower than the incidence of the disease
(C) It refers to the number of new cases over a given time period
(D) It describes the existence of a disease at a particular moment in time
(E) The denominator includes the total population at risk

31. A 20-year-old man is stabbed in the left chest, medial to the nipple. His blood pressure is 90/60 mm Hg, pulse is 130/minute, and respiratory rate is 32/minute. The jugular venous pulse increases on inspiration, whereas the peripheral pulse and blood pressure decrease on inspiration. Breath sounds are normal bilaterally. The patient's chest x-ray is unremarkable. After receiving 2 L of isotonic saline, the blood pressure remains low, whereas the central venous pressure rises to 32 cm H_2O. The first step in the management of this patient is to

(A) insert a chest tube placed under water seal and suction into the left pleural cavity
(B) increase parenteral fluids until the blood pressure increases
(C) order a stat echocardiogram
(D) decrease venous pressure by administering a venodilator
(E) decrease venous pressure by administering a loop diuretic

32. A 9-year-old boy presents with confusion and decreased school performance. He soon develops a spastic gait with dysarthria and dysphagia. He also develops visual loss. A magnetic resonance imaging (MRI) scan shows massive demyelination of the white matter in the posterior areas of the hemispheres. The most likely diagnostic laboratory test would be

(A) cerebrospinal fluid (CSF) for oligoclonal bands
(B) urine for arylsulfatase A
(C) plasma for very long-chain fatty acids
(D) amino acid screen
(E) urine for porphyrin screening

33. Which factor contributes most to the mechanism of the third stage of labor?

(A) Rapidly falling estrogen level after delivery
(B) Avulsion of anchoring villi by contracting myometrium
(C) Duration of the first two stages of labor
(D) Level of circulating placentally produced prolactin
(E) Lowering of P_{CO_2} in the umbilical vein

34. An otherwise normal 3-year-old child has recurrent right lower lobe pneumonia. Which condition is most likely responsible for this patient's disease?

(A) Primary B- or T-cell immunodeficiency disorder
(B) Cystic fibrosis
(C) Chédiak-Higashi syndrome
(D) Congenital lung abnormality
(E) Foreign body aspiration

35. A tender mass is present in the subareolar region of both breasts of an adolescent male. The masses should be

(A) excised
(B) incised and drained
(C) left alone
(D) aspirated for culture and cytology
(E) treated with topical steroids

36. The psychodynamic phenomenon of transference refers to

(A) the transfer of feelings from a feared object to a less feared object
(B) the means by which anxiety-provoking images are transformed into more acceptable thoughts
(C) a way of transforming oneself into a better adjusted person
(D) the transfer of conflict from one situation to another
(E) the shifting of feelings originally associated with one person to another individual

37. A 33-year-old woman who is 29 weeks pregnant with her fourth child presents to the obstetric unit with onset of painless vaginal bleeding 2 hours ago, accompanied by passage of significant blood and clots. Fetal heart rate is regular at 150 beats/min. She is having no uterine contractions. The best working diagnosis is

(A) placenta previa
(B) abruptio placentae
(C) vasa pracvia
(D) bloody show
(E) disseminated intravascular coagulation

38. A recently discovered treatment for acute leukemia extends the life span but does not either prevent the disease or lead to its cure. Which statement is true?

(A) The incidence of acute leukemia will increase
(B) The prevalence will decrease
(C) The incidence will decrease
(D) The prevalence will increase
(E) Both incidence and prevalence will increase

39. A 65-year-old smoker has a 40 pack-year history. A 20-pound weight loss over the last 3 months is associated with epigastric pain after eating, diarrhea, and jaundice. Physical examination reveals a palpable, nontender gallbladder and clay-colored stools. Laboratory studies show a total bilirubin of 8.0 mg/dl (normal is 0.1–1.0 mg/dl), a direct bilirubin of 6.0 mg/dl (normal is 0.0–0.3 mg/dl), a serum alkaline phosphatase of 450 U/L (normal is 20–70 U/L), a serum glutamic–pyruvic transferase (SGPT) of 150 U/L (normal is 8–20 U/L), and a urine dipstick that is positive for bilirubin (normal is negative) and negative for urobilinogen (normal is trace amounts). The primary process that is most likely responsible for this patient's findings is located in the

(A) common bile duct
(B) liver
(C) gallbladder
(D) duodenum
(E) pancreas

40. A 16-year-old woman who is 34 weeks pregnant with her first child presents on a routine prenatal visit with a blood pressure of 150/95 and 2+ protein on a dipstick. Repeat blood pressure after 2 hours is unchanged. Her initial 14-week blood pressure was 120/75. The most likely explanation for these findings is

(A) blunted angiotensin response
(B) elevated β endorphins
(C) acute diffuse vasoconstriction
(D) primary renal disease
(E) chronic hypertension

41. A 55-year-old woman with hypercalcemia discovered as an incidental finding on a normal routine physical examination (including pelvic and breast examination) most likely has

(A) an excessive dietary intake of calcium
(B) metastatic breast cancer
(C) a history of taking thiazide diuretics
(D) a benign parathyroid adenoma

42. A 40-year-old woman complains of an unmanageable fear of snakes. Although she knows that no poisonous ones inhabit her area, she cannot hike with her friends. What is the most commonly postulated psychodynamic defense in such situations?

(A) Dissociation
(B) Projection
(C) Displacement
(D) Conversion
(E) Resistance

43. In 1993 in Anytown, USA, there were 2100 live births, 100 stillbirths ($\geq$ 20 weeks' gestation), and 5 neonatal deaths (first 28 days of life). There were 25 sets of twins and 3 sets of triplets. Two mothers died. The perinatal mortality rate in Anytown, USA, in 1993 was

(A) 105/2200
(B) 100/2100
(C) 125/2205
(D) 100/2200
(E) 59/2205

44. A radical mastectomy differs from a modified radical mastectomy in that the former removes

(A) all of the breast tissue on the affected side
(B) the nipple-areolar complex
(C) the ipsilateral axillary nodes
(D) the pectoralis minor
(E) the pectoralis major

45. A 75-year-old man develops severe midabdominal pain associated with vomiting and abdominal distention approximately 30 minutes after eating. He has lost 25 pounds over the past few months because he is afraid of precipitating the pain after eating. Abdominal examination during an asymptomatic interval is normal. A bruit is heard over the right femoral artery, and distal pulses in both extremities are diminished. Stool guaiacs are negative as are colonoscopy and barium studies. The pathogenesis of this patient's condition is most likely

(A) psychogenic
(B) neoplastic
(C) inflammatory
(D) ischemic
(E) intermittent obstruction

46. In the United States, the most commonly used agent for seizure prophylaxis during labor in preeclamptic patients is

(A) phenobarbital
(B) diazepam
(C) magnesium sulfate
(D) diphenylhydantoin
(E) magnesium gluconate

47. A 75-year-old woman who has a history of coronary artery disease and who is using warfarin is brought into the emergency room with left-sided weakness and eye deviation to the right. The most appropriate emergent test to obtain is

(A) magnetic resonance imaging (MRI) of the brain
(B) computed tomography (CT) scan of the brain
(C) electroencephalogram (EEG)
(D) carotid duplex ultrasound
(E) spinal tap

48. A lumpectomy (segmental mastectomy) is best described as a

(A) total mastectomy with low axillary node dissection
(B) wide excision of a parenchymal lesion of the breast, with low axillary node dissection and postoperative radiation
(C) excision of all breast tissue including the nipple-areolar complex
(D) removal of breast tissue only, with nipple preservation

49. Which statement about hepatitis B and pregnancy is true?

(A) Pregnancy accelerates the course of acute maternal hepatitis B
(B) Mode of delivery has no impact on maternal–neonatal transmission
(C) Breast-feeding does not increase neonatal risk of hepatitis B
(D) Neonates can be protected from hepatitis B by passive immunization at birth
(E) Rapidity of disease progression is the same in mother and neonate

50. A very anxious 25-year-old man complains of severe right lower quadrant pain but experiences much relief after normal saline solution is administered. This situation most strongly suggests that

(A) the pain is psychogenic
(B) he has a histrionic personality disorder
(C) he was volume-depleted
(D) he has factitious disorder
(E) he is responding to placebo

52. A 65-year-old man presents with an acute onset of pain, paresthesias, pallor, and an absent dorsalis pedis pulse in his right leg. The skin is cool and pallor is increased on raising the leg. These symptoms most likely represent

(A) superficial thrombophlebitis
(B) herniation of a lumbar disc
(C) arterial occlusion
(D) deep venous insufficiency

53. Which drug class is most likely to cause depression?

(A) Oral hypoglycemic drugs
(B) Antiparasitic drugs
(C) Nonsteroidal anti-inflammatory drugs
(D) Selective serotonin reuptake inhibitory drugs
(E) Antihypertensive drugs

51. A research study investigated the relation between mean blood glucose values in pregestational diabetic women and major fetal malformations.

| | **Maternal Mean Plasma Glucose Values** | | |
Major Fetal Malformation	**<130 mg/dl**	**≥130 mg/dl**	**Totals**
Present	2	10	12
Absent	300	50	350
Totals	302	60	362

The odds ratio for this study is
(A) 300 divided by 50 = 6
(B) 50 divided by 10 = 5
(C) 60 divided by 2 + 10 = 5
(D) 300/2 divided by 60/10 = 25

54. A 58-year-old college professor had onset of a myocardial infarction 4 hours ago and is now in the intensive care unit (ICU). His electrocardiogram (ECG) shows an increasing incidence of short runs of ventricular tachycardia. The most appropriate drug to administer at this early time after his infarct is

(A) amiodarone
(B) flecainide
(C) lidocaine
(D) quinidine
(E) verapamil

55. A 27-year-old woman who is 15 weeks pregnant with her first child presents to the office with exquisitely painful, blister-like lesions on her labia. She had similar episodes before pregnancy. Her temperature is normal. Which statement about her pregnancy is true?

(A) She should undergo cesarean section to protect her infant from infection
(B) Her fetus has an increased risk of congenital malformations
(C) Transplacental transmission to her fetus is a significant concern
(D) Breast-feeding of her infant is probably unsafe
(E) Decisions regarding route of delivery are best made at onset of labor

56. A hard-driving, competitive 45-year-old attorney is hospitalized. Which condition is most likely to be seen in this patient?

(A) Cancer
(B) Coronary artery disease
(C) Bronchial asthma
(D) Obesity
(E) Diabetes mellitus

57. A 23-year-old woman with insulin-dependent diabetes presents to the emergency room with mental confusion, bizarre behavior, perspiration, increased salivation, restlessness, and tachycardia. The next step in the management of this patient is to

(A) order a complete blood count (CBC)
(B) do a stat blood glucose
(C) order serum electrolytes
(D) order a stat drug screen
(E) order arterial blood gases

58. In a woman under 40 years of age, which of the following breast abnormalities would have the highest predictive value for malignancy?

(A) Painful, moveable mass
(B) Painless, moveable mass
(C) Bloody nipple discharge
(D) Clear nipple discharge
(E) Breast skin edema with dimpling

59. A 33-year-old woman is seen for her first prenatal visit when she is 10 weeks pregnant. She had an infant previously who died on the second day of life from group B streptococcal infection. Which statement about the management of her current pregnancy is true?

(A) Most women with positive culture will have noninfected infants
(B) A negative vaginal culture means that her fetus will not be at risk at delivery
(C) Appropriate treatment for a positive culture can eradicate the bacteria
(D) The organism is a pathological bacteria in the female genital tract
(E) Rapid on-culture assay tests are highly specific for the organism

60. A 26-year-old woman presents with progressive writhing and jerking movements of the extremities. She has two brothers and two sisters, both normal; however, a first cousin with a similar problem died undiagnosed at 45 years of age. Her computed tomography (CT) scan of the brain was unremarkable, but the magnetic resonance imaging (MRI) scan revealed hypodense basal ganglia bilaterally. Her laboratory tests are unremarkable except for some elevated liver function tests. She is a nondrinker. The best diagnostic test would be

(A) spinal tap for glucose, protein, and oligoclonal bands
(B) urine for porphyrin screening
(C) urine for heavy metal screening (lead, mercury, arsenic)
(D) serum and urine copper and ceruloplasmin levels
(E) urine for amino acid screening

61. A right spontaneous pneumothorax would be associated with

(A) breath sounds on the right
(B) egophony on the right
(C) hyperresonance to percussion on the right
(D) increased width of intercostals on the right
(E) mediastinal structures shifted to the left

62. A 55-year-old man complains of increasing sadness and inability to find pleasure in anything. The risk of suicide is highest if the most prominent additional symptom is

(A) tearfulness
(B) feelings of hopelessness
(C) sleep disturbance
(D) lassitude
(E) anorexia

63. Which substance is associated with fetal and neonatal anomalies related to vascular disruptions from maternal prenatal use?

(A) Tobacco
(B) Alcohol
(C) Narcotics
(D) Amphetamines
(E) Cocaine

64. Patients who have been taking diuretics and who develop cardiac arrhythmias due to digitalis can often be treated by

(A) raising blood sodium concentration
(B) raising blood potassium concentration
(C) lowering blood magnesium concentration
(D) raising blood calcium concentration

65. A 75-year-old widow with $300,000 in savings develops Alzheimer's disease and will require nursing-home care for the rest of her life. This care will be paid for initially by

(A) Medicare
(B) Medicaid
(C) a health maintenance organization (HMO)
(D) an independent practice association (IPA)
(E) her savings

66. Which substance has a defined congenital anomaly syndrome associated with maternal prenatal use?

(A) Tobacco
(B) Alcohol
(C) Marijuana
(D) Amphetamines
(E) Narcotics

67. A 21-year-old man complains of morning back pain over the last 3 months. The pain improves as the day progresses and when he exercises. Physical examination shows diminished anterior flexion of the lumbar spine, muscle spasms in the lower back, and forward stooping when the patient walks. An x-ray shows bilateral sclerotic changes in the sacroiliac area. Which test would be most useful in arriving at the diagnosis?

(A) Erythrocyte sedimentation rate
(B) Rheumatoid factor
(C) Serum uric acid
(D) Serum antinuclear antibody test
(E) Human leukocyte antigen (HLA)-B27

68. A 10-year-old child with an upper respiratory infection treated with aspirin and antihistamines presents with fever, protracted vomiting, and lethargy. Physical examination reveals mild hepatomegaly. Total bilirubin, serum transaminases, and serum ammonia are increased. The most likely diagnosis is

(A) hepatitis A
(B) drug-induced hepatitis
(C) Reye's syndrome
(D) infectious mononucleosis
(E) Gilbert's disease

69. An 18-year-old woman who is 25 weeks pregnant with her first child has a history of repaired transposition of the great vessels. She has no symptoms at rest, but has minor limitation with physical activity. Based on the New York Heart Association's functional classification, what class of heart disease would she be assigned?

(A) Class 0
(B) Class I
(C) Class II
(D) Class III
(E) Class IV

70. Which one of the following pain relationships is correct?

(A) Mid–small bowel obstruction: constant, boring, midabdominal pain
(B) Acute pancreatitis: midepigastric transverse pain radiating into the back
(C) Retrocecal appendicitis: right lower quadrant colicky pain with obstipation
(D) Ruptured ovarian cyst: lower quadrant colicky pain with obstipation
(E) Posterior duodenal ulcer with penetration: flank pain with radiation to the right lower quadrant

71. Which one of the following fracture relationships is correct?

(A) Greenstick fracture: displaced fracture with angulation   *not displaced.*
(B) Pott's fracture: fracture of vertebral body
(C) Colles' fracture: fracture of proximal radius   *distal.*
(D) Intertrochanteric fracture of femur: high association with avascular necrosis
(E) Supracondylar fracture of humerus in child: predisposition for Volkmann's ischemic contracture of forearm

72. Which statement about thromboembolic disorders in pregnancy is true?

(A) Superficial thrombophlebitis requires anticoagulant therapy
(B) The best single test for deep venous thrombosis is a venogram
(C) Warfarin has a high molecular weight and does not cross the placenta
(D) Maternal heparin therapy has significant direct fetal effects
(E) Most thromboembolic problems in pregnancy occur antenatally

73. Which dependency is most clearly heritable?

(A) Alcohol
(B) Cocaine
(C) Heroin
(D) Tobacco
(E) Benzodiazepine

74. A patient with chronic glaucoma is also under treatment for chronic obstructive pulmonary disease. He is referred for evaluation of a sudden increase in intraocular pressure. Which drug used in pulmonary disease is most likely to be responsible?

(A) Atropine
(B) Epinephrine
(C) Timolol
(D) Pilocarpine
(E) Terbutaline

75. Which statement about human immunodeficiency virus (HIV) and pregnancy is true?

(A) Pregnancy accelerates maternal acquired immune deficiency syndrome (AIDS) or HIV-related disease
(B) Mode of delivery has no impact on maternal–neonatal transmission
(C) Breast-feeding does not increase neonatal risk of becoming HIV positive
(D) Neonates can be protected from HIV by passive immunization at birth
(E) Rapidity of disease progression is the same in mother and neonate

76. How does the number of visits made by patients to physicians in the United States compare with the number of visits made by people in countries with socialized medicine?

(A) Fewer
(B) The same
(C) Twice as many
(D) Three times as many
(E) Four times as many

77. A 23-year-old man with acquired immune deficiency syndrome (AIDS) has recurrent candidiasis and a *Pneumocystis carinii* pneumonia. The physician would expect this patient to have

(A) a normal skin reaction to intradermal injections of common antigens
(B) a low circulating CD8 suppressor T-cell count
(C) hypogammaglobulinemia
(D) an abnormal phytohemagglutinin assay
(E) intact cellular immunity

78. A 69-year-old man with a history of coronary artery disease and hypertension presents with acute onset of right facial weakness and numbness. On examination, his speech and extremity strength are normal, but he has significant weakness of the right face, including the orbicularis oculi. In addition, he complains of roaring in the right ear, and his taste sensation is absent on the right side of the anterior tongue. Sensation is normal to pinprick. Which choice would best explain the findings?

(A) Bell's palsy
(B) Brain-stem glioma
(C) Left middle cerebral artery stroke
(D) Lacunar stroke of the left internal capsule
(E) Parotid tumor

79. A 34-year-old woman who is 26 weeks pregnant with her third child had a positive 50-g glucose screen. Her 3-hour 100-g oral glucose tolerance test results are as follows: fasting, 102; 1 hour, 194; 2 hours, 170; 3 hours, 135. In White's Classification of Diabetes in Pregnancy, she meets the criteria for

(A) class A1
(B) class A2
(C) class B
(D) class C
(E) class D

80. The most common complication of measles in a child is

(A) acute appendicitis
(B) subacute sclerosing panencephalitis
(C) interstitial pneumonia
(D) keratoconjunctivitis
(E) otitis media

81. A 28-year-old woman complains that her mother is a "witch" and has only the worst intentions. On the other hand, she idealizes an aunt whom she describes as a "sage" and the source of strength in her life. Which defense mechanism is this woman using?

(A) Projection
(B) Idealization
(C) Conversion
(D) Splitting
(E) Symbolization

82. A patient in the intensive care unit has developed ventricular tachyarrhythmia. Treatment with intravenous boluses of lidocaine has controlled the arrhythmia only transiently—the arrhythmia disappeared within 1 minute and reappeared within 4 minutes of each bolus. Immediately after each injection the plasma lidocaine concentration was in the therapeutic range. Which statement is most accurate?

(A) Rapid metabolic inactivation of lidocaine is responsible for the short duration of its antiarrhythmic action
(B) Laboratory determinations of blood levels of lidocaine after IV administration are frequently in error
(C) The elimination half-life of lidocaine is approximately 2 minutes
(D) Lidocaine is rapidly redistributed to other tissues
(E) Cardiac cells rapidly develop tachyphylaxis to IV lidocaine

83. Compared with cow's milk, human breast milk contains significantly greater amounts of

(A) solute load
(B) vitamin C
(C) protein
(D) vitamin K
(E) iron

84. A 23-year-old woman who is 32 weeks pregnant with her first child comes in to the emergency department complaining of 12 hours of increasing right-upper abdominal pain radiating to the back. She also reports nausea and vomiting. Her temperature is 99.5° F. Which statement is true?

(A) Appendicitis can be ruled out because of the location of the pain

(B) Exploratory laparotomy should not be performed because of risk of preterm labor

(C) High estrogen levels in pregnancy predispose to cholelithiasis

(D) Peritoneal response to inflammation is unchanged in pregnancy

(E) Pancreatitis is common in pregnancy

85. An abnormal finding in a newborn girl would be

(A) a hemoglobin of 18 g/dl

(B) vaginal bleeding

(C) an increased cord blood immunoglobulin M (IgM) level

(D) gynecomastia

(E) a total bilirubin of 2 mg/dl

86. Which one of the following test relationships is correct?

(A) Finkelstein's test: chronic stenosing tenosynovitis

(B) Schoeber's test: osteoarthritis

(C) McMurray's test: dislocated hip

(D) Ortolani's test: rheumatoid arthritis

(E) Positive anterior draw sign: tear of posterior cruciate

87. Which dietary deficiency is most likely to cause dementia?

(A) Vitamin B_{12}

(B) Vitamin C

(C) Iron

(D) Magnesium

(E) Lecithin

88. Which disorder is most likely responsible for conjunctival irritation in a newborn 24 hours after an uneventful delivery?

(A) Gonococcal ophthalmia

(B) Chlamydial conjunctivitis

(C) *Staphylococcus aureus* conjunctivitis

(D) Chemical conjunctivitis

(E) Lacrimal duct obstruction

89. A sonogram is performed on a 22-year-old woman who is 30 weeks pregnant. A single fetus is noted, with head in the right-upper quadrant, back to the mother's left. Both fetal thighs are flexed, and both legs are extended. What is the fetal presentation?

(A) Frank breech

(B) Complete breech

(C) Incomplete breech

(D) Double footling breech

(E) Transverse breech

90. The following electrocardiogram (ECG) is from a 65-year-old man with ischemic heart disease. The most likely diagnosis is

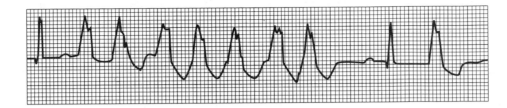

(A) premature atrial contractions
(B) atrial flutter
(C) paroxysmal atrial tachycardia
(D) ventricular tachycardia
(E) sinus tachycardia

91. Terbutaline is administered to a woman in her seventh month of pregnancy because of uterine contractions that began during the previous week. Which effect can be anticipated?

(A) Increased extracellular potassium
(B) Increased gastrointestinal motility
(C) Decreased blood glucose and insulin
(D) Increased heart rate and possible arrhythmias
(E) Constriction of bronchial smooth muscle

92. A 58-year-old man with widely disseminated small cell carcinoma of the lung has hypotension, decreased serum cortisol levels, and profound electrolyte disturbances. Which set of laboratory data is most closely associated with this patient's clinical abnormality?

	Serum sodium 135–147 mEq/L	Serum potassium 3.5–5.0 mEq/L	Serum chloride 95–105 mEq/L	Serum bicarbonate 22–28 mEq/L
(A)	118	3.0	88	21
(B)	152	2.8	110	33
(C)	125	2.9	80	36
(D)	126	5.8	86	18

93. The contraindication for preterm labor tocolysis is

(A) multiple gestation
(B) placenta previa
(C) severe preeclampsia
(D) pyelonephritis
(E) positive vaginal β-strep culture

94. A 1-day-old infant is noted to have an asymmetric Moro reflex. Physical examination reveals that the right arm is adducted and internally rotated. Which disorder best explains the infant's problem?

(A) Klumpke's paralysis
(B) Fractured right clavicle
(C) Todd's paralysis
(D) Erb-Duchenne paralysis
(E) Spinal injury with associated hemiparesis

95. Which one of the following hernia relationships is correct?

(A) Femoral hernia: high incidence of bowel strangulation in women
(B) Indirect hernia: hernia that goes through Hesselbach's triangle
(C) Ventral hernia: hernia through the linea semilunaris
(D) Direct hernia: hernia that descends into the scrotal sac
(E) Pantaloon hernia: hernia with incarceration of part of the bowel wall

96. A 62-year-old woman with a 35-year history of treatment with antipsychotic medications for schizophrenia complains of the insidious onset of peculiar movements. Such movements most resemble those of

(A) Parkinson's disease
(B) Huntington's disease
(C) hemiballismus
(D) hemiparesis
(E) Wilson's disease

97. A newborn examination of a 6-hour-old infant delivered with difficulty by low forceps reveals an asymmetric Moro reflex involving the right arm. The infant is cyanotic and has labored respiration. The abdomen does not bulge with inspiration, and there are decreased breath sounds in the right chest. Which diagnosis is the most likely in this infant?

(A) Respiratory distress syndrome
(B) Meconium aspiration
(C) Ipsilateral paralysis of the diaphragm
(D) Tracheoesophageal fistula
(E) Choanal atresia

98. A 24-year-old black woman with a seizure disorder treated with phenytoin is noted to have the following findings on complete blood count (CBC) when she is 15 weeks pregnant: hemoglobin (Hgb) 9.3, hematocrit (HCT) 29, mean corpuscular volume (MCV) 105. What is the most likely cause for these findings?

(A) Sickle cell trait
(B) Iron deficiency
(C) Physiologic anemia
(D) Folate deficiency
(E) Thalassemia

99. Medicare was designed primarily for

(A) poor people
(B) minor children of poor people
(C) people eligible for Social Security
(D) people without health insurance
(E) people who require nursing-home care

100. A 45-year-old woman presents with a diffuse, nonpainful enlargement of the thyroid gland and generalized malaise. Physical examination shows sinus bradycardia, puffiness of her face and eyelids, coarse dry skin, and a delayed recovery phase of her Achilles reflex. There is no cervical adenopathy. Which set of thyroid studies most closely matches this patient's disease?

	Serum T_4	Resin T_3 uptake	Free T_4 index	Serum TSH
(A)	Increased	Decreased	Normal	Normal
(B)	Increased	Increased	Increased	Low
(C)	Decreased	Increased	Normal	Normal
(D)	Decreased	Decreased	Decreased	Increased
(E)	Decreased	Decreased	Decreased	Decreased

101. A 28-year-old woman who is 34 weeks pregnant with her first child comes to the office complaining of intermittent watery vaginal discharge. Which diagnostic method will be most helpful in assessing ruptured membranes?

(A) Nitrazine paper on the perineum
(B) Speculum examination for vaginal pooling
(C) Sonogram for amniotic fluid volume
(D) Urinalysis for urinary tract infection
(E) Digital examination for cervical dilation

102. A newborn examination demonstrates severe hypotonia, generalized weakness, absent tendon stretch reflexes, fasciculations of the tongue, and preservation of the extraocular muscles. Which disorder is the most likely diagnosis in this infant?

(A) Myotonic dystrophy
(B) Werdnig-Hoffmann disease
(C) Infant botulism
(D) Infantile myasthenia gravis
(E) Duchenne's muscular dystrophy

103. Which one of the following injury relationships is correct?

(A) Dislocation: disruption of normal relationships between articular surfaces
(B) Sprain: complete or partial tear of ligaments that is confirmed by x-ray
(C) Strain: partial disruption of a musculotendinous unit short of rupture with weakness and impairment of muscle motion
(D) Tendon rupture: produces weakness, loss of muscle motion, and muscle fasciculations
(E) Avulsion fracture: fragment of bone pulled off by periosteum overlying the tibia

104. A patient with eye discharge, mild photophobia, a normal pupillary reaction to light, and normal intraocular pressure most likely has

(A) acute glaucoma
(B) optic neuritis
(C) acute conjunctivitis
(D) acute anterior uveitis
(E) central retinal artery occlusion

105. In the psychodynamic view, personality disorders are

(A) a response to environmental pressures
(B) dormant until the individual leaves the shelter of the family
(C) caused by childhood problems
(D) not responsive to treatment
(E) innate

106. The son of a 65-year-old woman whose husband died more than 2 years ago consults a physician about his mother's current behavior. Which behavior would the physician consider normal under these circumstances?

(A) Brief periods of painful longing
(B) Feelings of worthlessness
(C) A suicide attempt
(D) Inability to work
(E) Despair

107. Which set of arterial blood gases is most closely associated with an adult patient who has rheumatoid arthritis and clinical evidence of salicylate intoxication?

	pH 7.35–7.45	Paco$_2$ 33–44 mm Hg	Bicarbonate 22–28 mEq/L
(A)	7.29	53	25
(B)	7.38	22	12
(C)	7.53	49	39
(D)	7.43	70	46

108. A 28-year-old woman who is 30 weeks pregnant comes to the office because she is concerned about feeling no fetal movements for the past 2 days. The method of choice in assessing fetal death is

(A) persistent absence of fetal movements
(B) change of a positive serum pregnancy test to negative
(C) amniocentesis for examination of amniotic fluid
(D) real-time ultrasound assessment for cardiac motion
(E) abdominal x-ray examination of the fetus

109. A newborn develops cyanosis that occurs with feeding but is relieved by crying. The most likely diagnosis is

(A) a tracheoesophageal fistula
(B) bronchopulmonary dysplasia
(C) respiratory distress syndrome
(D) choanal atresia
(E) a patent ductus arteriosus

110. A 75-year-old man develops unilateral, painless loss of vision, associated with pallor of the optic disc, a cherry red fovea, and bloodless arterioles. These findings are most consistent with

(A) central retinal vein occlusion
(B) acute glaucoma
(C) acute anterior uveitis
(D) central retinal artery occlusion
(E) optic neuritis

111. An elderly patient develops painful swelling of the right parotid gland 10 days after a cholecystectomy. This is most likely secondary to

(A) *Staphylococcus aureus*
(B) duct obstruction by a stone
(C) a viral infection
(D) hemorrhage
(E) an immunological reaction

112. Behavioral psychotherapy is distinguished from cognitive psychotherapy by the

(A) view of behavior as a response to the environment
(B) use of desensitization
(C) use of patient education
(D) use of psychoactive medications as adjunctive treatments
(E) ability to account for the effect of organic lesions on behavior

113. Which combination of standard fetal measurements is used in second- and third-trimester sonographic assessments of fetal growth/weight: abdominal circumference (AC), biparietal diameter (BPD), crown–rump length (CRL), femur length (FL), head circumference (HC), humerus length (HL), transcerebellar diameter (TCD)?

(A) AC, BPD, CRL, FL

(B) HC, BPD, AC, FL

(C) BPD, HC, AC, CRL

(D) BPD, HC, AC, TCD

(E) BPD, CRL, FL, TCD

114. A child presents with circular areas of alopecia that are Wood's-lamp positive. Which pathogen is most likely responsible?

(A) *Epidermophyton floccosum*

(B) *Microsporum canis*

(C) *Candida albicans*

(D) *Trichophyton mentagrophytes*

(E) *Aspergillus* species

115. A 26-year-old medical student with a history of hepatitis A is immunized against hepatitis B. Which set of hepatitis serology data is most closely associated with this student's history?

	anti-HAV IgM	anti-HAV IgG	anti-HBc IgM	anti-HBs	HBsAg	HBeAg
(A)	−	+	+	−	−	−
(B)	−	+	−	+	−	−
(C)	−	+	+	−	+	+
(D)	+	−	−	+	−	−
(E)	+	−	−	−	−	−

HAV = hepatitis A; HBV = hepatitis B; c = core antigen; e = e antigen; HBsAg = surface antigen.

116. The most common cause of puerperal endomyometritis is

(A) manual removal of a retained placenta

(B) postpartum tubal sterilization

(C) retained products of conception

(D) scheduled cesarean delivery

(E) prolonged rupture of membranes (PROM)

117. A newborn with a normal physical examination passes blood with the meconium. Which test would be most indicated in this patient to determine the cause of the bloody stool?

(A) Apt test on the blood in the stool

(B) Hemoglobin electrophoresis of the blood from the stool

(C) Barium enema

(D) Clinitest examination of the stool

(E) Methylene blue stain of the stool

118. A 56-year-old woman on total parenteral nutrition develops alopecia, a maculopapular rash around the mouth and eyes, and taste and smell abnormalities most likely due to a deficiency of

(A) essential fatty acids
(B) zinc
(C) selenium
(D) magnesium
(E) copper

119. Which statement about the pathophysiology of bipolar disorder is the most accurate?

(A) Pathognomonic abnormalities in lithium transport may occur at the cellular membrane
(B) Antimanic drugs generally block central dopamine receptors
(C) The lesion does not appear to be heritable
(D) Abnormal levels of neurotransmitters have been reported during manic episodes
(E) Chromosomal abnormalities are common

120. A 35-year-old man is in an automobile accident. Physical examination reveals point tenderness over the left lower ribs and signs of hypovolemic shock. Breath sounds are normal in the lungs. These findings are most likely secondary to

(A) a pulmonary contusion with hemorrhage into the pleural cavity
(B) rupture of the spleen
(C) rupture of the colon
(D) transection of the abdominal aorta

121. A 35-year-old woman presents with moderate hypertension, muscle weakness, polyuria, and paresthesias with tetanic manifestations. There is no evidence of pitting edema. A 24-hour urine test for potassium and free cortisol shows increased loss of potassium and normal levels of free cortisol. A computed tomography (CT) scan of the adrenal glands shows a localized, encapsulated mass in the left adrenal gland. Which set of laboratory data would most likely be present in this patient?

	Serum aldosterone	Plasma renin	Serum potassium	Serum bicarbonate
(A)	Increased	Increased	Decreased	Increased
(B)	Normal	Decreased	Decreased	Increased
(C)	Increased	Decreased	Decreased	Increased
(D)	Decreased	Decreased	Increased	Decreased

122. A 35-year-old woman underwent an emergency cesarean delivery of her second child and hysterectomy at 34 weeks' gestation because of obstetric hemorrhage due to placenta accreta. She received 5 units of packed red blood cells. Her blood pressure was in the hypotensive range for 30 minutes during the procedure. Which pituitary hormone is most likely to be affected by her clinical course?

(A) Adrenocorticotropic hormone (ACTH)
(B) Prolactin
(C) Thyroid-stimulating hormone (TSH)
(D) Follicle-stimulating hormone (FSH)
(E) Antidiuretic hormone (ADH)

123. What is the most common cause of the anemia of prematurity?

(A) Folate deficiency
(B) B_{12} deficiency
(C) Iron deficiency
(D) α-Thalassemia minor
(E) β-Thalassemia minor

124. Which two maternal bony pelvis anatomic landmarks determine the diagonal conjugate?

(A) The upper margin of the symphysis and the coccyx
(B) The lower margin of the symphysis and the sacral promontory
(C) The upper margin of the symphysis and the sacral promontory
(D) The middle of the symphysis and the coccyx
(E) The middle of the symphysis and the ischial spine

125. Excluding the thyroid, which of the following statements best describes most instances of cervical adenopathy in the adult population?

(A) Most are primary cancers
(B) Most are benign
(C) Most are metastatic
(D) Most are cystic
(E) Most represent Hodgkin's disease

126. A 15-year-old boy develops symptoms of gonorrhea and comes to see the physician. Before treating him, the physician should

(A) obtain parental consent
(B) counsel him on safe sexual practices
(C) notify state health authorities
(D) notify his sexual partner
(E) notify his parents that treatment will start with or without their consent

127. Which anesthetic modality is most associated with myometrial relaxation?

(A) Inhaled halothane
(B) Paracervical block
(C) Thiopental sodium
(D) Subarachnoid block
(E) Pudendal block

Questions 128–129

A 30-year-old woman who is an executive seeks treatment for persistent anxiety, which has increased since she joined a law firm 4 years ago. She describes worry and rumination that she is inadequate in social situations, concerns that she will not be granted partnership next year, and fears that her life will turn out badly. She also complains of difficulty sleeping, trouble concentrating, tenseness, and irritability. She says that her worries get the better of her at times, but she just cannot make them go away. She denies any other significant medical problems, any substance abuse, or any history of psychosis. Mental status examination reveals an anxious woman. She is appropriately dressed, and her thought processes are logical. There is no evidence of hallucinations or delusions. She shows no psychomotor retardation. Her conversation includes no suicidal rumination or feelings of hopelessness.

128. The most likely diagnosis is

(A) adjustment disorder with anxious mood
(B) social phobia
(C) generalized anxiety disorder
(D) obsessive-compulsive disorder
(E) major depression, single episode

129. The most effective pharmacologic treatment for this patient would be

(A) fluphenazine (Prolixin)
(B) buspirone (BuSpar)
(C) thioridazine (Mellaril)
(D) alprazolam (Xanax)
(E) triazolam (Halcion)

130. Which pharmacologic agent given to the mother enhances fetal pulmonary maturity?

(A) Ritodrine
(B) Isoxsuprine
(C) Betamethasone
(D) Nifedipine
(E) Terbutaline

Questions 131–132

131. An 8-year-old boy, 1 week post–upper respiratory infection, develops petechial lesions over his entire body. A platelet count is 20,000 platelets/µl. The remainder of the complete blood count is normal. No hepatosplenomegaly is present. A bone marrow aspirate exhibits megakaryocytes, but platelet budding is poor. Which diagnosis is the most likely in this patient?

(A) Thrombotic thrombocytopenic purpura
(B) Idiopathic thrombocytopenic purpura
(C) Disseminated intravascular coagulation
(D) Henoch-Schönlein purpura
(E) Rocky Mountain spotted fever

132. All of the following statements concerning this 8-year-old boy are true EXCEPT

(A) intravenous gamma-globulin therapy is useful
(B) platelet-associated immunoglobulin G (IgG) is usually present
(C) 90% of patients recover within 1 year
(D) it is the most common bleeding disorder in childhood
(E) platelet concentrates should be given prophylactically to prevent bleeding

133. A 20-year-old man presents with a history of delayed developmental milestones, problems with impulse control, and an IQ of 65. A complete workup for the cause would probably show

(A) genetic or chromosomal abnormalities
(B) perinatal insults
(C) sociocultural deprivation
(D) maternal substance abuse
(E) mild mental retardation

134. A 35-year-old woman who is afraid of snakes is told to go to the snake house at the zoo and look at the snakes until she is no longer afraid. This patient's therapy is an example of the behavioral technique known as

(A) systematic desensitization
(B) flooding
(C) sensitization
(D) cognitive therapy
(E) biofeedback

135. A 42-year-old man presents with an acute onset of severe right ocular pain and blurry vision. Physical examination reveals the pupil to be mid-dilated and fixed. No discharge is present. The examining physician would expect

(A) blood in the anterior chamber
(B) an increased intraocular pressure
(C) a corneal erosion on slit-lip examination
(D) papilledema
(E) bloodless arterioles and a cherry red fovea

136. Which cause of intrauterine growth retardation (IUGR) leads to an asymmetric pattern on ultrasound?

(A) Chronic hypertension
(B) Trisomy 18
(C) Rubella infection
(D) Renal agenesis
(E) Toxoplasmosis

Questions 137–139

An 81-year-old man presents with left temporal pain of several days' duration. The pain is aching, and he notes night sweats. He has a mild leukocytosis (13,000 white blood cells, normal differential), as well as weight loss because of jaw pain induced by eating. Chest x-ray and computed tomography (CT) scan of the brain are normal. The sedimentation rate is 110.

137. What is the most likely diagnosis?

(A) Migraine headache
(B) Cluster headache
(C) Temporal arteritis
(D) Malignant otitis externa
(E) Major depression

138. What is a major complication of this condition?

(A) Myocardial infarction
(B) Pulmonary emboli
(C) Deep venous thrombosis
(D) Lacunar infarction
(E) Retinal artery ischemia

139. What is the treatment strategy of choice if this condition is suspected?

(A) Ergot for acute relief and β blockers for prophylaxis
(B) Admission to intensive care unit with intravenous nitroglycerin
(C) Intravenous steroids and temporal artery biopsy
(D) Admission with hourly neurologic checks
(E) Intravenous heparin with transition to warfarin for 6 months

Questions 140–142

A 35-year-old obese woman with a 20 pack-year history of smoking presents with the sudden onset of tachypnea, dyspnea, cough, and right-sided pleuritic chest pain 48 hours after a total hysterectomy for low-grade endometrial carcinoma. She has a low-grade fever, sinus tachycardia, and a blood pressure of 100/70 mm Hg. Examination of the chest shows scattered, bilateral expiratory wheezes and dullness to percussion at the right lung base. No calf tenderness is present. A chest x-ray shows a small pleural effusion at the right lung base as well as a wedge-shaped area of hypovascularity and atelectasis in the right lower lobe. An electrocardiogram (ECG) shows nonspecific ST- and T-wave abnormalities. An arterial blood gas drawn with the patient breathing room air reveals a pH of 7.50 (7.35–7.45), Pa_{CO_2} of 29 mm Hg (normal is 33–44 mm Hg), a Pa_{O_2} of 70 mm Hg (normal is 75–105 mm Hg), and a bicarbonate of 21 mEq/L (normal is 22–28 mEq/L).

140. The first step in the management of this patient is to

(A) perform a pleural tap
(B) order a perfusion scan of the lungs
(C) order a sputum for Gram's stain, culture, and sensitivity
(D) order pulmonary function tests
(E) order a consultation for bronchoscopy

141. The arterial blood gases are consistent with

(A) an abnormal alveolar–arterial gradient
(B) a primary metabolic acidosis
(C) respiratory failure
(D) a compensatory respiratory alkalosis

142. The most likely diagnosis in this patient is

(A) atelectasis secondary to a mucous plug
(B) adult respiratory distress syndrome
(C) acute bronchial asthma
(D) a pulmonary embolus with infarction
(E) a bacterial pneumonia

143. Which factor is common to all psychotherapies?

(A) An explanation for pathological behavior
(B) A firm concept of the unconscious
(C) A long duration of treatment
(D) A warning to avoid drug treatment as much as possible
(E) A belief that the privacy of the interpersonal experience must take precedence over other considerations

DIRECTIONS: Each of the numbered items or incomplete statements in this section is negatively phrased, as indicated by a capitalized word such as NOT, LEAST, or EXCEPT. Select the ONE lettered answer or completion that is BEST in each case.

144. Complications of otitis media include all of the following EXCEPT

(A) brain abscess
(B) cholesteatoma
(C) "malignant" external otitis
(D) conductive hearing loss
(E) facial nerve paralysis

145. All of the following factors are causal theories of depression EXCEPT

(A) double-bind communication
(B) inadequate exposure to light
(C) faulty cognitive framework
(D) object loss
(E) learned helplessness

146. Normal reflex reactions in the newborn include all of the following EXCEPT

(A) rooting reflex
(B) parachute reflex
(C) stepping reflex
(D) Moro embrace reflex
(E) Babinski reflex

147. The cardinal movements of labor that enable the fetus to adapt to the maternal pelvis include all of the following EXCEPT

(A) descent
(B) external rotation
(C) extension
(D) internal rotation
(E) extraction

148. Normal hematologic parameters in the newborn include all of the following EXCEPT

(A) slight prolongation of the prothrombin time
(B) hemoglobin ranging from 16–18 g/dl
(C) mean corpuscular volume (MCV) above 100 μm^3
(D) absolute lymphocytosis
(E) presence of 3 to 10 nucleated red blood cells (RBCs) per 100 white blood cells (WBCs)

149. A 72-year-old man complains that he is having significant difficulty concentrating on tasks and remembering recent events. The LEAST likely cause of his problems is

(A) normal aging
(B) alcoholic dementia
(C) Alzheimer's disease
(D) cerebrovascular disease
(E) depression

150. A typical commercially prepared fortified formula versus either human or cow milk contains a greater concentration of all of the following EXCEPT

(A) vitamin D
(B) vitamin K
(C) linoleic acid
(D) fat
(E) iron

151. Which occurrence is NOT a sign of placental separation?

(A) Gush of vaginal bleeding
(B) Umbilical lengthening outside vagina
(C) Fundus of uterus rising
(D) Uterus becoming firm and globular
(E) Cervix visible at the introitus

152. A 6-year-old patient has a platelet count of 10,000 cells/μl (150,000–350,000, normal range) after a recent upper respiratory infection. Petechiae and ecchymoses are scattered over the skin, but splenomegaly is absent. A bone marrow examination reveals adequate numbers of megakaryocytes that appear to be generating platelets. Based on these findings, the clinician then orders a platelet-associated immunoglobulin G (IgG) test, which returns a positive result. All of the following statements are true EXCEPT

(A) the patient has a platelet destruction problem
(B) immunologic destruction of platelets is likely present
(C) this patient's condition is a good example of a type III hypersensitivity reaction
(D) the child has idiopathic thrombocytopenic purpura (ITP)
(E) most patients recover platelet function

153. All of the following illnesses are more common in black than in white persons EXCEPT

(A) obesity
(B) hypertension
(C) bipolar illness
(D) diabetes
(E) heart disease

154. Capabilities of a 3-year-old child usually include all of the following EXCEPT

(A) becoming toilet-trained
(B) copying a cross
(C) copying a circle
(D) putting short sentences together
(E) copying a square

155. Which condition is NOT a diagnostic criterion for severe preeclampsia?

(A) Hyperemesis
(B) Blurred vision
(C) Cyanosis
(D) Thrombocytopenia
(E) Epigastric pain

156. *Streptococcus pneumoniae* (pneumococcus) is LEAST likely to be a common pathogen in which disorder in the pediatric population?

(A) Bruton's agammaglobulinemia
(B) Chronic granulomatous disease (CGD) of childhood
(C) Sickle cell disease
(D) Splenectomized patient with hereditary spherocytosis
(E) Spontaneous peritonitis in nephrotic syndrome

157. Which of the following is LEAST likely to interfere with normal wound healing?

(A) Hemoglobin of 10 g/dl
(B) Diabetes mellitus
(C) Corticosteroids
(D) Zinc deficiency
(E) Malnutrition

158. A normal 6- to 9-month-old child can do all of the following EXCEPT

(A) transfer an object from hand to hand
(B) maintain a seated position
(C) repeat vowel sounds
(D) rise independently and walk a few steps alone
(E) grasp objects between the thumb and forefinger

159. Myasthenia gravis might be treated acutely or chronically by all of the following measures EXCEPT

(A) steroids
(B) anticholinergic medications
(C) plasmapheresis
(D) thymectomy
(E) immunoglobulin

160. Clinical features associated with a tracheoesophageal fistula include all of the following EXCEPT

(A) cyanosis that occurs at rest but is relieved by crying
(B) cyanotic episodes associated with feeding
(C) a history of polyhydramnios during pregnancy
(D) stomach filled with air
(E) inability to pass a catheter into the stomach

161. Which of the following surgical procedures for peptic ulcer disease is LEAST likely to be associated with the dumping syndrome?

(A) Truncal vagotomy with pyloroplasty
(B) Parietal cell vagotomy
(C) Vagotomy and antrectomy
(D) Subtotal gastrectomy
(E) Selective vagotomy

162. Absence, or petit mal, seizures are characterized by all of the following EXCEPT

(A) sudden onset
(B) gradual cessation
(C) an approximately 10-second duration; duration rarely longer than 45 seconds
(D) mild clonic jerking
(E) fluttering of the eyelids

163. According to the 1993 report of the National Cholesterol Education Panel (NCEP), major risk factors for coronary artery disease include all of the following EXCEPT

(A) man 45 years and older
(B) family history of premature coronary artery disease
(C) diabetes mellitus
(D) current cigarette smoking
(E) sedentary lifestyle

164. Live vaccines include all of the following EXCEPT

(A) Salk polio vaccine
(B) bacille Calmette-Guérin (BCG) vaccine
(C) measles vaccine
(D) mumps vaccine
(E) rubella vaccine

165. Which characteristic is NOT a component of the Apgar score?

(A) Skin color
(B) Muscle tone
(C) Body temperature
(D) Heart rate
(E) Respiratory effort

166. All of the following statements concerning diphtheria-tetanus-pertussis (DTP) vaccine are true EXCEPT

(A) an acute febrile illness is a contraindication to administering the vaccine
(B) an evolving or suspected neurologic illness is a contraindication to administering the vaccine
(C) the vaccine is contraindicated in an immuno-compromised patient
(D) acute encephalopathy is rarely associated with the pertussis component of the vaccine
(E) a shock-like state may occur as a complication of immunization

167. All of the following statements about clozapine are true EXCEPT that

(A) it is effective in one-third of patients with schizophrenia who are unresponsive to other antipsychotic medications
(B) it has significant renal toxicity
(C) it causes significant sedation
(D) it cannot be used unless weekly white blood cell counts are obtained
(E) it has a dose-related risk for causing seizures

168. All of the following statements concerning the measles-mumps-rubella vaccine are true EXCEPT

(A) pregnancy is a contraindication for immunization
(B) immunodeficiency is a contraindication for immunization
(C) it is contraindicated in patients who have just received gamma globulin
(D) subacute sclerosing panencephalitis is a rare complication attributed to the measles component of the vaccine
(E) arthralgias, arthritis, or both are possible complications of the mumps component of the vaccine

169. All of the following conditions suggest a diagnosis of neurofibromatosis EXCEPT

(A) bilateral acoustic neuromas
(B) Lisch nodules in the iris
(C) six or more café au lait spots greater than 1.5-cm diameter
(D) autosomal recessive pattern
(E) intracranial hamartomas

170. *Haemophilus influenzae* type B is LEAST likely to be a common pathogen in which disease in the pediatric population?

(A) Acute epiglottitis
(B) Otitis media
(C) Septic arthritis
(D) Neonatal meningitis
(E) Orbital cellulitis

171. Which condition is NOT likely to be associated with multiple sclerosis (MS)?

(A) Bilateral trigeminal neuralgia (tic douloureux) in a 45 year old
(B) Progressive gait spasticity and visual loss with no other evidence of cerebral involvement
(C) Bilateral intranuclear ophthalmoplegia
(D) Aphasia and right arm weakness resolving over 1 week
(E) A magnetic resonance imaging (MRI) scan revealing multiple white matter lesions confluent at the angles of the lateral ventricles of a 30 year old

172. All of the following statements concerning specialized vaccines are true EXCEPT

(A) *Haemophilus influenzae* B vaccine is recommended for those patients with recurrent otitis media or a history of acute epiglottitis

(B) influenza vaccine is not recommended for normal children

(C) pneumococcal vaccine should be administered, after 2 years of age, to those children who have functional or anatomic asplenia (e.g., sickle cell disease)

(D) it is generally recommended that all newborns be immunized with hepatitis B virus (HBV) vaccine

(E) newborns of mothers carrying HBV antigen should receive hepatitis B immune globulin at birth and should be actively immunized with HBV vaccine

173. All of the following statements about low-density lipoprotein (LDL) are true EXCEPT

(A) LDL is the best screen for primary prevention of coronary artery disease

(B) the level determines whether drug therapy is required

(C) oxidized LDL is more atherogenic than native LDL

(D) LDL contains the majority of cholesterol circulating in blood

(E) LDL is calculated with the following formula: LDL = (cholesterol − HDL) − (triglyceride II 5)

174. All of the following pairings of accidents with the most common age-group in which they occur are accurate EXCEPT

(A) suffocation—6 months old

(B) baby-walker injury—1 year old

(C) drowning in a swimming pool—2 years old

(D) pedestrian injury—6 years old

(E) accidental poisoning—7 years old

175. The following ejection fractions (EFs) are from three patients who represent different types of people

Patient	EF
Patient A	0.30
Patient B	0.66
Patient C	0.80

All of the following statements about the data are true EXCEPT

(A) patient A could have a large left ventricular aneurysm

(B) patient B could have severe aortic stenosis

(C) patient C could be an Olympic long-distance runner

(D) increasing cardiac contractility could increase the ejection fraction in patient B

(E) a β-blocker could decrease the ejection fraction in patient B

176. All of the following immunizing agents initiate passive immunity EXCEPT

(A) rabies vaccine

(B) immune globulin

(C) Rh immune globulin

(D) diphtheria antitoxin

(E) crotalin antivenin

177. All of the following are considered normal findings in a 75-year-old man EXCEPT

(A) mild glucose intolerance

(B) increased serum alkaline phosphatase

(C) increased autoantibody production

(D) decreased creatinine clearance

(E) slight increase in hemoglobin concentration

178. All of the following pulmonary function tests and arterial blood-gas findings in restrictive lung disease are different from those in obstructive lung disease EXCEPT

(A) total lung capacity
(B) tidal volume
(C) residual volume
(D) FEV_1/FVC ratio
(E) partial pressure of arterial CO_2 ($Paco_2$)

179. A 3-month-old infant should be able to perform all of the following EXCEPT

(A) babble and make cooing sounds
(B) when supine, follow an object 90 degrees from the midline through an arc of 180 degrees
(C) when prone, lift the head 45 degrees
(D) form a fully developed social smile
(E) roll from the prone to the supine position

180. All of the following poison–antidote relationships are correct EXCEPT

(A) methanol—ethanol infusion
(B) gold—dimercaprol
(C) organophosphates—pralidoxime
(D) β-adrenergic blockers—glucagon
(E) tricyclic antidepressants—atropine

DIRECTIONS: Each set of matching questions in this section consists of a list of four to twenty-six lettered options (some of which may be in figures) followed by several numbered items. For each numbered item, select the ONE lettered option that is most closely associated with it. To avoid spending too much time on matching sets with large numbers of options, it is generally advisable to begin each set by reading the list of options. Then, for each item in the set, try to generate the correct answer and locate it in the option list, rather than evaluating each option individually. Each lettered option may be selected once, more than once, or not at all.

Questions 181–182

Match each drug with the corresponding graph.

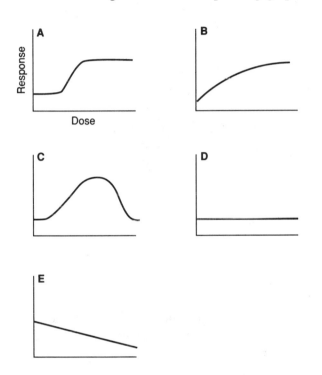

181. Nortriptyline

182. Lithium

Questions 183–184

A patient presents with polycythemia. For diagnostic purposes, oxygen saturation, red blood cell (RBC) mass, plasma volume, and plasma erythropoietin levels are obtained. For each set of laboratory results, select the diagnosis it best represents.

(A) Polycythemia rubra vera
(B) Chronic obstructive pulmonary disease (COPD)
(C) Stress polycythemia
(D) Renal adenocarcinoma

183. Low oxygen saturation, increased RBC mass, normal plasma volume, and increased erythropoietin levels

184. Normal oxygen saturation, normal RBC mass, decreased plasma volume, and normal erythropoietin levels

Questions 185–187

For each description of a cardiac drug, select the agent that it most closely describes.

(A) Nifedipine
(B) Lidocaine
(C) Nitroprusside
(D) Hydralazine
(E) Guanethidine

185. This drug blocks the release of catecholamines and slowly depletes stores of norepinephrine at sympathetic postganglionic nerve terminals. Its effects on blood pressure may be decreased if tricyclic antidepressants are coadministered.

186. This orally active vasodilator acts mainly on arterioles. In some patients, the drug may cause a reversible systemic lupus erythematosus–like syndrome.

187. This orally effective agent is used in the management of angina and hypertension. Compared with most other agents in its class, it is safer in patients with atrioventricular conduction abnormalities. However, it can cause worsening of heart failure because of its negative inotropic actions.

Questions 188–189

Match each addictive substance with the corresponding bar.

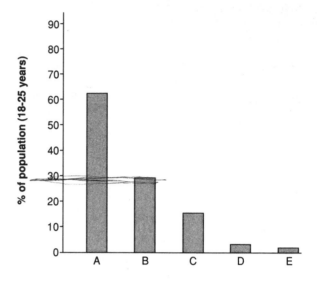

188. Cocaine

189. Tobacco

Questions 190–191

Using the following table, match each description of an inhalational anesthetic with its appropriate properties.

Anesthetic	Blood:Gas Partition Coefficient	Minimal Alveolar Concentration (%)
(A)	0.47	> 100
(B)	12.00	0.16
(C)	1.40	1.4
(D)	2.30	0.8
(E)	1.8	1.68

190. The agent with the slowest rate of onset of anesthetic action

191. The agent that is likely to be least potent as an inhalational anesthetic

Questions 192–195

For characteristics of renal disease given below, select the urinary finding most closely associated.

(A) Red blood cell (RBC) casts
(B) White blood cell (WBC) casts
(C) Hyaline casts
(D) Renal tubular casts
(E) Waxy casts
(F) Fatty casts

192. Urinary finding in an 8-year-old boy with anasarca and a 24-hour urine protein greater than 3.5 g

193. Urinary finding that distinguishes acute pyelonephritis from acute cystitis

194. Urinary finding that indicates a patient with end-stage renal disease

195. Urinary finding that would be expected in a 12-year-old child who develops hypertension, periorbital edema, and smoky-colored urine 2 weeks after recovering from scarlet fever

Questions 196–197

The goal of therapy in hypertension is to prevent cardiovascular complications, with minimal adverse effects on the quality of life. The diagram represents the four primary sites in which drugs can act to control blood pressure.

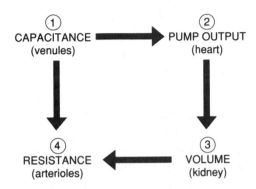

For each description of an antihypertensive drug, choose the drug most closely associated.

(A) Propranolol
(B) Captopril
(C) Minoxidil
(D) Hydrochlorothiazide
(E) Diazoxide

196. This orally active drug acts mainly at site 4 and is usually reserved for management of moderate to severe hypertension. Tachycardia and edema may occur, as may hypertrichosis, which is particularly bothersome to female patients.

197. Acting at site 3, initial doses of this drug may cause severe hypotension in hypovolemic patients. Although adverse effects are rare, hematotoxicity and proteinuria may occur. The antihypertensive effects of this drug may be impaired by use of nonsteroidal anti-inflammatory drugs (NSAIDs).

Questions 198–200

For each clinical description below, select the anemia most closely associated.

(A) Iron deficiency

(B) Anemia of chronic disease

(C) Thalassemia minor

(D) Lead poisoning

(E) B_{12} deficiency

(F) Folate deficiency

(G) Congenital spherocytosis

(H) Sickle cell anemia

(I) Autoimmune hemolytic anemia

198. A 3-year-old black child presents with abdominal colic and a history of pica. Physical examination shows pale conjunctiva and palmar creases, but no localizing signs are present on abdominal examination. Bone x-rays show densities in the epiphyses. A complete blood count (CBC) shows a hemoglobin of 7.0 g/dl (mean 11 g/dl), a mean corpuscular volume (MCV) of 55 μm^3 (normal is 80–100 μm^3), and a normal leukocyte and platelet count. Red blood cell (RBC) morphology is reported to show microcytic cells with hypochromasia and coarse basophilic stippling. The corrected reticulocyte count is 9%.

199. A 32-year-old woman with systemic lupus erythematosus (SLE) presents with generalized weakness and malaise. Physical examination shows pale palmar creases, generalized lymphadenopathy, and hepatosplenomegaly. The CBC is reported to have a hemoglobin of 5.0 g/dl (normal is 12–16 g/dl), MCV of 103 μm^3 (normal is 80–100 μm^3), a leukocyte count of 3000 cells/μl (normal is 4500–11,000 cells/μl), and a platelet count of 120,000 cells/μl (normal is 150,000–450,000 cells/μl). Numerous spherocytes are noted on the smear. The uncorrected reticulocyte count is 27%. The direct Coombs' test is positive.

200. A 42-year-old male alcoholic presents with hepatosplenomegaly and ascites. Additional findings include spider angiomata and bilateral gynecomastia. The neurologic and mental status examination are normal. A CBC exhibits a hemoglobin of 7.0 g/dl (normal is 13.5–17.5 g/dl), an MCV of 120 μm^3 (normal is 80–100 μm^3), a leukocyte count of 2500 cells/μl (normal is 4500–11,000 cells/μl), and a platelet count of 75,000 cells/μl (normal is 150,000–450,000 cells/μl). Macro-ovalocytes and hypersegmented neutrophils are noted on the peripheral smear. The corrected reticulocyte count is 1%.

ANSWER KEY

1-C	30-D	59-A	88-D	117-A
2-C	31-C	60-D	89-A	118-B
3-B	32-C	61-C	90-D	119-D
4-D	33-B	62-B	91-D	120-B
5-A	34-E	63-E	92-D	121-C
6-D	35-C	64-B	93-C	122-B
7-A	36-E	65-E	94-D	123-C
8-E	37-A	66-B	95-A	124-B
9-D	38-D	67-E	96-B	125-C
10-E	39-E	68-C	97-C	126-B
11-D	40-C	69-C	98-D	127-A
12-B	41-D	70-B	99-C	128-C
13-D	42-C	71-E	100-D	129-B
14-A	43-A	72-B	101-B	130-C
15-B	44-E	73-A	102-B	131-B
16-D	45-D	74-A	103-A	132-E
17-A	46-C	75-B	104-C	133-E
18-E	47-B	76-A	105-C	134-B
19-B	48-B	77-D	106-A	135-B
20-D	49-D	78-A	107-B	136-A
21-C	50-E	79-A	108-D	137-C
22-A	51-E	80-E	109-D	138-E
23-C	52-C	81-D	110-D	139-C
24-A	53-E	82-D	111-A	140-B
25-A	54-C	83-B	112-A	141-A
26-D	55-E	84-C	113-B	142-D
27-C	56-B	85-C	114-B	143-A
28-A	57-B	86-A	115-B	144-C
29-D	58-E	87-A	116-E	145-A

146-B	157-A	168-E	179-E	190-B
147-E	158-D	169-D	180-E	191-A
148-D	159-B	170-D	181-C	192-F
149-A	160-A	171-D	182-A	193-B
150-D	161-B	172-A	183-B	194-E
151-E	162-B	173-A	184-C	195-A
152-C	163-E	174-E	185-E	196-C
153-C	164-A	175-B	186-D	197-B
154-E	165-C	176-A	187-A	198-D
155-A	166-C	177-E	188-D	199-I
156-B	167-B	178-B	189-A	200-F

ANSWERS AND EXPLANATIONS

1. The answer is C. *(Hematology; congenital spherocytosis and gallstones)*
Young patients with gallstones, anemia, and splenomegaly are always suspect for an extravascular hemolytic anemia, particularly congenital spherocytosis. Gallstones are best recognized by ultrasound (gold standard test), whereas hemolytic anemias are identified by an elevated reticulocyte count reflecting increased marrow turnover of red blood cells (RBCs) in response to the hemolysis.

The patient has congenital spherocytosis, which is an autosomal dominant disease, with a deficiency of spectrin in the RBC membrane. Spectrin deficiency results in the formation of spherocytes that have less membrane than a normal RBC. This condition renders them extremely susceptible to rupture when placed in hypotonic saline solution, which is the basis for the osmotic fragility test. In the peripheral smear, spherocytes do not have a central area of pallor, as opposed to normal RBCs, which are a biconcave disc (doughnut without a hole) with a central area of pallor where hemoglobin is less concentrated. In addition, their spheroidal shape causes them to be trapped and destroyed in the splenic sinusoids by macrophages, thus the term extravascular hemolysis. Macrophages degrade the heme of hemoglobin into indirect bilirubin, which is released into the bloodstream, taken up by the hepatocyte, conjugated into direct bilirubin, and excreted in the bile. The increased bilirubin load in the bile precipitates as jet black calcium bilirubinate stones (pigment stones), predisposing the patient to cholecystitis. Splenectomy is the treatment of choice.

Iron deficiency and anemia associated with inflammation are not hemolytic anemias and do not predispose to gallstones. Bile salt deficiency does predispose to gallstones but is not associated with a hemolytic anemia. Although sickle cell disease, the most common hemoglobinopathy in black persons, is commonly associated with gallstones, no sickle cells are reported in the peripheral smear, thus excluding that diagnosis. Sickle cell trait does not predispose a person to a hemolytic anemia or stone formation.

2. The answer is C. *(Neurology; acute medical management)*
In all cases of acute medical management, airway, breathing, and circulation (the ABCs) should be addressed first. Insertion of a tongue blade in the convulsing patient does nothing to improve management and may lacerate the tongue. A 50% dextrose bolus may be appropriate, but would clearly follow, in importance, the establishment of a patent airway; in addition, the bolus should be preceded by intravenous (IV) thiamine. The diazepam–phenytoin combination is an excellent means of acute medical management of status, but would still follow establishment of the ABCs. Pentobarbital coma is a "last resort" to stop status epilepticus and would follow all other measures, especially IV phenytoin.

3. The answer is B. *(Obstetrics; gestational age calculation)*
A good menstrual history is essential for calculating the estimated due date. Nägele's rule is a convenient method of using the last menstrual period and arriving at an estimated date calculation. All the statements are true, but only (B) is related to Nägele's rule. Here, 3 months are subtracted from—and 7 days are added to—the last normal menstrual period. Adjustments must be made for longer or shorter cycle lengths.

4. The answer is D. *(Orthopedics; pathologic bone fractures)*
The most common causes of pathologic fractures are metastatic bone disease and primary diseases of bone. They are called pathologic because there is a disease in the bone, as opposed to trauma resulting in a fracture of normal bone. Among the primary tumor sites that metastasize to bone are breast (most common), lung (small cell carcinoma) and thyroid (follicular carcinoma). Multiple myeloma, the most common primary hematologic malignancy of bone, is also associated with pathologic fractures due to the presence of lytic lesions secondary to the secretion of osteoclast activating factor by the malignant plasma cells. Benign diseases causing pathologic fractures include bone cysts, Paget's disease of

bone, and osteoporosis. A pathologic fracture secondary to infection (e.g., osteomyelitis) is uncommon.

5. The answer is A. *(Psychiatry; psychodynamics)*
Undoing refers to the performance of an activity that symbolically reverses some previous behavior or thought. This defense mechanism is commonly present in individuals who feel either conscious or unconscious guilt. Denial, sublimation, dissociation, and intellectualization are other mechanisms of defense.

6. The answer is D. *(Laboratory medicine; establishing reference intervals for a test)*
A laboratory test shows how often the test is positive in patients with a disease; that is, the sensitivity of the test ("positivity in disease") and how often the test is negative (normal) in people who do not have the disease; that is, the specificity of the test ("negativity in health"). A test that is performed on people with a disease can return with a positive or negative test result. A positive test result is called a true-positive (TP), whereas a negative test result is called a false-negative (FN). An FN misclassifies the patient as normal. Similarly, a test that is performed on a normal person can return with a negative or positive test result. A negative test result is called a true-negative (TN), whereas a positive test result is called a false-positive (FP). An FP misclassifies the person as having the disease.

The sensitivity of the test is established by testing only patients with known disease, who may have positive (TP) or negative (FN) test results. The formula is as follows:

$$\text{Sensitivity} = TP / TP + FN \times 100$$

A test with 100% sensitivity has no FNs; that is, every person in the known disease population has a positive test. Therefore, a negative (normal) test result must be a TN rather than an FN, since the test has no FNs. This test then qualifies as being useful in screening for disease because normal test results exclude disease. However, a positive test result may represent a TP or an FP, so another test must be performed to decide whether it is a TP or an FP. Note that the formula for sensitivity says nothing about the FP rate, because it deals only with the disease population.

The specificity of a test applies only to normal people, who can have negative (TN) or positive (FP) test results. The formula is as follows:

$$\text{Specificity} = TN / TN + FP \times 100$$

A test with 100% specificity has no FPs; that is, this test is always normal in normal people. Therefore, the test result must be a TP. However, a normal test result can represent a TN or an FN, because nothing in the formula relates to findings in the diseased population (e.g., the FN rate). A test with 100% specificity is useful for confirming disease because a positive test result must be a TP and not an FP.

Ideally, a test with 100% sensitivity is first used on a patient who is suspect for a particular disease. If the test result is negative, that patient does not have that disease. However, if the test result is positive, a test with 100% specificity is used. If that test result is positive, the screening test result is a TP. However, if that test result is negative, the screening test result is an FP. For example, if the physician thinks that a patient is human immunodeficiency virus (HIV)-positive, the first test to order is an enzyme-linked immunosorbent assay (ELISA) screening test. If the test result is negative, the patient is not HIV-positive. However, if the test result is posi-, a Western blot assay is automatically performed. If this test result is also positive, the ELISA screen is a TP. If the test result is negative (normal), the ELISA screen is an FP. In this example, the ELISA test has a high sensitivity and can screen for HIV, whereas the Western blot assay has a high specificity and can confirm HIV positivity.

The reference interval for the test can be adjusted to create a test with high sensitivity or high specificity.

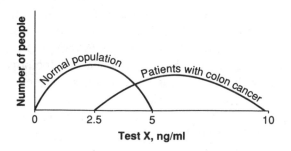

Note that this test shows an overlap of the normal cancer populations between 2.5 and 5 ng/ml; this area includes normal people and people with disease. Establishing a test with 100% sensitivity (no FNs) means setting the upper limit of the reference interval at that value at the beginning of the disease curve. In this case, the reference interval is 0–2.5 ng/ml. This range has no FNs. However, a positive test result (> 2.5 ng/ml) does not necessarily mean that the patient has the disease. Note, for example, that some normal people are in the overlap area between 2.5 and 5 ng/ml. These patients are considered FPs. Thus, creating a test with 100% sensitivity automatically lowers the specificity of the test because some people with a positive test result are FPs.

Establishing a test with 100% specificity (no FPs) means setting the value at the end of the normal curve as the upper limit of normal. In this case, it is 0–5 ng/ml. Note that test results greater than 5 ng/ml are all TPs. However, a normal test result (0–5 ng/ml) does not mean that the patient is normal. The overlap area between 2.5 and 5 ng/ml contains some people with the disease. These patients are classified as FNs. Thus, creating a test with 100% specificity automatically lowers the sensitivity of the test because the number of FNs is increased.

With this information, if the reference interval is 0–5 ng/ml (100% specificity) and a test result is 4 ng/ml, the test result is either a TN or an FN. The sensitivity of the test is decreased at this interval because there are more FNs, but the specificity of the test is 100% because there are no FPs beyond 5 ng/ml. A reference interval of 0–2.5 ng/ml creates a test with 100% sensitivity. Test results between 2.5 and 5 ng/ml are either TPs or FPs because some normal people are in that overlap area.

7. The answer is A. *(Obstetrics; gestational age calculation)*
The duration of gestation can be estimated by uterine size. The earlier in pregnancy that the assessment of uterine size is made, the more accurate it is because the proportionate change in detectable uterine size from week to week is greater earlier in the pregnancy than it is later. As

pregnancy progresses, the accuracy of estimation from uterine size is progressively less precise.

8. The answer is E. *(Pulmonology; bronchogenic carcinoma, obstructive lung disease)*
Patients with a smoking history, weight loss, clubbing of the fingers, hemoptysis, and hilar adenopathy are strongly suspect for a primary bronchogenic carcinoma, particularly squamous and small cell carcinoma (oat cell carcinoma). Cough is the most common presenting symptom of lung cancer (75%), followed by weight loss (40%) and hemoptysis (25%–30%).

The physical findings indicate chronic obstructive lung disease. The bronchitic component consists of productive cough, rhonchi, wheezes, and dilated tubular shadows representing thickened bronchial walls. The emphysematous component is represented by an increased anteroposterior diameter, distant heart sounds, and flattened diaphragms.

Cytology is the gold standard test for bronchogenic carcinoma and has its highest diagnostic yield in centrally located cancers like squamous and small cell carcinoma. The sputum cytology using Papanicolaou's stain test reports cells with deeply eosinophilic staining cytoplasm and irregular, hyperchromatic nuclei. Because keratin becomes bright red with this stain, the patient most likely has a primary squamous cell carcinoma. Small cell carcinomas have small, lymphocyte-sized, basophilic staining cells in cytology smears.

Tuberculosis, bronchiectasis, and pulmonary embolism can all be associated with hemoptysis but would have a different clinical presentation and absence of neoplastic cells in sputum.

9. The answer is D. *(Pediatrics; Henoch-Schönlein purpura)*
Henoch-Schönlein purpura typically presents with a rash on the lower extremities and buttocks. Systemic lupus erythematosus (SLE), although accompanied by arthritis and fever, usually involves a malar rash. The rash of Rocky Mountain spotted fever begins peripherally and spreads to the entire body. Idiopathic thrombocytopenic purpura (ITP) is associated with a

petechial rash, primarily on pressure points such as where the elastic band of underwear touches the skin. Also, the platelet count is depressed in ITP. Poststreptococcal glomerulonephritis does not typically involve a rash, although hematuria is present.

10. The answer is E. *(Neurosurgery; acoustic neuroma)*

An acoustic neuroma is associated with tinnitus, nausea and vomiting, vertigo, nystagmus, and eighth-nerve deafness. It is most commonly a neurilemoma (schwannoma), which is a benign encapsulated tumor arising from Schwann cells. Untreated mastoiditis that erodes through bone to produce acoustic nerve damage is rare. Cerebellar tumors and vertebral-basilar artery insufficiency produce ataxia but are not usually associated with eighth-nerve damage. A glioblastoma multiforme is the most common primary malignancy of the brain in adults and usually involves the frontal lobes. It would not be expected to produce eighth-nerve damage.

11. The answer is D. *(Obstetrics; pelvic examination)*

The astute observer can identify the irreversible changes that pregnancy brings to the reproductive tract. A transverse-appearing external os is more typical of a multiparous than a nulliparous cervix. Increased bluish hue is true of pregnancy but is unrelated to parity. Purulent discharge is characteristic of cervicitis but is unrelated to parity. A retracted squamocolumnar junction is found in postmenopausal women but is unrelated to parity. Absence of scarring is a characteristic of nulliparous not multiparous women.

12. The answer is B. *(General surgery; Boerhaave's syndrome and bulimia)*

Boerhaave's syndrome refers to a full thickness rupture of the distal thoracic esophagus or stomach and is associated with vomiting or retching. In most cases, this syndrome is associated with alcoholics who have forceful vomiting or retching. However, it is also the most serious complication of bulimia, an eating disorder associated with bingeing on excessive amounts of food and self-induced vomiting.

Mallory-Weiss syndrome is a closely related disorder, except for the presence of a tear rather than a rupture. Gastroesophageal reflux, tension pneumothorax, and gastric ulcer disease are not associated with Boerhaave's syndrome.

13. The answer is D. *(Psychiatry; psychodynamics)*

Rationalization refers to the distortion of reality so that the actual act or event seems to be desirable. This mechanism is often used when an individual cannot accept the implications of a particular outcome of events. Derealization, compensation, displacement, and projection are other mechanisms of defense.

14. The answer is A. *(Obstetrics; vital statistics)*

Vital statistics facilitate an understanding of the impact of human reproduction on a population. Fertility rate is the number of live births per 1000 women between 15 and 44 years of age. Reproductive rate, perinatal rate, and obstetric rate do not define any official rates. Birth rate is the number of live births per 1000 population.

15. The answer is B. *(Biostatistics; case–fatality rate)*

The case–fatality rate expresses the probability of death from a disease over a specified period of time. The number of deaths from a disease is divided by the number of new cases diagnosed over the time period. In the scenario described, the number of rabies cases diagnosed last year was 100. Even though 7 deaths occurred from this group, the calculation is based only on the 5 deaths that occurred during the year under consideration. Therefore, the answer is 5/100.

16. The answer is D. *(Pulmonology; primary pulmonary hypertension)*

Primary pulmonary hypertension (PH) occurs in middle-aged women, who present with progressive onset of dyspnea (most common symptom), fatigue, chest pain, syncopal episodes, and a universally poor prognosis (candidate for heart–lung transplantation). The majority of cases of PH are secondary, so other causes must be ruled out before considering it a primary disease.

Mechanisms of PH include: (1) a reduction in the cross-sectional area of the pulmonary artery bed by loss of pulmonary vasculature (e.g., emphysema), vasoconstriction (e.g., chronic hypoxemia, chronic respiratory acidosis), or obstruction of vessels (e.g., recurrent pulmonary emboli); (2) increased pulmonary venous pressure (e.g., left heart disease—mitral stenosis, pulmonary venous disease); (3) increased pulmonary blood flow (e.g., left-to-right shunts—ventricular septal defect, patent ductus arteriosus); and (4) increased blood viscosity (e.g., polycythemia rubra vera).

Vessel lesions seen in all types of PH include intimal fibrosis and medial hypertrophy of smooth muscle. Tufts within capillary channels resembling a vascular plexus (plexogenic arteriopathy) are commonly seen in primary PH. Accentuation of P_2 is a characteristic finding in PH. Right ventricular hypertrophy (left parasternal heave) and increased jugular venous pulse are caused by increased resistance to pulmonary blood flow. Decreased pulmonary blood flow to the left heart results in a decreased cardiac output, reflected by syncopal episodes, chest pain, and a decreased carotid pulse. Hypoxemia arises from a mismatch of ventilation and perfusion in the lungs, which serves as a stimulus for erythropoietin release and subsequent secondary polycythemia.

Mitral stenosis (most commonly secondary to chronic rheumatic fever), pickwickian syndrome (obesity associated with respiratory acidosis), obstructive lung disease, and polycythemia rubra vera, although secondary causes of PH, are ruled out by the history, physical examination, and laboratory studies given in the case study. The combination of PH and right ventricular hypertrophy of noncardiac origin is called cor pulmonale.

17. The answer is A. *(Neurology; acute medical management)*
Although some physicians might argue that heparin would add little in the case of an acute, stable stroke, in a young person with no medical contraindication and no computed tomography (CT) evidence of bleeding, the risk should be very small, and the heparin might treat a coagu-

lopathy unrecognized in the acute stages. Carotid enterectomy would be useless, because the patient's symptoms relate to a posteroinferior cerebellar artery infarct (in the distribution of the lateral medulla), and an infarct usually relates to ipsilateral vertebral artery disease. Outpatient follow-up is inappropriate in the case of an acute stroke, especially because there is a risk of edema in the cerebellum and herniation after a few days. In this event, emergent surgery would be appropriate, but not as acute medical management.

18. The answer is E. *(Obstetrics; vital statistics)*
A maternal death is death of the mother as the result of the reproductive process. The first four choices are erroneous because the denominator must be per 100,000 live births.

19. The answer is B. *(Pediatrics; epistaxis)*
Nose-picking is the most common cause of epistaxis in the pediatric population. Trauma and irritation (colds, allergic rhinitis) are other causes. Bleeding disorders are much less common causes of epistaxis and usually have other manifestations.

20. The answer is D. *(General surgery; hyperthyroidism due to Plummer's disease)*
Plummer's disease refers to hyperthyroidism associated with a multinodular goiter, where one or more of the nodules become autonomous and secrete excessive amounts of thyroxine. Graves' disease is the most common cause of hyperthyroidism and is associated with a diffuse goiter. Hashimoto's thyroiditis is the most common cause of hypothyroidism and is characterized by a diffusely enlarged gland. Follicular adenomas are solitary nodules that are rarely functional. Papillary adenocarcinoma is the most common primary cancer of the thyroid and is nonfunctional.

21. The answer is C. *(Obstetrics; vital statistics)*
The perinatal mortality rate is the number of stillbirths and neonatal deaths per 1000 live births. The first two options are identical answers but do not include live births in the denominator. The last two options include abortions, which are not included in perinatal mortality rate calculations.

22. The answer is A. *(Psychiatry; schizophrenia)* In such cases, a premorbid history of social withdrawal is predictive of more severe and long-lasting psychopathology. A family history of schizophrenia is commonly found in second-degree relatives and has little prognostic significance. Sudden onset of psychotic symptomatology has a more favorable prognosis. Magnetic resonance imaging (MRI) changes are associated with more severe symptoms and clinical course in schizophrenia. The presence of catatonic symptomatology is not associated with any particular clinical course.

23. The answer is C. *(Biostatistics; incidence of disease)* Incidence is defined as the number of new cases of a disease over a specified period of time divided by the population at risk for that disease over that same time period, which is option C. Option A is incorrect because it refers to a moment in time (prevalence) rather than a period of time. Option B is incorrect because the numerator and denominator must be related. Option D is false because the numerator in an incidence calculation is a subset of the denominator; therefore, the numerator can never exceed the denominator. Option E is wrong because it is the denominator, not the numerator, that includes the total population at risk.

24. The answer is A. *(Infectious disease; endotoxic (septic) shock)* Endotoxic shock (septic shock) is commonly secondary to gram-negative septicemia (most commonly *Escherichia coli*) from a urinary tract abnormality, such as acute pyelonephritis or urinary tract obstruction. Endotoxin released from the cell walls of gram-negative bacteria produces characteristic hemodynamic findings that significantly differ from those associated with shock caused by hypovolemia (fluid loss), cardiac dysfunction (cardiogenic shock), and reflex vagal stimulation (neurogenic shock). Endotoxins activate the complement pathway, resulting in the release of anaphylatoxins C3a and C5a, which cause vasodilation of peripheral vessels, resulting in warm skin. In addition, increased arteriolar dilatation increases venous return to the heart, with a subsequent increase in cardiac output (high-output failure). Endotoxins also stimulate macrophages/monocytes to release tumor necrosis factor-alpha and interleukin-1, which damage endothelial cells and also increase neutrophil adhesion to endothelial cells, thus decreasing the peripheral neutrophil count. Endothelial damage in the lungs commonly predisposes to adult respiratory distress syndrome and also to disseminated intravascular coagulation.

Hypovolemic and cardiogenic shock characteristically are associated with a decreased cardiac output, sinus tachycardia with a weak pulse, and cold, clammy skin because of peripheral vasoconstriction. Neurogenic shock is caused by reflex vagal stimulation, with decreased cardiac output, hypotension, and decreased cerebral blood flow, causing the patient to faint.

25. The answer is A. *(Obstetrics; pelvic shapes)* Based on the general bony architecture, the female pelvis may be classified into four basic types. Gynecoid occurs in approximately 50% of women. Android, anthropoid, and platypelloid occur with frequencies of 30%, 20%, and 3%, respectively. Obstetroid is not a formally defined pelvic shape.

26. The answer is D. *(Pediatrics; renal solute load of protein in cow's milk)* Cow's milk is not recommended for children until 1 year of age. The high level of protein presents an increased solute load to the kidneys, and this overload can lead to dehydration.

27. The answer is C. *(General surgery; Hirschsprung's disease)* An absence of ganglion cells in the myenteric plexus of the rectum is known as Hirschsprung's disease. Stool is unable to pass the aganglionic segment, thus producing a "functional obstruction" with proximal dilatation of normal bowel and constipation. Newborns with this disorder are frequently unable to pass their meconium. Rectal examination reveals an absence of stool in the rectal vault. There is an association with Down syndrome and Chagas' disease due to

Trypanosoma cruzi. Necrotizing enterocolitis is the most common cause of death. Toxic mega-colon and perforation can also occur. Hirsch-sprung's disease is not associated with fecal soil-ing (present in functional constipation), bleeding, or excessive mucus in the stool.

28. The answer is A. *(Psychiatry; conversion disorder)*
Conversion disorder is often associated with blandness, which is sometimes referred to as "la belle indifférence." Simple phobias, obsessive-compulsive disorder, and hypochondriasis are often associated with anxiety. Melancholic depression may be associated with decreased psychomotor activity.

29. The answer is D. *(Obstetrics; first stage of labor)*
The first stage of labor (onset of true labor to complete cervical dilation) has two phases: a latent phase, during which cervical effacement and early dilation occur; and an active phase, dur-ing which more rapid cervical dilation occurs. The first three options are frequently noted in active labor but can occur in early labor. Membrane rupture is not essential for active labor diagnosis. Cervical dilation of at least 4 cm marks the active phase.

30. The answer is D. *(Biostatistics; prevalence of disease)*
Prevalence describes the disease at a specific time, which is option D. Option A is incorrect because it describes incidence, not prevalence. Option B is incorrect because prevalence is a function of incidence multiplied by duration of time. Therefore, it can never be lower than inci-dence. As the duration of a disease decreases, prevalence may approach incidence, but it will never be less. Option C is false because preva-lence is the number of cases at a point in time rather than over a time period. Option E is irrele-vant because calculation does not include a denominator.

31. The answer is C. *(Cardiology; cardiac tam-ponade)*
Cardiac tamponade is characterized by a de-crease in cardiac output and an increase in central venous pressure owing to restriction of blood flow into and out of the heart as fluid in the peri-cardial sac restricts filling of all the cardiac chambers. Echocardiography is the most sensi-tive and specific noninvasive test to establish the presence of fluid in the pericardial sac. Once the diagnosis is established, pericardiocentesis should be performed to immediately reduce intrapericardial sac pressure. Surgery follows to locate the source of the tamponade in those cases that are associated with trauma.

Distention of the neck veins on inspiration is called Kussmaul's sign. Normally, the increase in negative intrathoracic pressure on inspiration sucks blood from the jugular venous system into the right heart. However, if the right heart is restricted by fluid in the pericardial sac, the blood regurgitates into the jugular veins on inspiration.

A drop in the pulse or the blood pressure greater than 10 mm Hg on inspiration is called pulsus paradoxus. It reflects the drop in inflow of blood into the right heart on inspiration, which automatically decreases the outflow from the left ventricle. An increase in central venous pressure without an increase in blood pressure further documents the inability of the heart to receive fluid and pump it out into the systemic circula-tion; therefore, giving additional fluid would exacerbate the condition.

32. The answer is C. *(Neurology; plasma test for fatty acids)*
Adrenoleukodystrophy is marked by disorder of peroxisomes, which leads to the accumulation of very long-chain fatty acids in the tissues. X-linked, it affects males, usually beginning at 7 or 8 years of age. It is characterized by demyelina-tion of the central nervous system (CNS), as well as adrenal insufficiency. Although multiple scle-rosis (MS) is also a CNS demyelinating disease and can be suggested by oligoclonal bands, the clinical scenario with posterior hemisphere pre-dominance best fits adrenoleukodystrophy. Another disorder, metachromatic leukodystro-

phy, can be demonstrated by arylsulfatase A deficiency, but generally presents with weakness and decreased reflexes instead of spasticity, and with symmetric CNS demyelination. Amino acid screening is useful in the younger age-groups, but less fruitful especially in demyelinating disorders. Urine for porphyrin screening is helpful for peripheral demyelination, but less likely for central demyelination.

33. The answer is B. *(Obstetrics; third stage of labor)*
The third stage of labor starts from delivery of the infant and ends with the delivery of the placenta. The factor that contributes most to the mechanism of the third stage of labor is avulsion of anchoring villi by contracting myometrium. Although it is true that the estrogen level falls after delivery of the placenta, this decrease does not contribute to the third stage. The length of the first and second stages of labor is unrelated to the duration of the third stage. The levels of prolactin and umbilical vein P_{CO_2} are not involved in placental separation.

34. The answer is E. *(Pediatrics; recurrent pneumonia, foreign body aspiration)*
Foreign body aspiration is the most common cause of recurrent pneumonia in an otherwise healthy 3-year-old child. Because of the lung's anatomy, the right side is more common for aspiration. Many times when a child presents with pneumonia, a history of choking can be elicited. Immunodeficiency disorders are characterized by recurrent infections, usually by opportunistic organisms and failure to thrive. Cystic fibrosis similarly results in failure to thrive. Pneumonia is usually caused by *Pseudomonas*. Malabsorption and clubbing are often seen. Chédiak-Higashi syndrome is autosomal recessive, and partial albinism is a key to diagnosis. Giant granules are seen in neutrophils. Recurrent infections are common. Congenital lung abnormalities present at a much earlier age.

35. The answer is C. *(General surgery; gynecomastia)*
The patient has gynecomastia. Gynecomastia, the development of breast tissue in males, is normal in the neonate, pubertal boy, and elderly male. Increased estrogen stimulation (hyperestrinism) of breast tissue is the common factor in all cases of gynecomastia.

Adolescent gynecomastia is usually bilateral, and the tissue averages 2 to 3 cm in diameter. The breast enlargement is transient and most often subsides within a year. It is usually left alone unless it is greater than 5 cm and does not regress by 16 to 17 years of age. In the latter situation, a subcutaneous mastectomy is performed. Incision, aspiration, and topical steroids are not indicated.

In an adult male, hyperestrinism producing gynecomastia can be due to increased synthesis secondary to an adrenal/testicular tumor; increased human chorionic gonadotropin (hCG) from a testicular tumor; the hyperplastic Leydig cells in Klinefelter's syndrome; decreased catabolism of estrogen, as in cirrhosis of the liver (most common cause of pathologic gynecomastia); decreased androgen activity, which leaves estrogen unopposed (e.g., caused by cimetidine, spironolactone, hypothalamic/pituitary disorder); unknown mechanisms (e.g., marijuana, digitalis).

36. The answer is E. *(Psychiatry; psychodynamics)*
Transference often occurs in psychotherapy. By observing the way the patient interacts with the therapist, the therapist can gain insight into the patient's past conflicts with others. None of the other answers are related to the phenomenon of transference.

37. The answer is A. *(Obstetrics; placenta previa)*
Placenta previa is bleeding arising from a placenta abnormally implanted in the lower uterine segment. Abruptio placentae usually involves painful bleeding from a normally implanted placenta. Bleeding from vasa praevia is usually of fetal origin, leading to exsanguination of the fetus. Normal fetal heart rate would rule out this diagnosis. A bloody show is usually blood-tinged

mucus from cervical dilation and would not have significant clots. Disseminated intravascular coagulation is usually secondary to another pathological process rather than a primary diagnosis.

38. The answer is D. *(Biostatistics; incidence versus prevalence of disease)*
As the length of survival from acute leukemia increases (assuming the rate of new cases diagnosed remains unchanged), the number of cases at any point in time increases. Incidence, based on number of new cases only, remains unchanged. However, prevalence, based on number of active cases at a particular point in time, increases.

39. The answer is E. *(Gastroenterology; pancreatic carcinoma with obstructive jaundice)*
Carcinoma of the head of the pancreas is most common in men over 50 years of age. It produces an extrahepatic obstructive jaundice (65%) by blocking off the common bile duct. Additional findings include weight loss (60%), postprandial epigastric pain (75%) that is relieved by leaning forward, diarrhea owing to malabsorption, and a palpable gallbladder (Courvoisier's sign—50%) secondary to distention of the gallbladder by pressure in the bile duct. Smoking, diabetes, and chronic pancreatitis have been implicated in the genesis of pancreatic carcinoma.

Obstruction to bile flow (cholestasis) produces characteristic laboratory findings. Because bile predominantly contains direct (conjugated) bilirubin, the backflow of bile into the liver eventually results in regurgitation of direct bilirubin into the blood, which results in a direct hyperbilirubinemia (direct fraction > 50% of the total) and bilirubinuria because direct bilirubin is water-soluble. Absence of bile in the intestine results in clay-colored stools; usually, bilirubin is converted into urobilinogen (stercobilinogen), which provides the normal stool color. Absence of urobilinogen in the stool is associated with its absence in the urine as well, because a small proportion is normally reabsorbed via the enterohepatic circulation and recycled back to the liver (90%) and kidneys (10%) for filtration into the urine. Alkaline phosphatase and γ-glutamyltrans-

ferase are excellent markers for cholestasis and preferred over transaminases such as alanine and aspartate aminotransferases (ALT and AST, respectively), which are better indicators of diffuse liver cell necrosis.

Although a stone in the common bile duct, intrahepatic cholestasis, primary adenocarcinoma of the ampulla of Vater in the duodenum, and gallbladder disease can produce obstructive jaundice, the age, history of weight loss, and palpable gallbladder are more commonly associated with carcinoma of the head of the pancreas.

40. The answer is C. *(Obstetrics; hypertensive disorders of pregnancy)*
The case presentation describes the findings in a patient with preeclampsia, which typically occurs in primigravidas in the last trimester of pregnancy. Preeclampsia is characterized by an enhanced angiotensin response rather than a blunted one. This condition is usually unrelated to endorphin level, primary renal disease, or chronic hypertension.

41. The answer is D. *(General surgery; hypercalcemia in asymptomatic people; primary hyperparathyroidism)*
In an asymptomatic woman with a normal exam and no history of bone pain, hypercalcemia is most likely due to primary hyperparathyroidism.

Primary hyperparathyroidism is due to an adenoma in one of the inferior parathyroid glands in approximately 85% of cases. Hypercalcemia, hypophosphatemia, and elevated parathormone levels are present. A renal stone is the most common symptomatic presentation for primary hyperparathyroidism.

Hypercalcemia in a hospitalized patient is most likely due to cancer (most commonly breast cancer). Hypercalcemia in malignancy is either due to local production of factors that activate osteoclasts (interleukins, prostaglandin) or, most commonly, to secretion of a parathyroidlike peptide by breast carcinoma, squamous cell carcinoma of the lung, or renal adenocarcinoma. The peptide causes hypercalcemia and hypophosphatemia, but the parathormone level is decreased due to suppression by hypercalcemia (negative feedback). Thiazide diuretics produce hypercalcemia by increasing renal absorption of calcium and by enhancing osteoclast activity. Primary hyperparathyroidism is commonly present in thiazide-induced hypercalcemia. Excessive intake of calcium is a rare cause of hypercalcemia.

42. The answer is C. *(Psychiatry; psychodynamics)*
Displacement occurs when the emotions associated with a psychologically unacceptable object, idea, or activity are transferred to another object or situation, which is often symbolically related to the original one. An example of this proposed psychodynamic explanation for simple phobias is snakes, which are often said to symbolize a penis. The other responses are not postulated as mechanisms for simple phobia.

43. The answer is A. *(Biostatistics; mortality rate)*
The perinatal mortality rate is calculated by adding the number of fetal deaths ($\geq$ 20 weeks' gestation) and the number of neonatal deaths (within first 28 days of life), then dividing by the total number of births. In the scenario presented, 100 + 5 is divided by 2100 + 100, which equals 105/2200.

44. The answer is E. *(General surgery; radical mastectomy versus modified radical mastectomy)*
The difference between a radical (Halsted) and a modified radical mastectomy is that the latter spares the pectoralis major muscle. Both operations remove all ipsilateral breast tissue, the nipple-areolar complex, and the axillary lymph nodes below the axillary vein. A radical mastectomy has the disadvantage of being the most disfiguring of the available treatments for management of primary breast cancer.

45. The answer is D. *(Gastroenterology; mesenteric angina)*
Mesenteric angina most commonly occurs in elderly men who have evidence of atherosclerotic disease. It is characterized by severe midabdominal pain associated with vomiting and abdominal distention approximately 30 minutes after eating. The pain is so great that patients are fearful of eating and experience subsequent weight loss.

If infarction occurs, which is not present in this patient, patients may have peritoneal signs (rebound tenderness), absent bowel sounds, and hypotension. In addition, a striking neutrophilic leukocytosis with a left shift (> 10% band neutrophils). The serum amylase is increased, and this change is frequently misinterpreted as acute pancreatitis. Barium studies reveal "thumbprinting" of the mucosa caused by submucosal hemorrhages and edema.

Chronic ischemic disease of the bowel may result in ischemic strictures in the splenic flexure of the colon where the superior and inferior mesenteric arteries overlap, leaving a watershed area with an inadequate blood supply. Ischemic strictures do not occur in the small bowel because it does not have an overlapping blood supply. Strictures are associated with obstructive signs and symptoms.

Although left-sided colon carcinoma, with obstruction, inflammation (diverticulitis, Crohn's disease), and other causes of obstruction (adhesions, hernias, volvulus), produces abdominal pain, the age of the patient, the relationship of the pain with eating, physical findings of atherosclerotic peripheral vascular disease, absence of blood in the stool, and negative colonoscopy and barium studies favor an ischemic origin for the disease. Angiography would be helpful in confirming the diagnosis.

46. The answer is C. *(Obstetrics; preeclampsia)*
Prevention of seizures is a crucial aspect of the care of any woman with a hypertensive disorder of pregnancy; and, in the United States, magnesium sulfate is the most commonly used preventive agent for this condition. Phenobarbital, diazepam, and diphenylhydantoin are standard anticonvulsant medications, but are not used primarily for seizure prophylaxis. Magnesium gluconate has no anticonvulsant activity.

47. The answer is B. *(Neurology; emergent test, computed tomography)*

A computed tomography (CT) scan immediately shows any blood present—the most pressing concern in a patient who is anticoagulated and has a new neurologic deficit. A magnetic resonance imaging (MRI) scan, although helpful, is less sensitive for acute bleeds, takes longer, and is less likely to be available on an emergent basis. The electroencephalogram (EEG) would be expected to show focal slowing on the right but cannot differentiate between an ischemic and hemorrhagic stroke. Carotid duplex ultrasonography would be useful in the course of the workup, but is not justified on an emergent basis. Finally, a spinal tap not only would be unhelpful diagnostically, but also might put an anticoagulated patient at risk for a spinal epidural hematoma.

48. The answer is B. *(General surgery; lumpectomy)*

The majority of patients with potentially curable breast cancer are given the choice between a lumpectomy (segmental mastectomy), which includes excision of the lesion, low axillary node dissection, and postoperative radiation therapy, and a modified radical mastectomy, which removes all of the breast tissue on the affected side, the nipple-areolar complex, the pectoralis minor, and the axillary nodes below the axillary vein. Lumpectomy is usually limited to women with small tumors (< 4 cm). Simple lumpectomy without low axillary dissection and postoperative radiation is not considered adequate treatment for breast cancer. A low axillary node resection is useful for planning therapy and staging of the patient. Postoperative radiation kills any remaining tumor in the breast tissue. Adjuvant systemic therapy must be considered for nearly all patients with potentially curable breast cancer.

49. The answer is D. *(Obstetrics; hepatitis B and pregnancy)*

The neonate can gain protection from hepatitis B by passive immunization at birth. The hepatitis B virus is a DNA virus that is transmitted via blood, saliva, vaginal secretions, semen, and breast milk, as well as across the placenta. Pregnancy does not appear to accelerate acute hepatitis B in the mother. The main route of neonatal infection is by vaginal delivery. The virus can be transmitted through breast milk. Neonatal infection can be fulminant and lethal.

50. The answer is E. *(Psychiatry; pain)*

The normal saline solution is unlikely to have corrected the patient's underlying pathology. However, it is common for patients to respond to the placebo effect inherent in many medical interventions. Such responses do not suggest that pain or discomfort is factitious, exaggerated, or nonphysiologic.

51. The answer is E. *(Biostatistics; odds ratio and relative risk)*

The odds ratio is a method of estimating relative risk in retrospective studies. It is calculated by dividing the odds of exposure among the diseased group (the numerator) by the odds of exposure among the disease-free group (denominator). Using the data from the table, the numerator is 10/2 and the denominator is 50/350.

52. The answer is C. *(General surgery; peripheral arterial occlusion)*

The patient has an acute arterial occlusion. Acute arterial occlusion is associated with pain, absence of the pulse, paresthesias, paralysis, and pallor of the extremity, which is accentuated when the extremity is raised. The popliteal artery is the most susceptible vessel for occlusion, since it is commonly affected by atherosclerosis and is a small calibre artery. A herniated disc would not be expected to involve the whole leg, nor would it present with the given symptom/sign complex. There would be an absence of deep tendon reflexes and various motor and sensory signs as well. Superficial thrombophlebitis in the saphenous system of the legs presents with pain and tenderness along the course of the vessel. Deep venous insufficiency is associated with superficial varicose veins and stasis dermatitis around the ankle.

53. The answer is E. *(Psychiatry; depression)*
Of the drugs listed, antihypertensive drugs are most likely to cause depression. Other drugs that are strongly associated with depression are steroids and hypnotics. Psychostimulants can also precipitate depression during drug withdrawal.

54. The answer is C. *(Pharmacology; cardiac drugs)*
Lidocaine is a class I_B antiarrhythmic agent, blocking both activated and inactivated sodium channels. It is the drug of choice for suppression of ventricular tachycardia after acute myocardial infarction. Given intravenously, lidocaine has a rapid onset and reduces the incidence of ventricular fibrillation. It is the least cardiotoxic of the currently available antiarrhythmic agents, but in high doses may depress myocardial contractility and cause hypotension.

55. The answer is E. *(Obstetrics; herpes simplex and pregnancy)*
The description is that of recurrent genital herpes. The herpes simplex virus has potential for significant adverse impact on the fetus, neonate, or both. If no lesions are present at the start of labor, this woman can safely undergo labor and vaginal delivery. Because she has protective antibodies against herpes, she does not experience viremia; therefore, there is no risk of transplacental viral passage. If she has no breast lesions after delivery, she can safely breast-feed.

56. The answer is B. *(Behavioral science; coronary artery disease and type A personality)*
Coronary artery disease is closely associated with the "type A" personality shown by this patient. Other medical illnesses associated with psychological factors are cancer (separation and loss), bronchial asthma (dependency), obesity (oral fixation and regression), and diabetes mellitus (stress and passivity).

57. The answer is B. *(Endocrinology; hypoglycemia in diabetes mellitus)*
The most common overall cause of hypoglycemia is excessive insulin in a person with insulin-dependent diabetes. Hypoglycemia is precipitated by administration of an excessive dose of insulin, increased physical activity, delay in eating a meal, fluctuations in absorption in various administration sites, and autonomic neuropathy impairing counterregulatory mechanisms. The adrenergic symptoms of hypoglycemia include perspiration, tachycardia, increased salivation, and restlessness. These symptoms can be blunted if the patient is taking a beta-blocker (e.g., propranolol), thus making the diagnosis more difficult. Lack of Kussmaul's breathing (deep respirations) and no smell of ketones on the breath are clues that ketoacidosis is not present in this patient. Immediate measurement of blood glucose with glucose-oxidase–impregnated paper strips or a glucometer is easily accomplished in the emergency room, so therapy can be initiated. Patients who are conscious should be given oral feedings of fruit juice. Comatose patients are usually given an intravenous infusion of 50% dextrose in water. If intravenous glucose is not available, 1 mg of glucagon is given intramuscularly.

The history that this patient has insulin-dependent diabetes and the classic adrenergic symptoms of hypoglycemia argue against the need for a complete blood count (CBC), serum electrolytes, a drug screen, or arterial blood gas determination as the initial step in management.

58. The answer is E. *(General surgery; physical findings in breast cancer)*
Breast skin edema with dimpling resembling orange peel or pigskin is called "peau d'orange." This is due to the obstruction of subcutaneous lymphatics by a tumor. This finding is almost pathognomonic of cancerous involvement of the breast.

The most common presenting symptom of breast cancer is a painless, moveable mass usually located in the upper outer quadrant of the breast. Painful masses in the breast are usually benign (e.g., traumatic fat necrosis, fibrocystic change). An exception to the rule is inflammatory carcinoma, which is painful.

Bloody nipple discharge in a woman under 40 years of age is most commonly due to a benign intraductal papilloma, whereas malignancy is the most common cause after 50 years of age. A clear nipple discharge is not associated with cancer.

Other physical findings that suggest malignancy are dimpling of the skin on movement of the arms, vascular engorgement overlying the breast, diffuse "inflammation" of the breast (inflammatory carcinoma), nipple erosions (Paget's disease), and presence of a mass in a woman over 50 with axillary node enlargement.

59. The answer is A. *(Obstetrics; group B streptococcus and pregnancy)*
The group B streptococcus has potential for significant adverse impact on the fetus, neonate, or both. A positive culture tends to indicate infants who are not infected. A negative culture does not rule out the organism being present at delivery because the majority of carriers are so only intermittently or transiently. Treating carriers is ineffective for eradicating the organism. The organism is part of normal female genital tract flora. Current nonculture tests are specific but not very sensitive.

60. The answer is D. *(Neurology; diagnostic test)*
This patient likely has Wilson's disease, an autosomal recessive disorder of the lenticular nuclei (globus pallidus and putamen) and the liver, hence the name hepatolenticular degeneration. The positive but spotty family history would be an argument for the autosomal recessive pattern rather than autosomal dominant (such as Huntington's disease), and the abnormal liver functions and positive magnetic resonance imaging (MRI) would confirm the autosomal recessive pattern. Copper and ceruloplasmin screening confirms the diagnosis. Porphyrin screening is helpful in the patient with acute mental status changes, abdominal pain, and ascending paralysis (mimicking Guillain-Barré syndrome). Although multiple sclerosis might be shown by spinal tap (but is unlikely with a negative MRI), it could not explain the abnormal liver functions. Likewise, the heavy metal screening would not explain the clinical situation (but patients with disorders of iron deposition, such as hemachro-

matosis, can have deposition of iron in the basal ganglia). Aminoacidurias are unlikely in this age-group, although not impossible.

61. The answer is C. *(General surgery; spontaneous pneumothorax)*
A spontaneous pneumothorax is most commonly the result of a ruptured bleb within the pleura which causes an ipsilateral collapse of the lung. If located on the right side, this would result in decreased breath sounds and hyperresonance to percussion. In addition, the intercostal width would be decreased, since there is less volume of air in the cavity and the mediastinal structures would shift to the right side.

A tension pneumothorax refers to an accumulation of air in the pleural cavity that increases with each inspiration. This is analogous to air entering a tire but not leaking out. A tension pneumothorax results in decreased breath sounds on the affected side, hyperresonance to percussion and widening of the intercostals on the affected side (increased air in the cavity) but shifting of the mediastinal structures and trachea to the opposite side.

In either a spontaneous or a tension pneumothorax, treatment requires the insertion of a chest tube placed under water seal. Egophony is a physical finding associated with a lung consolidation such as pneumonia. When the patient says "eeeeeee," it sounds like "aaaaaaa" through the stethoscope.

62. The answer is B. *(Psychiatry; depression)*
The presence of hopelessness as a component of depression greatly increases the chance of suicide. Another high risk finding would be a suicide plan. The other choices are associated with the syndrome of depression, but are not as strongly associated with suicidal behavior.

63. The answer is E. *(Obstetrics; substance abuse)*
A frequent adverse effect associated with maternal prenatal use of many substances is intrauterine growth retardation and preterm delivery. Each substance listed has an adverse impact on pregnancy outcome, but only cocaine has clearly

defined vascular-disruption anomalies such as intestinal atresia, limb-reduction defects, and brain anomalies.

64. The answer is B. *(Pharmacology; cardiac drugs)*

The concentrations of certain ions in the extracellular compartment influence sensitivity to digitalis. Potassium competes with digitalis for binding to Na^+-K^+-adenosinetriphosphatase (ATPase) [the initial "target" of cardiac glycosides] and also inhibits abnormal cardiac automaticity. Therefore, moderate hyperkalemia can reverse the cardiotoxic actions of digitalis. The suggested changes in serum calcium, magnesium, and sodium tend to enhance the toxicity of the cardiac glycosides.

65. The answer is E. *(Behavioral science; long-term nursing-home care)*

Long-term nursing-home care is paid for by an individual's private funds. Only after most of this woman's $300,000 are exhausted (the amount which can remain is dictated by state law) will she be declared indigent and become eligible for Medicaid. Medicare pays for nursing-home care for people 65 years of age and older, only for a limited time period and only after a patient has been hospitalized for a specific illness.

66. The answer is B. *(Obstetrics; substance abuse)*

Substance use by an expectant mother can affect reproduction, from fertility through pregnancy and lactation. Tobacco, alcohol, marijuana, amphetamines, and narcotics have an adverse impact on pregnancy outcome, but only alcohol has a clearly defined syndrome with intrauterine growth restriction, central nervous system effects, and facial anomalies.

67. The answer is E. *(Rheumatology; ankylosing spondylitis)*

Ankylosing spondylitis is a seronegative (negative rheumatoid factor), human leukocyte antigen (HLA)-B27–positive (95%) spondyloarthropathy that occurs primarily in young men between 15 and 30 years of age. Characteristic features include an insidious onset of morning stiffness in the lower back that persists for more than 3 months and improves as the day progresses or when the person exercises. Sclerotic changes in the sacroiliac area are the first x-ray evidence of the disease. Patients have diminished anterior flexion of the spine, which is documented with the Schoeber test. Eventually, the vertebral column fuses to produce the classic "bamboo spine." Additional complications include restriction of chest movement and subsequent restrictive-type lung disease, iridocyclitis (25%), aortic valve insufficiency (3%–10%), and reactive amyloidosis. Indomethacin is the drug of choice.

The serum antinuclear antibody test is negative in ankylosing spondylitis because it is not a collagen vascular disease or a variant of rheumatoid arthritis. Gout does not present with lower back pain, so a uric acid level is not indicated. The erythrocyte sedimentation rate is a nonspecific indicator of inflammation that has little clinical usefulness in either diagnosing or following disease activity in patients with joint diseases.

68. The answer is C. *(Pediatrics; Reye's syndrome)*

Reye's syndrome shows a very high association with the ingestion of aspirin-containing medicines during influenza-like illnesses or varicella. Reye's syndrome usually presents in a previously healthy child who suffers an upper respiratory infection (90%) or varicella (5%–7%). After the child seems to have recovered, the symptoms of vomiting, lethargy, and confusion can appear and progress quickly. Liver enzymes and ammonia are elevated. Treatment requires early recognition and control of increased intracranial pressure. Prognosis depends on duration of disordered cerebral function.

69. The answer is C. *(Obstetrics; heart disease and pregnancy)*

The New York Heart Association's functional classification of heart disease is of value in both assessing the risk of pregnancy for a patient with cardiac disease and determining the optimal management during pregnancy, labor, and delivery. Class 0 is not part of the New York classification. Class I shows no signs or symptoms at any time. Class III has no symptoms at rest, but marked limitation with physical activity. Class IV has symptoms even at rest. Class II is the classification of this 18-year-old pregnant woman. She has no symptoms at rest, but minor limitation with physical activity.

70. The answer is B. *(General surgery; abdominal pain, acute pancreatitis)*
Acute pancreatitis produces midepigastric pain that is steady, boring, and often penetrates straight through into the back or radiates to the periumbilical area. Colicky pain is a feature of obstruction and would not be expected in retrocecal appendicitis or a ruptured ovarian cyst. Obstipation refers to constipation and inability to pass gas. It is associated with obstruction. Therefore, a mid–small bowel obstruction would have a colicky pain rather than a steady, boring type of pain. A retrocecal appendicitis is associated with diarrhea. A ruptured ovarian cyst, particularly on the right side, simulates the pain of acute appendicitis with right lower quadrant pain and rebound tenderness due to irritation of the peritoneum from the cyst fluid. A posterior penetrating duodenal ulcer would extend into the pancreas, producing a localized type of pancreatitis with pain radiating into the back rather than the right lower quadrant.

71. The answer is E. *(Orthopedics; fractures)*
A supracondylar fracture of the humerus often entraps the brachial artery and the median nerve. There is a danger of developing Volkmann's ischemic contracture in the forearm muscles due to the ischemia. A fasciotomy is often necessary to release the pressure in the tight forearm muscle compartment. Greenstick fractures are commonly seen in children and refer to a break in the cortex on the convex side of the shaft but an intact concave side. A Pott's fracture occurs when the foot is forced into eversion and abduction resulting in fractures of both malleoli (bimalleolar fracture). A Colles' fracture involves the distal end of the radius at the suprastyloid level, plus a fracture of the styloid process of the ulnar. It produces a "dinner fork" deformity. It is caused by falling on an outstretched hand.

Fracture of the femoral neck is not only the most common fracture of the femur in the elderly but also the fracture most often associated with avascular necrosis and increased nonunion. Osteoporosis, due to estrogen deficiency in the female, is the most common cause of these fractures. Intertrochanteric fractures do not have the same risk for avascular necrosis.

72. The answer is B. *(Obstetrics; thromboembolic disorders and pregnancy)*
The best single test for deep venous thrombosis is a venogram. Thromboembolic disorders are one of the major causes of maternal mortality in the United States. Superficial thrombophlebitis does not require anticoagulant medication. Warfarin crosses the placental barrier freely and is identified with a unique embryopathy. On the other hand, heparin does not cross the placenta and therefore has no direct fetal effects. Approximately 80% of thromboembolic pregnancy complications occur in the postpartum period.

73. The answer is A. *(Psychiatry; substance abuse)*
Many studies have demonstrated a component of heritability for alcohol dependency, especially in male offspring of male alcoholics, even if the child is not raised by the parent. Although there is speculation about heritability of other substance dependencies, the data are much less compelling. Social factors appear to be of great significance in causing opiate, stimulant, and tobacco dependency.

74. The answer is A. *(Pharmacology; autonomic drugs)*
Drugs that block muscarinic receptors (e.g., atropine) are effective bronchodilators and may be as useful as beta$_2$-receptor agonists (e.g., terbutaline) in patients with chronic obstructive pulmonary disease. However, the mydriatic action of atropine increases intraocular pressure and causes acute angle closure in patients with glaucoma. Epinephrine, timolol (a beta blocker), and pilocarpine are all used in the management of glaucoma.

75. The answer is B. *(Obstetrics; HIV and pregnancy)*
Infection with the human immunodeficiency virus (HIV) results in the development of the acquired immune deficiency syndrome (AIDS), which has been a recognized disease in the United States since 1981. Pregnancy does not appear to accelerate HIV. Neonates can be infected from breast-feeding mothers. There is no current effective immunization for neonates. Disease progression in neonates and infants is more rapid than in adults. Mode of delivery does not affect maternal–neonatal transmission.

76. The answer is A. *(Behavioral science; visits to physicians)*
People in the United States make significantly fewer visits to physicians than do people in developed countries with socialized medicine.

77. The answer is D. *(Infectious disease; acquired immune deficiency syndrome)*
Acquired immune deficiency syndrome (AIDS) is the most common acquired immunodeficiency in the United States. It is caused by human immunodeficiency virus-1 (HIV-1), which is an RNA retrovirus containing reverse transcriptase. The virus attacks and destroys CD4 helper T cells, thus lowering the CD4 helper T-cell count (less than 200 cells/μl) and reversing the CD4 helper T-cell/CD8 suppressor T-cell ratio from a normal of 2/1 to less than 0.5.

Because helper T cells are integral to normal cellular immunity (type IV hypersensitivity), tests that evaluate cellular immunity are impaired. Intradermal injections of common antigens do not elicit the expected immune response. This lack of immune response is called anergy. In vitro stimulation of T-cell response to phytohemagglutinin, a potent T-cell mitogen, is also impaired. Epstein-Barr virus and cytomegalovirus infections are common in AIDS. They are potent polyclonal stimulators of B cells, which produce a polyclonal gammopathy. However, because patients are unable to mount an antibody response to new antigen, they are still susceptible to bacterial infections. Defective cellular immunity is responsible for *Pneumocystis carinii* lung infection,

which is the most common initial presentation in AIDS, and other opportunistic infections.

78. The answer is A. *(Neurology; Bell's palsy)*
Bell's palsy is idiopathic and nearly always acute. All the patient's deficits are referable to the peripheral nervous system, including the loss of taste (chorda tympani branch of the facial nerve) and hyperacusis (branch to the stapedius muscle of the ear). The strokes are unlikely because of sparing of the rest of the right body and no other central signs. A brain-stem glioma and parotid tumor, although commonly presenting with facial nerve weakness, are unlikely when the acuteness of the event is considered.

79. The answer is A. *(Obstetrics; diabetes mellitus and pregnancy)*
The incidence of diabetes mellitus in pregnancy is less than 0.5%, but if present, it can adversely affect both mother and fetus. The case presentation describes abnormal 1- and 2-hour glucose values, but a normal fasting level. This description meets the criteria for class A1, and the disorder can be treated with diet alone. The other classes listed require additional insulin therapy.

80. The answer is E. *(Pediatrics; complications of measles)*
Otitis media is the most common complication of measles, occurring in 8500 to 15,000 per 100,000 cases. Because of mesenteric node involvement, diffuse lymphadenopathy can cause abdominal pain mimicking appendicitis. Subacute sclerosing panencephalitis is a rare neurologic complication, occurring in 0.5 to 2 per 100,000 cases. Interstitial pneumonia is caused by the measles virus itself and is more common in immunocompromised patients. Bronchopneumonia is more common than interstitial pneumonia and is usually caused by pneumococcus. The keratoconjunctivitis seen in measles is asymptomatic and can persist up to 4 months.

81. The answer is D. *(Psychiatry; psychodynamics)*
Splitting is described as the psychological separation of all good qualities into one individual and

all bad qualities into another. This separation occurs when an individual cannot tolerate ambivalent feelings toward a particular individual. Children and persons with borderline personality disorder often manifest evidence of splitting.

82. The answer is D. *(Pharmacology; cardiac drugs and pharmacokinetics)*
Rapid control of the arrhythmia follows achievement of a therapeutic blood level of lidocaine. Although lidocaine is metabolized extensively by the liver, the elimination half-life of the drug is 1 to 2 hours, which cannot account for such a rapid reappearance of the arrhythmia. There is no evidence that cardiac cells are capable of rapid (and reversible) changes in sensitivity to any antiarrhythmic drug. In this situation, the reappearance of the arrhythmia reflects the rapid redistribution of lidocaine to other tissues, resulting in a decrease in plasma concentration of the drug below therapeutic levels. A similar process, involving redistribution of thiopental from the brain to other tissues, is responsible for termination of the anesthetic effects of the intravenous barbiturate.

83. The answer is B. *(Pediatrics; cow's milk versus human breast milk)*
Human breast milk contains approximately four times as much vitamin C as does cow's milk. Both milks contain approximately the same amount of water and solids. Cow's milk contains approximately twice the protein of human milk and four times the amount of vitamin K. Both milks contain similar amounts of iron, but iron in human milk is better absorbed.

84. The answer is C. *(Obstetrics; cholelithiasis and pregnancy)*
The high estrogen levels during pregnancy may predispose the woman to cholelithiasis. The right-lower quadrant location of the appendix may be altered by the enlarging uterus. Although preterm labor is a concern, laparotomy should not be deferred when indicated. Peritoneal response is blunted during pregnancy, therefore making assessment of the degree of inflammation more difficult. Pancreatitis is uncommon in reproductive-age women, compared with older individuals.

85. The answer is C. *(Pediatrics; findings in a newborn girl)*
Cord blood immunoglobulin M (IgM) is the lowest at birth than any other stage of life. Mean hemoglobin at birth is 16.8 g/dl and can be as high as 22 g/dl. Vaginal bleeding (pseudomenses) and gynecomastia are not uncommon and are probably secondary to maternal hormones transferred through the placenta. Bilirubin levels of 2 mg/dl or higher are common in newborns.

86. The answer is A. *(Orthopedics; orthopedic tests)*
Finkelstein's test is used to diagnose chronic stenosing tenosynovitis (deQuervain's disease). The patient is asked to make a tight fist over the flexed thumb. The examiner pushes the base of the flexed thumb in an ulnar direction and the patient feels pain in the region of the radial styloid process.

Schoeber's test is for ankylosing spondylitis, an HLA-B27–positive arthritis that begins in the sacroiliac area and involves the vertebral column. It tests for the limited anterior flexion of the spine, which is a characteristic finding in these patients.

McMurray's test evaluates the knee for meniscus tears. If a click is felt along the posteromedial margin of the knee while it is being rotated, this indicates a medial meniscus tear. If a click is felt along the posterolateral margin, a lateral meniscus tear is present.

Ortolani's test evaluates newborns for congenital hip dislocation. A positive test is when abduction of the affected thigh produces a palpable click as the dislocated femoral head slips back into the acetabulum.

The anterior draw sign is used to test for a tear in the anterior cruciate ligament of the knee. It is performed by moving the knee forward, while the lower leg is stabilized. Increased mobility of the knee in a forward direction indicates a tear of the anterior cruciate in the knee. A posterior draw sign indicates a tear of the posterior cruciate ligament.

87. The answer is A. *(Psychiatry; cognitive disorder)*
Vitamin B$_{12}$ deficiency causes neurodegeneration and dementia. Causes of B$_{12}$ deficiency include strict vegetarianism, alcoholism, and pernicious anemia. This condition is relatively more common in the elderly and should be investigated as part of any workup for dementia.

88. The answer is D. *(Pediatrics; conjunctival irritation in newborn)*
Chemical irritation (e.g., AgNO$_3$, or silver nitrate) is the most common cause of conjunctivitis in the first 24 hours after birth. Gonococcal ophthalmia presents as a purulent conjunctivitis approximately 2 to 3 days after birth—or up to 21 days if prophylaxis is given. Chlamydial conjunctivitis is the most common infectious cause and occurs 5 to 23 days after birth. *Staphylococcus aureus* conjunctivitis is less common. Congenital lacrimal duct obstruction appears days to weeks after birth and is usually unilateral. It generally resolves over time with gentle massage of the duct.

89. The answer is A. *(Obstetrics; fetal malpresentation)*
Breech presentation occurs when the fetal buttocks or lower extremities present into the maternal pelvis, a finding in 3% of deliveries. In frank breech, thighs are flexed, legs extended. Complete breech has both thighs and knees flexed. Incomplete breech occurs when one or both thighs are extended and one or both knees lie below the buttocks. Transverse breech is not a medical term.

90. The answer is D. *(Cardiology; ventricular tachycardia)*
Ventricular tachycardia is defined as three or more beats of ventricular origin that occur in succession at a rate in excess of 100 beats/min (usually between 120 and 220 beats/min). The rhythm may be regular or irregular. P waves may be present, with no fixed relationship to the QRS complexes, or absent, depending on the ventricular rate. The width of the QRS is 0.12 second or

greater, and the morphology is bizarre, with notching frequently present.

This patient's ventricular rate is approximately 150 beats/min and the rhythm is slightly irregular. A burst of seven consecutive wide complexes follows a normal sinus rhythm and ends with a premature ventricular complex coupled to a sinus complex. The configuration of the premature complex is similar to that of the tachycardia complexes, so this configuration represents a ventricular tachycardia. When prompt therapy is indicated, lidocaine is the treatment of choice.

Premature atrial contractions originate in the atria outside of the sinus node. The rhythm is irregular because ventricular activation may not occur (nonconduction), resulting in a pause in the cardiac rhythm.

Atrial flutter is a regular atrial rhythm that results from reentry at the atrial level. The atrial rate varies from 220 to 350 beats/min, whereas the ventricular rate varies from 150 to 175 beats/min, indicating atrioventricular conduction ratios ranging from 2:1 to 4:1. The atrial waves have a "sawtooth" or "picket fence" configuration.

Paroxysmal (supraventricular) tachycardia has a regular atrial rate of 160 to 220 beats/min and a similar ventricular rate if the atrial rate is under 200 beats/min (atrioventricular conduction ratio of 1:1). The atrial rhythm is usually regular. P waves are frequently difficult to identify; but when present, they may have different contours than sinus P waves. The P-R and QRS intervals are variable. The QRS complexes are of normal configuration. Carotid sinus massage or the Valsalva maneuver (patients hold their breath) is frequently used to convert paroxysmal tachycardia to normal sinus rhythm.

Sinus tachycardia is caused by an increased rate of discharge from the sinus node. The rate is regular and greater than 100 beats/min. Each QRS is preceded by an upright P wave in leads I and II, and aV$_F$.

91. The answer is D. *(Pharmacology; autonomic drugs)*
Activators of beta$_2$ adrenoceptors (e.g., terbutaline), which cause relaxation of respiratory,

uterine, and vascular smooth muscle, are used to treat asthma and to suppress premature labor. Beta$_2$ activation promotes uptake of potassium (decreased extracellular level) and glycogenolysis (increased blood glucose). Parasympathomimetic (not sympathomimetic) drugs increase gastrointestinal motility. Reflex tachycardia is likely in response to vasodilation and also from direct cardiostimulant actions because terbutaline is not totally selective for beta$_2$ receptors.

92. The answer is D. *(Endocrinology; Addison's disease)*
A patient with small cell carcinoma of the lung with disseminated disease, hypotension, decreased serum cortisol, and electrolyte abnormalities most likely has adrenal insufficiency, or Addison's disease. Metastatic carcinoma must destroy greater than 90% of both adrenal glands before symptoms and signs of adrenal insufficiency are manifested.

The loss of cortisol, mineralocorticoids, and catecholamines has profound effects on body homeostasis. Hypocortisolism results in hypoglycemia, because cortisol is a gluconeogenic hormone. Hypoaldosteronism affects the distal tubule exchange of sodium for potassium or hydrogen ions. This condition results in a hypertonic loss of sodium in the urine and subsequent hyponatremia and hypotension from volume depletion. The retention of potassium produces hyperkalemia, which alters cardiac function. Inability to secrete hydrogen ions causes them to combine with chloride ions in the extracellular fluid to form hydrochloric acid (HCl). This acid produces a metabolic acidosis, which is manifested by a drop in serum bicarbonate. Loss of catecholamines has the potential for affecting heart rate, cardiac contractility, and vascular tone by decreasing beta-receptor stimulation.

Choice A with hyponatremia, hypokalemia, hypochloremia, and a low bicarbonate could be due to the inappropriate antidiuretic hormone syndrome. Excess release of antidiuretic hormone causes an increase in the reabsorption of free water, which has a dilutional effect on sodium, chloride, potassium, and bicarbonate.

Choice B with hypernatremia, hypokalemia, hyperchloremia, and metabolic alkalosis is commonly associated with mineralocorticoid excess states, such as primary aldosteronism. In this disease, autonomous (unregulated) production of aldosterone by the adrenal gland results in an excess reabsorption of sodium to produce hypernatremia. The increased exchange of sodium for potassium produces a hypokalemia. In addition, the excess exchange of sodium for hydrogen ions leaves bicarbonate behind in the tubules because the hydrogen ions came from the dissociation of carbonic acid into hydrogen ions and bicarbonate. The excess bicarbonate that is left behind produces a metabolic alkalosis.

Choice C with hyponatremia, hypokalemia, hypochloremia, and metabolic alkalosis is commonly seen with diuretic therapy using either loop diuretics or thiazides. As sodium reabsorption is blocked by these drugs, the excess delivery of sodium to the distal tubule increases the exchange of sodium for potassium, which produces hypokalemia, and hydrogen ions, which leave unneutralized bicarbonate behind, resulting in metabolic alkalosis.

93. The answer is C. *(Obstetrics; preterm labor)*
Even though less than 10% of all infants born in the United States are preterm, they account for up to 70% of neonatal morbidity and mortality. Multiple gestation, placenta previa, and pyelonephritis are indications for tocolysis. However, if severe preeclampsia is present, the mother's life and health are jeopardized by prolonging the pregnancy; therefore, tocolysis is inappropriate. A positive β-strep culture is not a contraindication for tocolysis.

94. The answer is D. *(Pediatrics; Erb-Duchenne paralysis)*
Erb-Duchenne paralysis is a brachial plexus injury. It usually occurs during delivery as a consequence of traction of the head. C5 and C6 are involved. Ipsilateral diaphragmatic paralysis occurs with involvement of C4. The position of the arm and hand is referred to as the "waiter's tip." Klumpke's paralysis involves C7, C8, T1 and is characterized by a "claw hand." Clavicular

fracture causes an asymmetric Moro, and crepitus is felt over the clavicle. Todd's paralysis is a hemiparesis occurring after a seizure and resolves within 24 hours. Spinal cord injuries occur most commonly at the level of C7, T1. Complete paralysis of voluntary motion occurs below that level. Signs can appear at birth or within the first week.

95. The answer is A. *(General surgery; hernia types)*
Femoral hernias are more common in women. The hernias protrude small bowel through the femoral canal beneath the inguinal ligament and medial to the femoral artery. The neck of the hernia is narrow, thus predisposing the bowel to strangulation and infarction in 30%–40% of cases.

Indirect hernias are the most common type of hernia. In children, they represent the persistence of the peritoneal communication between the abdominal cavity and the tunica vaginalis. In adults, they are secondary to a protrusion of a new peritoneal process that progresses obliquely through the internal inguinal ring, out the external ring, and into the scrotum. Small bowel extends into the scrotal sac and hits the side of the examining finger when the patient strains. There is a danger of strangulation, but not as great as that associated with a femoral hernia. The Bassini repair is the most common surgical procedure used in adults. It approximates the transversalis fascia to Poupart's ligament and leaves the spermatic cord in its normal anatomic position. The Marcy repair is used in children. It involves high ligation of the sac and tightening of the internal ring.

Direct hernias protrude through Hesselbach's triangle. They protrude directly at the examining finger on examination and appear as a symmetrical, circular swelling at the external ring. There is very little risk of strangulation. Reinforcement of the defective fascia in Hesselbach's triangle is essential in its repair. A pantaloon hernia is a combination of a direct and indirect hernia.

Ventral hernias (incisional hernias) refer to the herniation of bowel into a previous surgical site. Factors predisposing to these hernias include obesity, old age, debilitation, the need for surgical drains, postoperative wound infections, poor surgical technique, and violent coughing in the postoperative period.

A spigelian hernia refers to bowel that herniates through the linea semilunaris located above the level of the inferior epigastric artery.

96. The answer is B. *(Psychiatry; antipsychotics, tardive dyskinesia)*
Tardive dyskinesia emerges in a substantial number of patients who have had long-term treatment with antipsychotics. This dyskinesia consists of choreoathetoid movements, which are reminiscent of those of Huntington's disease. The condition often is first evident in the fingers and tongue, but later becomes more generalized.

97. The answer is C. *(Pediatrics; ipsilateral paralysis of the diaphragm)*
Phrenic nerve injury with ipsilateral diaphragmatic paralysis must be suspected in this infant. The abdomen does not bulge because the breathing is mostly thoracic. Diagnosis is made by ultrasound or fluoroscopy. Respiratory distress syndrome is more common in preterm infants and presents with cyanosis, respiratory distress, and grunting respirations. The mother usually has no history of difficult delivery. Chest x-ray reveals a ground-glass appearance. Meconium aspiration syndrome appears at birth, and there is a history of meconium-stained amniotic fluid. Tracheoesophageal fistula presents as choking and cyanosis with feeding. Again, there is no history of difficult delivery or signs of brachial palsy. Choanal atresia is suspected in a cyanotic newborn who becomes pink on crying, and the diagnosis is made by failure to pass a catheter through the nasal passages.

98. The answer is D. *(Obstetrics; seizure disorder and pregnancy)*
Maternal megaloblastic anemia and fetal congenital malformations due to folic acid deficiency can occur as rare complications of anticonvulsant therapy, specifically phenytoin (Dilantin). All the options listed except folate deficiency are associated with either normal or low mean corpuscular

volume (MCV), whereas phenytoin can diminish absorption of folate, resulting in macrocytosis, as seen in this patient.

99. The answer is C. *(Behavioral science; Medicare)*
Medicare was designed primarily for people eligible for Social Security (i.e., those 65 years of age and older and those with chronic disabilities). Medicaid was designed primarily for poor people. Long-term nursing-home care is not covered by either Medicare or Medicaid unless the patient is indigent.

100. The answer is D. *(Endocrinology; Hashimoto's thyroiditis with hypothyroidism).*
A woman with diffuse, nonpainful enlargement of the thyroid and clinical evidence of hypothyroidism most likely has Hashimoto's thyroiditis, which is a chronic thyroiditis in which autoimmunity plays a prominent role. Clinical signs and symptoms of hypothyroidism reflect a generalized hypometabolic state. They include

- sinus bradycardia
- coarse dry skin
- cold intolerance
- macroglossia
- congestive cardiomyopathy
- pretibial nonpitting edema
- gastric atrophy and hypomotility
- severe depression
- puffiness of the face and eyelids
- a delayed recovery phase of the Achilles reflex
- raspy voice (vocal cord edema)
- proximal muscle weakness
- constipation
- menstrual irregularities
- slow mentation

Thyroid profiles usually include a serum T_4, resin T_3 uptake (RTU), free T_4 index (FT_4-I), and thyroid-stimulating hormone (TSH). The serum T_4 reflects hormone that is bound to thyroid-binding globulin (TBG) and hormone that is free. Therefore, changes in either the free hormone level or the concentration of TBG affect the total T_4. For example, a low T_4 could represent a low free T_4 (hypothyroidism) or a low TBG, whereas an increased T_4 could represent an increase in free T_4 (hyperthyroidism) or an increase in TBG. Factors that increase TBG are commonly associated with an increase in estrogen, such as in women who are taking birth control pills or estrogen, or are pregnant. A low TBG is seen in patients receiving androgens or anabolic steroids, in the nephrotic syndrome (protein is lost in the urine), and with high doses of aspirin.

Although TBG measurements are available, the RTU, reported as a percentage, reflects TBG levels. If the concentration of TBG is normal, the RTU moves in the same direction as the T_4 and the FT_4-I, which is the multiplication of the serum T_4 by the RTU. For example, a patient with hypothyroidism would have a low serum T_4, low RTU, and a low FT_4-I. However, if the TBG concentration is altered, the RTU moves in the opposite direction, so that the multiplication of the serum T_4 by the RTU "normalizes" the FT_4-I. For example, if a patient has a low concentration of TGB, there would be a low serum T_4 (decreased TBG), high RTU, and a normal FT_4-I. The serum TSH, secreted from the anterior pituitary, has a negative feedback relationship with circulating T_4 and T_3. Therefore, if the serum T_4 is increased or decreased, serum TSH is decreased or increased, respectively. TSH is normal if there are alterations in TBG.

With this background, this patient with primary hypothyroidism would be expected to have a low T_4, low RTU, low FT_4-I, and high TSH. The TSH is the most sensitive test for diagnosing primary hypothyroidism, because it is increased even when the serum T_4 is on the low side of normal, indicating a gland that is on the verge of failing.

Choice A with an increased T_4, decreased RTU, normal FT_4-I, and normal TSH represents a person with an increase in TBG.

Choice B with an increased T_4, increased RTU, increased FT_4-I, and low TSH is a patient with hyperthyroidism, most commonly Graves' disease.

Choice C with a decreased T_4, increased RTU, and normal FT_4-I, and normal TSH is a person with a decrease in TBG.

Choice E with a decreased T_4, decreased RTU, decreased FT_4-I, and a decreased TSH is a patient with a problem in either the anterior pituitary (secondary hypothyroidism) or the hypothalamus (tertiary hypothyroidism), with a decreased release of thyrotropin-releasing hormone (TRH).

101. The answer is B. *(Obstetrics; premature rupture of membranes)*
Accurate assessment of premature rupture of membranes (PROM) is essential because the outcome of pregnancy can be adversely impacted by a positive diagnosis. This question addresses confirmation of PROM by examination, rather than with historic data. Nitrazine paper and sonographic oligohydramnios have low specificity and sensitivity for ruptured membranes. Urinalysis is not relevant. Digital examination should never be done until membrane rupture is ruled out, because of the increase in infectious morbidity. A speculum examination is helpful in determining the extent of vaginal pooling.

102. The answer is B. *(Pediatrics; Werdnig-Hoffmann disease)*
Werdnig-Hoffmann disease is a spinal muscular atrophy of unknown cause. It is inherited in an autosomal recessive fashion. Infants can be symptomatic at birth. Sparing of the extraocular muscles and sphincters is characteristic. Fasciulations are a sign of denervation of muscle and are best seen in the tongue. Infants assume a flaccid "frog-leg" posture. Most die by 2 years of age. A neonatal form of myotonic dystrophy appears in infants born to mothers with myotonic dystrophy. Clubfoot and contractures are common. Fasciculations are not seen. Infant botulism has a peak onset at 2 to 6 months of age. Infantile myasthenia gravis can be transient—as in those infants born of mothers with myasthenia gravis—or, very rarely, congenital. Fasciculations are not seen and the extraocular muscles are not spared. Duchenne's muscular dystrophy is rarely symptomatic at birth.

103. The answer is A. *(Orthopedics; ligament and tendon tears)*
A dislocation is a disruption of normal relationships between articular surfaces. A sprain is a complete or partial tear of ligaments associated with swelling and tenderness. Physical exam

rather than x-rays confirms the diagnosis, since x-rays are normal. A tendon rupture causes weakness and loss of ability to produce the characteristic motion of the muscle. Muscle fasciculations are a sign of lower motor neuron disease and would not be expected in tendon injuries. An avulsion fracture is usually located near a joint. A fragment of bone is pulled off by the tendon or ligament.

104. The answer is C. *(Ophthalmology; conjunctivitis)*
In acute conjunctivitis, the patient has a purulent eye discharge with matting of the eyelashes. There is mild photophobia, a normal pupillary reaction to light and normal intraocular pressure. It is most commonly secondary to *Staphylococcus aureus, Streptococcus pneumoniae,* or *Haemophilus aegypti* (pink eye). Topical polymyxin B, neomycin, and bacitracin are effective therapies.

Acute anterior uveitis refers to inflammation of the uveal tract, which is formed by the iris, ciliary body, and choroid. Etiologies include sarcoidosis and HLA-B27–positive spondyloarthropathy (e.g., ankylosing spondylitis). Patients have blurred vision, no conjunctival discharge, moderate pain, severe photophobia, a ciliary flush (engorgement of the deep pericorneal blood vessels), a constricted, irregular pupil, normal intraocular pressure, and a poor pupillary light reflex. Acute anterior uveitis usually responds to topical corticosteroids.

Acute glaucoma is characterized by elevation of intraocular pressure. Optic neuritis refers to inflammation of the optic nerve, which may be secondary to infection (tuberculosis, syphilis), multiple sclerosis, or glaucoma. There is a sudden unilateral loss of vision and pain on eye movements. The optic disc frequently appears swollen and associated with flame-shaped pericapillary hemorrhages. Intravenous and oral steroid therapies are used for treatment.

Central retinal artery occlusion is characterized by a sudden, complete, painless loss of vision in one eye, most commonly in an elderly patient. Retinal examination reveals pallor of the optic disc; edema of the retina; a cherry red fovea; bloodless, constricted arterioles; and a "boxcar" segmentation of blood in the retinal veins. Surgical decompression of the anterior chamber in less than 1 hour following occlusion prevents permanent damage to the eye.

105. The answer is C. *(Psychiatry; personality disorder)*
Psychodynamic theory postulates that the adult personality is, in large part, the product of early childhood experiences. Personality pathology results from various kinds of emotional traumas and conflicts that occur during development. Specific kinds of childhood trauma result in specific kinds of personality disorders.

106. The answer is A. *(Behavioral science; bereavement)*
Brief periods of painful longing are seen in normal bereavement even many years after the event, especially on holidays or on the anniversary of the death. Although the woman may feel that she has not done enough for the dead person, feelings of worthlessness or evilness, suicide attempts, despair, and inability to work for more than 2 years indicate depression rather than a normal grief reaction.

107. The answer is B. *(Emergency medicine; salicylate intoxication)*
To interpret arterial blood-gas disorders, respiratory abnormalities must be defined by comparing the patient's measured $Paco_2$ to the reference interval in the laboratory, which, in this case, is 33–44 mm Hg. Respiratory alkalosis, or increased clearing of CO_2, results in a $Paco_2$ less than 33 mm Hg. Respiratory acidosis, or hypoventilation, results in a $Paco_2$ greater than 44 mm Hg. Similarly, metabolic acidosis and alkalosis are defined by the reference limit for bicarbonate, in this case 22–28 mEq/L. Metabolic acidosis is defined as a bicarbonate less than 22 mEq/L, whereas metabolic alkalosis is defined as a bicarbonate greater than 28 mEq/L. The pH (normal range 7.35–7.45) defines whether the primary process is an acidemia (pH less than 7.35) or an alkalemia (pH greater than 7.45). Compensation for an alkalosis is always acidosis and vice versa, as depicted in the table. With rare exceptions, compensation does not bring the pH back into the normal range. The pH reflects the primary process in the patient.

Disorder	pH	Bicarbonate	Paco$_2$	Compensation
Metabolic alkalosis	Alkalemia	Increased	Increased	Respiratory acidosis
Metabolic acidosis	Acidemia	Decreased	Decreased	Respiratory alkalosis
Respiratory alkalosis	Alkalemia	Decreased	Decreased	Metabolic acidosis
Respiratory acidosis	Acidemia	Increased	Increased	Metabolic alkalosis

For example, a patient presents with a Pa_{CO_2} less than 33 mm Hg (respiratory alkalosis), a bicarbonate less than 22 mEq/L (metabolic acidosis), and a pH greater than 7.45 (alkalemia). This patient has a primary respiratory alkalosis, because the pH is alkalemic, with a compensatory metabolic acidosis. If the bicarbonate were normal, it would be an uncompensated respiratory alkalosis. Salicylate intoxication in adults commonly results in a mixed blood-gas disorder rather than a single blood-gas abnormality. There can be a primary metabolic acidosis, resulting from addition of salicylic acid to the blood. There can also be a primary respiratory alkalosis, secondary to the overstimulating effect of salicylates on the respiratory center (hyperventilation) in the brain. The presence of two primary blood-gas disorders that have opposing effects on the pH results in a normal pH. Compensation does not correct the pH into the normal range; therefore, a normal pH indicates the presence of a mixed disorder. If the person had only a primary metabolic acidosis, with respiratory alkalosis as compensation, the pH would be acidemic. This is usually the case with salicylate intoxication in children, who appear to go through the primary respiratory alkalosis phase and plunge into profound metabolic acidosis as the primary process. Similarly, if the patient had a primary alkalosis with metabolic acidosis as compensation, the pH would be alkalemic. This combination is a less common manifestation of salicylate intoxication.

With this background, the best choice for salicylate intoxication is B, because of a normal pH (7.38), respiratory alkalosis (Pa_{CO_2} of 22 mm Hg), and metabolic acidosis (bicarbonate of 12 mEq/L), indicating a mixed disorder.

Choice A has a respiratory acidosis (Pa_{CO_2} of 53 mm Hg), a normal bicarbonate (25 mEq/L), and an acid pH (7.29). This combination represents a primary respiratory acidosis without compensation.

Choice C has a respiratory acidosis (Pa_{CO_2} of 49 mm Hg), metabolic alkalosis (bicarbonate of 39 mEq/L), and an alkaline pH (7.53). This combination is a primary metabolic alkalosis with compensatory respiratory acidosis.

Choice D has a respiratory acidosis (Pa_{CO_2} of 70 mm Hg), a metabolic alkalosis (bicarbonate of 46 mEq/L), and a normal pH (7.43). This combination must be a mixed disorder, both primary respiratory acidosis and primary metabolic alkalosis. The opposing effects on pH of respiratory acidosis and metabolic alkalosis cause the pH to be normal.

108. The answer is D. *(Obstetrics; fetal death)*
Intrauterine fetal death is fetal demise after 20 weeks' gestation and complicates approximately 1% of pregnancies. Real-time ultrasound examination for cardiac motion is the method of choice for assessing fetal death. Maternal assessment of fetal movement is not accurate in sensitivity or specificity. The pregnancy test remains positive for a considerable time because the placenta continues to produce human chorionic gonadotropin. Amniocentesis is an invasive test that relies on dark, turbid fluid, which is a late development. Exposure of a possibly live fetus to x-rays is not recommended.

109. The answer is D. *(Pediatrics; choanal atresia)*
Choanal atresia should be suspected in any infant who develops cyanosis that occurs with feedings or at rest, but is relieved by crying. The cyanosis occurs because newborns are obligate nose-breathers. Diagnosis is made by failure to pass a catheter through the nasal passages. Tracheo-esophageal fistula is characterized by choking with feeding. An orogastric tube curls up and does not pass to the stomach. Bronchopulmonary dysplasia is a complication of respiratory distress syndrome and appears later. Cyanosis is not relieved by crying in either entity. A patent ductus arteriosus is a left-to-right shunt and is not associated with cyanosis.

110. The answer is D. *(Ophthalmology; central retinal artery occlusion)*
The patient has central retinal artery occlusion. This is characterized by a sudden, complete, painless loss of vision in one eye, most commonly in an elderly patient. Retinal exam reveals pallor of the optic disc, edema of the retina, a

cherry red fovea, bloodless, constricted arterioles, and a "boxcar" segmentation of blood in the retinal veins. Surgical decompression of the anterior chamber in less than 1 hour following occlusion prevents permanent damage to the eye.

Central retinal vein occlusion is characterized by a sudden, painless, unilateral loss of vision in patients with hypercoagulable states (polycythemia rubra vera), diabetes mellitus, or glaucoma. Retinal exam reveals swelling of the optic disc, venous dilatation and tortuosity, widespread retinal hemorrhages, and cotton-wool exudates. Acute anterior uveitis, optic neuritis, and acute glaucoma are all associated with eye pain.

111. The answer is A. *(General surgery; acute sialadenitis)*
The patient most likely has acute surgical parotitis (sialadenitis). Surgical parotitis usually occurs 1 week postoperatively in elderly patients who have poor dental hygiene and have been intubated. *Staphylococcus aureus* is the most common organism isolated. Surgical drainage and antibiotics are required.

Acute and chronic sialadenitis can also be a result of sialolithiasis, which refers to calculi in the major salivary gland ducts, most commonly in Wharton's duct draining the submandibular gland.

Parotid gland enlargement is also associated with Sjögren's syndrome, a collagen vascular disease characterized by immunologic destruction of minor salivary glands with subsequent development of dry eyes and dry mouth. Rheumatoid arthritis is frequently present as well.

Hemorrhage into the parotid is rare. Mumps is a common cause of viral parotitis.

112. The answer is A. *(Psychiatry; psychotherapy)*
Behavioral psychotherapy rests on a belief that behavior occurs in response to the environment. Therapy can alter behavior by changing the rewards and punishments found in the environment. Cognitive psychotherapy postulates that behavior occurs in response to the perception of the environment, not necessarily to the environment itself. Therefore, therapy can alter behavior by changing environmental perceptions through behavioral techniques, teaching, and assignments.

113. The answer is B. *(Obstetrics; intrauterine growth disorder)*
One of the most effective tools in diagnosing intrauterine growth retardation (IUGR) is sonographic evaluation of the fetal parameters. Option B correctly includes the four standard measurements combined to assess fetal weight. Crown–rump length (CRL) is a first-trimester parameter. Humerus length (HL) is similar to femur length (FL) but is not a standard formula. Transcerebellar diameter (TCD) is used for estimating gestational age, but not fetal weight.

114. The answer is B. *(Pediatrics; alopecia, Microsporum canis)*
Tinea capitis is most commonly caused by *Microsporum canis* and *Trichophyton* species, particularly *tonsurans*. *Microsporum* species fluoresce a bright blue–green color whereas *Trichophyton* do not. *Epidermophyton floccosum* is a cause of tinea cruris. *Candida albicans* is responsible for oral thrush and a diaper dermatitis in infants. *Aspergillus* does not cause alopecia, and it is an inhaled agent rather than a skin pathogen.

115. The answer is B. *(Gastroenterology; hepatitis B immunization, hepatitis A)*
People who have been immunized against hepatitis B (HBV) with Heptavax-B or Recombivax-HB develop protective antibodies only against surface antigen (anti-HBs) in 90% of cases. Patients who have recovered from hepatitis A (HAV) have anti-HAV immunoglobulin G (IgG) antibodies, which offer lifelong protection against HAV.

In HAV infections, the first antibody is anti-HAV immunoglobulin M (IgM) [the IgM indicating active infection], which appears after the prodrome and persists for 6 weeks or longer. Recovery is marked by a switch over to IgG.

In HBV infections, the first marker is surface antigen (HBsAg), which is noninfective. This marker is followed by "e" antigen (HBeAg), which is an infective particle. The first antibody to appear is an IgM antibody against core antigen (anti-HBc IgM), which may persist if the infection becomes chronic (presence of HBsAg beyond 6 months), but usually switches over to an IgG antibody, indicating recovery. If the patient is going to recover (90%), HBeAg disappears first, then HBsAg disappears (usually after 4 months). Between the fourth and fifth month (serologic gap, or window), when HBsAg and HBeAg are gone, the only serologic marker for infection is the anti-HBc IgM antibody. In the fifth to sixth month, anti-HBs develops, conferring immunity against future attacks of that particular HBV serotype.

Choice A is consistent with someone with a history of HAV (anti-HAV IgG) and who is presently recovering from HBV in the serologic gap (anti-HBc IgM only present).

Choice C is consistent with a patient with a history of HAV (anti-HAV IgG) who now has active HBV in the first 4 months of the disease, because HBsAg, HBeAg, and anti-HBc IgM are present.

Choice D represents a patient who has active HAV and either had HBV or was immunized against HBV, because anti-HBs is present. Presence of anti-HBc IgG would indicate that the patient had recovered from HBV, whereas a negative result would be consistent with immunization.

Choice E represents a patient who has active HAV and no evidence of HBV.

116. The answer is E. (Obstetrics; puerperal sepsis)
Puerperal sepsis accounts for significant postpartum maternal morbidity and mortality. Manual placental removal, retained products of conception, and cesarean delivery are risk factors for puerperal genital tract infection, but prolonged rupture of membranes (PROM) is the most frequent cause listed. Tubal sterilization is not a risk factor.

117. The answer is A. (Pediatrics; Apt test)
The most common cause of blood in the stool of a newborn is swallowed maternal blood. The Apt test helps distinguish adult hemoglobin from fetal hemoglobin. It is easier and less expensive than electrophoresis. If adult hemoglobin is detected, the blood is swallowed maternal blood. If fetal hemoglobin is found, a search begins for the cause of the bleeding.

118. The answer is B. (General surgery; zinc deficiency)
Zinc deficiency is characterized by alopecia, a maculopapular rash around the mouth and eyes, taste and smell abnormalities, and problems with healing of wounds. Essential fatty acid deficiency is characterized by an eczematous rash and thrombocytopenia. Selenium deficiency produces muscle pain and a type of cardiomyopathy. Magnesium deficiency is associated with resistance to activity of parathormone with subsequent hypocalcemia and tetany. Muscle weakness, irritability, delirium, and convulsions are also noted. Alcoholism is the most common cause of hypomagnesemia. Copper deficiency is associated with iron deficiency anemia, dissecting aortic aneurysm, and Menkes' kinky hair syndrome.

119. The answer is D. (Psychiatry; bipolar disorder)
Evidence of elevated levels of several central nervous system neurotransmitters has been reported during manic episodes in bipolar disorder. Although genetic variations occur in several lithium transport mechanisms, no particular abnormality has been clearly associated with bipolar disorder. The reasons for the antimanic properties of lithium and carbamazepine are unknown.

120. The answer is B. (General surgery; ruptured spleen)
Blunt trauma to the upper left abdomen or lower left chest, especially if associated with rib fractures, is frequently complicated by a ruptured spleen. This can be diagnosed by radionuclide scan, computed tomography (CT), or peritoneal lavage, if the diagnosis is equivocal. However, the presence of shock in this patient is an indication for immediate surgical intervention. The

location of the injury and the presence of hypovolemic shock would argue against rupture of the colon or transection of the abdominal aorta. A pulmonary contusion with hemorrhage into the pleural cavity is unlikely in the presence of normal breath sounds.

121. The answer is C. *(Endocrinology; primary aldosteronism)*
Primary aldosteronism is characterized by autonomous (unregulated) production of aldosterone from an adrenal adenoma and, less frequently, bilateral adrenal hyperplasia of the zona glomerulosa. Aldosterone normally acts on the distal tubules to increase sodium reabsorption in exchange for either potassium or hydrogen ions. Excessive aldosterone would be expected to result in an increased reabsorption of sodium to produce hypernatremia and an increase in plasma volume. Increased plasma volume plus the effect of sodium on increasing peripheral vascular resistance lead to hypertension. Furthermore, the increased plasma volume results in increased hydrostatic pressure in the peritubular capillaries, which shuts off the reabsorption of sodium in the proximal tubules, leading to a loss of sodium in the urine. This "escape mechanism" for sodium is enough to prevent clinical evidence of pitting edema. Increased plasma volume also decreases the plasma renin concentration.

Hypokalemia also results from the enhanced sodium exchange and loss in the urine. It is associated with proximal muscle weakness and, if chronic, can render the tubules resistant to the action of antidiuretic hormone (acquired nephrogenic diabetes insipidus), leading to polyuria.

In addition, the excess exchange of sodium for hydrogen ions leaves bicarbonate behind in the tubules because the hydrogen ions come from the dissociation of carbonic acid into hydrogen ions and bicarbonate. The excess bicarbonate produces a metabolic alkalosis.

Clinical evidence of tetany in this patient is due to the effect of alkalosis (metabolic or respiratory) on ionized calcium levels in the blood. Serum calcium is the sum total of calcium bound to proteins (40%), calcium bound to nonproteins (13%), and free, ionized calcium (47%), which is the metabolically active form of calcium. Alkalosis increases the negative charges on binding proteins, like albumin, which increases the binding of the divalent ionized calcium to albumin, leading to clinical evidence of tetany, without altering the total serum calcium.

Choice A represents either a patient on diuretics or a patient with Bartter's syndrome. Loop diuretics and thiazides block sodium reabsorption, leading to excess delivery of sodium to the distal tubule. Excessive exchange of sodium for potassium and hydrogen ions leads to hypokalemia and metabolic alkalosis by the mechanisms previously discussed. Volume depletion from sodium loss decreases the effective arterial blood volume, which is a stimulus for renin release and, ultimately, aldosterone (secondary aldosteronism).

Bartter's syndrome is caused by a defect in chloride reabsorption in the ascending tubules, which essentially results in the same series of events as with a loop diuretic, which blocks the chloride pump. Chronic volume depletion results in hyperplasia of the juxtaglomerular apparatus, release of renin, and subsequent release of aldosterone. Features of Bartter's syndrome and diuretics can be differentiated from primary aldosteronism by absence of hypertension and increase in plasma renin levels.

Choice B with a normal aldosterone, decreased plasma renin, hypokalemia, and metabolic alkalosis represents Liddle's syndrome. This syndrome is exactly the same as primary aldosteronism except for the presence of normal serum aldosterone levels. It is thought to be secondary to increased sensitivity of the tubules to normal levels of aldosterone.

Choice D with a low aldosterone, low renin, hyperkalemia, and metabolic acidosis (low bicarbonate) is hyporeninemic hypoaldosteronism. This condition is due to destruction of the juxtaglomerular apparatus, which synthesizes renin. Low renin ultimately results in low aldosterone, with subsequent loss of sodium in the urine, hypotension from volume depletion, hyperkalemia, and retention of hydrogen ions, leading to metabolic acidosis. Diabetes mellitus and tubulointerstitial diseases of the kidney are associated with this disease, otherwise known as type IV renal tubular acidosis. This disease should offer no confusion with primary aldosteronism.

122. The answer is B. *(Obstetrics; Sheehan's syndrome)*
This patient is a candidate for developing Sheehan's syndrome because of hypoperfusion of her anterior pituitary gland. Although all pituitary trophic hormones are at risk, the one that is most likely to be affected is prolactin.

123. The answer is C. *(Pediatrics; anemia of prematurity)* Iron def.
The majority of preterm infants have a "physiologic" anemia at approximately 6 weeks of age. Hemoglobin levels dip to approximately 7–10 g/dl. Term infants have the same phenomenon at 8–12 weeks, with hemoglobin levels of approximately 11 g/dl. Iron stores reach their low at approximately the same time.

124. The answer is B. *(Obstetrics; pelvic diameters)*
The diameters of the pelvic planes represent the amount of space available at each level. The plane of the pelvic inlet is the major consideration. The diagonal conjugate is determined by the lower margin of the symphysis and the sacral promontory. The coccyx and the ischial spine are not involved in measuring the diagonal conjugate; therefore, A, D, and E are not options. Because the diagonal conjugate is a dimension that can be measured by pelvic examination, it cannot include the upper margin of the symphysis; therefore, C is incorrect.

125. The answer is C. *(General surgery; neck masses)*
Excluding thyroid cancer, cervical adenopathy is most commonly due to metastatic disease, usually from a primary squamous carcinoma or adenocarcinoma. Malignant lymph nodes are frequently stony hard, nontender, and fixed. Malignant lymphomas (non-Hodgkin's and Hodgkin's) are also common primary causes of cervical adenopathy. Adenocarcinoma in the left supraclavicular node is frequently associated with metastatic stomach

adenocarcinoma (Virchow's node, or sentinel node). Cystic lesions in the neck could represent a thyroglossal duct cyst (midline location) or a branchial cleft cyst (located in the anterolateral neck).

126. The answer is B. *(Behavioral science; consent for minors)*
Parental consent or notification is not required for minors with sexually transmitted diseases. Good medical practice would include counseling the patient on prevention. Although parents usually must give consent for medical procedures involving minor children, parental consent or notification is not required when minor children are in emergency situations, show drug and alcohol dependence, or need medical care in pregnancy.

127. The answer is A. *(Obstetrics; obstetric anesthesia)*
The goal of obstetric anesthesia is to optimize maternal and neonatal outcome. Each anesthetic agent has risks and benefits. All the cited options are obstetric anesthetic modalities, but only halothane provides significant myometrial relaxation.

128–129. The answers are: 128-C, 129-B. *(Psychiatry; anxiety)*
Generalized anxiety disorder is characterized by excessive anxiety, which is difficult to control, along with such symptoms as restlessness, irritability, and sleep disturbances. No clear-cut stressor suggests adjustment disorder, the anxiety does not appear related to specific social situations, and there is no evidence of specific obsessions or compulsions. Although the patient may be very unhappy, as in major depression, her symptoms are better accounted for by generalized anxiety disorder.

Buspirone is an effective treatment for generalized anxiety disorder, especially for people who are sensitive to cognitive impairment. Longer acting benzodiazepines such as diazepam (Valium) are also very useful. Alprazolam and triazolam are shorter acting benzodiazepines, with a higher potential for inducing dependence.

Fluphenazine and thioridazine are antipsychotic medications, which should be reserved for treatment of psychosis.

130. The answer is C. *(Pharmacology; fetal pulmonary maturity)*
Fetal pulmonary maturity may be enhanced by maternal administration of corticosteroids that cross the placenta. Ritodrine and terbutaline are used as tocolytic agents; isoxsuprine is no longer used for tocolysis. Nifedipine has the potential for fetal adverse effects. Of this group of medications, only betamethasone has been shown to increase fetal synthesis of pulmonary surfactant and decrease neonatal respiratory distress syndrome.

131–132. The answers are: 131-B, 132-E. *(Pediatrics; idiopathic thrombocytopenic purpura)*
Idiopathic (immune) thrombocytopenic purpura is the most common thrombocytopenic purpura of childhood. The disease usually follows a viral infection. The infection seems to trigger an immune mechanism that starts platelet destruction. This destruction is manifested as acute onset of bruising and petechiae. Other than this condition, the patient looks well. Bleeding into tissues can occur. Platelet counts are depressed, and bleeding time is prolonged, but the white count is normal. Platelet antibodies are commonly seen. Bone marrow examination reveals normal megakaryocytes. The disease is self-limited, with resolution of the petechiae over 1 or 2 weeks, although thrombocytopenia may persist longer.

The prognosis for idiopathic thrombocytopenic purpura is excellent. Most patients recover within 2 or 3 months. Approximately 90% of children regain normal platelet counts within 9 to 12 months. Intravenous gamma-globulin infusions have shown a sustained rise in platelet counts. Platelet concentrates are recommended only in life-threatening situations because the rise in platelet count is only temporary and reflects their short life span.

133. The answer is E. *(Psychiatry; mental retardation)*
The case suggests a diagnosis of mild mental retardation. The cause of mild mental retardation is usually idiopathic, with no clear physical or social pathology. More severe mental retardation results from known physiologic lesions.

134. The answer is B. *(Behavioral science; behavioral therapy)*
In flooding, the person is exposed to the feared object until the fear subsides. In systematic desensitization, a person is exposed to the feared object in increasing doses. In sensitization, a person becomes hypersensitive to a stimulus so that even a weak exposure to the stimulus elicits a response. In cognitive therapy, a person is taught to use self-enhancing thoughts. In biofeedback, a person is taught control over autonomic activity.

135. The answer is B. *(Ophthalmology; acute glaucoma)*
The patient has acute glaucoma, which refers to an increase in intraocular pressure. Tonometer pressures greater than 21 are considered above normal. Glaucoma is due to a defect in Schlemm's canal, which normally drains the aqueous humor. Open-angle glaucoma is the most common type. Clinically, the onset is sudden with blurry vision, pain, minimal photophobia, ciliary injection, a steamy appearing cornea, an absent pupillary light reflex, and a pupil that is mid-dilated, fixed, and irregular. No discharge is present. Prompt treatment is required to prevent blindness. Therapies that reduce intraocular pressure include glycerin, pilocarpine, mannitol, and acetazolamide. A peripheral iridectomy or laser iridectomy is usually performed.

Blood in the anterior chamber is called a hyphema and is associated with acute visual loss. Corneal erosions produce blurry vision, pain, moderate photophobia, watery discharge, mild to moderate conjunctival injection, a hazy cornea, a positive fluorescein stain, a normal or constricted pupil, a poor to normal pupillary light reflex, and normal intraocular pressure. Papilledema refers to swelling of the optic disc due to increased intracranial pressure. There are venous stasis, prominent disc vessels, a swollen disc with blurred margins, and absence of the physiologic cup.

136. The answer is A. *(Obstetrics; intrauterine growth disorder)*
Intrauterine growth retardation (IUGR) is a term that describes small-for-dates fetuses who are at increased risk for perinatal morbidity and mortality. Only maternal chronic hypertension is associated with fetal brain-sparing but decreased abdominal size (asymmetric IUGR). Trisomy 18, rubella infection, renal agenesis, and toxoplasmosis result in symmetric IUGR, with inadequate growth of both the head and the body.

137–139. The answers are: 137-C, 138-E, 139-C. *(Neurology; temporal arteritis)*
Temporal arteritis generally affects the elderly population and is associated with severe, unremitting headache over the course of the temporal artery, associated with fever, malaise, jaw claudication, leukocytosis, and elevated sedimentation rate. A feared complication is central retinal artery thrombosis leading to blindness. The risk is so high that if the diagnosis is suspected on clinical grounds, it is best to begin intravenous steroids even before the diagnostic temporal artery biopsy is obtained. Migraine headaches, cluster headaches, otitis, and depression can be associated with lateralized headaches, but clearly do not fit the clinical picture. It is worth noting that the disease eventually fades, but the opposite temporal artery is also at risk for involvement.

140–142. The answers are: 140-B, 141-A, 142-D. *(Pulmonology; pulmonary embolus with infarction)*
Pulmonary embolism with infarction is most commonly seen in the setting of postoperative recovery associated with stasis of the venous circulation in the deep saphenous veins of the leg, which is the most common location (90%) for thromboembolism. Signs and symptoms depend on the size of the embolus. Large, saddle emboli that block four of the five pulmonary artery orifices result in sudden death because of acute right heart strain. Small emboli lodge peripherally, where they produce an infarction in fewer than

10% of patients. Infarction is more likely in patients with preexisting lung disease, such as heart failure or chronic obstructive lung disease.

Sudden onset of tachypnea is the most common presentation (92%) in a pulmonary embolism. Additional findings include

- dyspnea
- pleuritic chest pain (75%), because of a sterile inflammation of the pleura overlying the infarct
- hemorrhagic pleural effusions (35%–50%)
- fever (40%)
- sinus tachycardia (45%)
- wheezing (< 50%) related to the release of bronchoconstrictors from platelets in the embolus material
- hemoptysis (30%), because the majority of infarctions in the lung are hemorrhagic
- cough (50%)
- accentuation of P_2 (50%) secondary to pulmonary hypertension related to vessel constriction from hypoxemia and the release of thromboxane A_2 (TXA_2) from the platelets in the thrombus

Consequences of pulmonary infarctions include

- sudden death
- secondary pulmonary hypertension from small, recurrent pulmonary emboli, with or without cor pulmonale
- paradoxical embolization because of increased right atrial pressure opening up the foramen ovale and allowing thromboemboli to pass into the systemic circulation
- lung abscess, if the embolus is septic

Pulmonary angiography is the gold standard test for diagnosing a pulmonary embolus, particularly when other studies give conflicting results. However, most clinicians begin with a perfusion scan, which has a high probability of indicating an infarction if a lobar perfusion defect accompanies ventilation mismatch, the latter demonstrated by a ventilation scan. Perfusion defects last 7 to 14 days.

Calculation of the alveolar–arterial gradient (A-a gradient) has a sensitivity of 100% for indicating a ventilation or perfusion defect in the lungs. Normally, there is a slight mismatch between ventilation and perfusion in the lungs; therefore, the partial pressure of alveolar oxygen (P_{AO_2}) is not exactly the same as the partial pressure of arterial oxygen (Pa_{O_2}). A medically significant A-a gradient is any gradient 30 mm Hg or higher. It is easily obtained by first calculating the P_{AO_2} and then subtracting the measured Pa_{O_2}. The formula for the P_{AO_2} is the amount of oxygen inspired (% oxygen × 713) minus the amount of oxygen exchanged in the lungs ($Pa_{CO_2}/0.8$). In this case, the P_{AO_2} is 0.21 (concentration of oxygen in room air) × 713 − 29/0.8 = 114 mm Hg. Since the Pa_{O_2} is 70 mm Hg, the A-a gradient is 44 mm Hg, which is medically significant. In 10% of cases of pulmonary embolization, the Pa_{O_2} is normal, but the A-a gradient is always abnormal. If a patient is on oxygen, the percent oxygen is substituted in the preceding formula to calculate the P_{AO_2}.

Arterial blood gases usually reveal an acute respiratory alkalosis related to tachypnea from the pain induced by inflammation of the pleura. This patient has respiratory alkalosis (Pa_{CO_2} 29 mm Hg), a metabolic acidosis (bicarbonate 21 mEq/L), and an alkalemia (pH 7.50), so the proper interpretation is a primary respiratory alkalosis with a compensatory metabolic acidosis. The Pa_{O_2} of 70 mm Hg indicates hypoxemia, but the definition of respiratory failure is a Pa_{O_2} less than 60 mm Hg, with or without an elevation of Pa_{CO_2}.

Pulmonary function studies, Gram's stain with culture and sensitivity of sputum, and bronchoscopy are noncontributory in the workup of a pulmonary embolus.

A chest x-ray is abnormal in 50% of patients with a pulmonary infarction. Hamman's sign is a wedge-shaped density based in the pleura that points to the hilum. Westermark's sign is an area of hypovascularity and atelectasis distal to the occlusion, which is evident in this patient. Hemorrhagic pleural effusions occur in 35% to 50% of patients but are not diagnostic of a pulmonary infarction. Fluid analysis reveals an exudate with numerous red blood cells, neutrophils, and increased protein (greater than 3 g/dl).

An electrocardiogram (ECG) is abnormal in 50% of cases and can exhibit sinus tachycardia, nonspecific ST- and T-wave changes, a right ventricular strain pattern (S_1Q_3, T-wave inversion in leads V_{1-3}), atrial flutters, or right bundle branch block.

Patients should be anticoagulated with heparin to prevent further clot formation. The prognosis relates to the size of the embolus, the condition of the underlying lungs, and the proper diagnosis and treatment. The mortality is 30% in patients with undiagnosed pulmonary thromboembolism.

Regarding the other differentials listed in the question, atelectasis (localized collapse of the alveoli) is the most common cause of fever 24 to 48 hours after surgery, but it would not be expected to produce a sudden onset of tachypnea, the blood-gas changes of respiratory alkalosis, or a pleural effusion.

The adult respiratory distress syndrome is characterized by an acute onset of dyspnea, tachypnea, and severe hypoxemia 12 to 24 hours after an initiating event such as endotoxic shock, aspiration of gastric contents, pneumonia, or pulmonary embolism. Unlike this case, however, the chest x-ray reveals diffuse, bilateral infiltrates with both an interstitial and alveolar pattern.

Wheezing is not always an indication of bronchial asthma. Both heart failure with peribronchiolar edema and pulmonary embolism with bronchoconstriction secondary to the release of platelet factors from the embolus can produce wheezing.

A bacterial pneumonia is an unlikely cause of this patient's findings, because of the lack of cough productive of sputum, the suddenness of the onset of tachypnea, and the chest x-ray finding of hypovascularity rather than a parenchymal consolidation.

143. The answer is A. (*Psychiatry; psychodynamics*)
All effective psychotherapies have specific theories about the genesis of pathological behavior. Each theory explains the efficacy of the particular psychotherapy associated with it. Each school of psychotherapy may have a different theory about pathological behavior, and different techniques for treatment of the behavior.

144. The answer is C. *(Pediatrics; otitis media)*
Malignant external otitis (mastoid osteomyelitis) is a complication of external otitis. It is rare, and occurs in young immune-deficient patients. Although meningitis is the most common intracranial complication of otitis media, brain abscesses can also occur. Cholesteatomas result when squamous epithelium grows into the middle ear during the healing of a perforated tympanic membrane. Reversible conductive hearing loss occurs when an effusion is present. Facial nerve paralysis (partial or complete) can also occur.

145. The answer is A. *(Psychiatry; depression)*
Double-bind communication refers to incongruity between spoken and unspoken communication. This description of family dynamics in schizophrenia is no longer accepted. The other choices describe biologic, cognitive, psychodynamic, and behavioral theories of depression.

146. The answer is B. *(Pediatrics; reflex reactions in newborns)*
The parachute reflex, although not present in the newborn, appears at 6 to 8 months of age and never disappears. When the parachute reflex occurs, the infant is in the sitting position. Tilting the infant to either side results in a protective reaction—extension of the ipsilateral arm. The rooting, stepping, and Moro reflexes of the newborn disappear by 4 to 6 months. The Babinski reflex disappears by 12 to 16 months; if it reappears, it is abnormal, indicating an upper motor neuron lesion.

147. The answer is E. *(Obstetrics; labor stages)*
Six movements of the fetus during labor enable it to adapt to the maternal pelvis. Descent, external rotation, extension, and internal rotation are parts of the mechanism of labor, which also includes flexion and expulsion. Extraction, however, is part of an operative breech delivery.

148. The answer is D. *(Pediatrics; hematologic parameters in newborns)*
Lymphocytosis is not usually seen before 3 months of age and persists until approximately 6 years. Neonates have prolongation of the pro-

thrombin time because they have low levels of clotting factors. The mean hemoglobin at birth is 16.8 g/dl, with a range of 13.7 to 20. The mean corpuscular volume (MCV) of newborns is high, usually 110 to 128 μm^3. Nucleated red blood cells (RBCs) are commonly seen on a smear.

149. The answer is A. *(Psychiatry; aging)*
Aging alone does not cause significant difficulty with everyday cognitive function. It does, however, place a person at risk for development of illnesses that interfere with mentation. Alcoholic dementia, Alzheimer's disease, and cerebrovascular disease can all cause such disturbances. Depression can also interfere with concentration.

150. The answer is D. *(Pediatrics; nutrition of milk and formula)*
Human milk and cow milk contain a higher amount of fat than do commercially prepared formulas, approximately 45 g/L in breast milk versus 36 g/L in formula. Formula contains much higher levels of vitamin D (10 μg/L vs 0.5), vitamin K (54 μg/L vs 2.1), and iron (12 mg/L vs 0.5).

151. The answer is E. *(Obstetrics; third stage of labor)*
The cervix may be seen at the introitus when uterine ligament support relaxes, but its appearance is not a sign of placental separation. The other four choices are frequent signs of the start of placental separation.

152. The answer is C. *(Pediatrics; idiopathic thrombocytopenic purpura)*
Examples of type III hypersensitivity include serum sickness and immune complex pericarditis. Idiopathic thrombocytopenic purpura (ITP) is the most common thrombocytopenic purpura of childhood. In 70% of cases of ITP, a viral infection precedes the reaction. It is felt to have an immune basis. Increased platelet immunoglobulin G (IgG) has been found. Platelet destruction occurs peripherally, as evidenced by low platelet counts and normal megakaryocytes in the bone marrow. The disease is usually self-limited, with eventual normalization of the platelet count.

153. The answer is C. *(Behavioral science; race and illnesses)*
Obesity, hypertension, diabetes, and heart disease are more common in black than in white individuals. No significant racial difference exists in the occurrence of the affective disorders.

154. The answer is E. *(Pediatrics; stages of child development)*
Most 3-year-old children are toilet-trained. They can copy a cross and a circle. A 2-year-old child can form sentences consisting of three words. At 4 years of age, the child can copy a square.

155. The answer is A. *(Obstetrics; severe preeclampsia)*
Severe preeclampsia is characterized by significant alterations in physiologic function or end-organ involvement. Hyperemesis is a common pregnancy complication, but is not a criterion for severe preeclampsia. Hyperemesis is in contradistinction to blurred vision, cyanosis, thrombocytopenia, and epigastric pain, which are characteristic of severe preeclampsia.

156. The answer is B. *(Pediatrics;* Streptococcus pneumoniae*)*
Chronic granulomatous disease (CGD) is primarily an X-linked disorder of neutrophil function. The bacteria are ingested, but killing is impaired. Repeated infections by unusual bacteria are the hallmark. *Staphylococcus epidermidis, S. aureus,* and *Candida* are commonly isolated. Bruton's agammaglobulinemia also is X-linked, and all three major classes of immunoglobulins are decreased. Recurrent pneumococcal infections are common. Sickle cell disease causes altered splenic function, increasing the risk of pneumococcal infections. Peritonitis is the most common infection in nephrotic syndrome; pneumococcus is the most common organism. Pneumococcus is responsible for 60% of infections in splenectomized patients.

157. The answer is A. *(General surgery; wound healing)*
Only severe anemia (hemoglobin < 5 g/dl) significantly interferes with normal wound healing.

Diabetes mellitus imposes a significant risk for wound healing due to small vessel disease (ischemia), increased tissue levels of glucose (enhances bacterial growth), and defects in chemotaxis associated with hyperglycemia.

Corticosteroids impair collagen synthesis, resulting in delayed wound healing. In addition, they decrease neutrophil adhesion, thus preventing their emigration from vascular channels to the site of infection. This decreases the number of neutrophils in tissue, which impairs the healing process. Zinc deficiency impairs wound healing, since it is a cofactor for enzymes involved in collagen metabolism. Malnutrition decreases the nutrients necessary for normal wound healing. Other factors that interfere with wound healing are infection, foreign bodies, vitamin C deficiency, and neutropenia.

158. The answer is D. *(Pediatrics; stage of child development)*
Transferring objects occurs at 6 to 9 months of age. Most 9-month-old children can get to a sitting position. Repetitive vowels are present at 6 months of age, repetitive consonants by 9 months. Pincer grasp is seen by 6 to 7 months. Independent rising and walking usually are not seen until 11 to 12 months of age.

159. The answer is B. *(Neurology; myasthenia gravis)*
Anticholinergic medications would certainly not help in myasthenia gravis, a postsynaptic disorder of the neuromuscular junction, but cholinergic medicines can be beneficial. Immunosuppressants such as steroids can be helpful in suppressing the antibody production that leads to the generalized weakness of myasthenia gravis. Similarly, plasmapheresis and immunoglobulin can optimize the immune system by filtering and boosting, respectively, thereby overcoming the symptomatology, at least temporarily. Many patients are cured from removal of the thymus gland, although the benefit may be delayed for months or years.

160. The answer is A. *(Pediatrics; tracheo-esophageal fistula)*
Cyanosis that occurs at rest but is relieved by crying is characteristic of choanal atresia. Infants are obligate nose-breathers; but when they cry, air is inhaled and the cyanosis resolves, albeit temporarily. The condition is diagnosed by the inability to pass a catheter through the nose.

161. The answer is B. *(General surgery; parietal cell vagotomy)*
Surgical treatment in peptic ulcer disease is indicated if the patient is unresponsive to medical therapy; there is refractory hemorrhage; there is perforation; or if the patient has Zollinger-Ellison syndrome.

Three types of vagotomies are available: truncal, selective, and parietal (highly selective). Surgical options for a duodenal ulcer include antrectomy plus vagotomy (Billroth I or II), vagotomy plus pyloroplasty, or parietal cell vagotomy. Parietal cell vagotomies spare the nerve of Laterjet and are least likely to be associated with the dumping syndrome. This syndrome consists of reactive hypoglycemia, dizziness, flushing, and diarrhea 30 minutes after a meal.

Types of anastomoses include the Billroth I, where the stomach is reconnected to the duodenum, and the Billroth II, where the duodenum is closed at the pylorus and the stomach is anastomosed with the jejunum (gastrojejunostomy).

162. The answer is B. *(Pediatrics; petit mal seizures)*
Petit mal seizures cease as quickly as they commence. Motor activity stops abruptly, and patients develop a blank stare with fluttering of the eyelids. The seizures are brief (10–30 seconds), but may occur many times throughout the day. They end abruptly and have no postictal stage. Complex absence seizures have some myoclonic activity. Absence seizures can be triggered by hyperventilation. Electroencephalogram (EEG) shows a typical three-per-second spike-and-wave pattern.

163. The answer is E. *(Cardiology; major risk factors for coronary artery disease)*
The National Cholesterol Education Panel (NCEP) states that the major risk factors for coronary artery disease are being a man 45 years or older or a woman 55 years or older, hypertension ($\geq$ 140/90), current cigarette smoking, high-density lipoprotein (HDL) lower than 35 mg/dl, low-density lipoprotein (LDL) equal to or greater than 160 mg/dl, diabetes mellitus, and a family history of premature coronary artery disease. A negative risk factor is an HDL greater than 60 mg/dl. Sedentary lifestyle, obesity, birth control pill use, hyperuricemia, increased fibrinogen, and hostile personality are soft criteria for increased coronary artery disease risk.

164. The answer is A. *(Pediatrics; vaccines)*
Two types of polio vaccines are available. The Salk vaccine is a killed (inactivated) vaccine. It is recommended in patients with immune deficiency or if the vaccine recipient is in close household contact with an immunosuppressed individual (who has a significant degree of viral shedding). The Sabin vaccine is a live vaccine given orally.

165. The answer is C. *(Obstetrics; newborn evaluation)*
The Apgar score is an excellent tool for assessing the overall status of the newborn soon after birth. A normal score is 7 or greater at 1 minute, and 9 at 5 minutes. Skin color, muscle tone, heart rate, and respiratory effort are parts of the Apgar score used at 1 minute after birth to evaluate the degree of neonatal resuscitation that will be appropriate. Body temperature of the neonate is an important physiologic concern but is not a component of the Apgar score.

166. The answer is C. *(Pediatrics; diphtheria-tetanus-pertussis vaccine)*
Diphtheria-tetanus-pertussis (DTP) vaccine is not contraindicated in immunocompromised patients, nor does it put them at higher risk for any of the diseases. Acute febrile illnesses and unstable or evolving neurologic conditions are contraindications because it becomes difficult to distinguish symptoms of the disease from reac-

tions to the vaccine. An upper respiratory infection is not a contraindication. Acute encephalopathy, although rare, can be associated with the pertussis component. Also rare is an acute shock-like state that can last for a few hours. Because most serious side effects are attributed to the pertussis component, it should be deleted from subsequent immunizations, and only DT should be given.

167. The answer is B. *(Psychiatry; antipsychotic medication)*
Use of clozapine does not cause significant renal toxicity. It does have the other effects listed. Its value is its effectiveness in patients who have not responded to safer antipsychotic medications.

168. The answer is E. *(Pediatrics; measles-mumps-rubella vaccine)*
No reactions to the mumps component have been described. Pregnancy and immunodeficiency states are contraindications for vaccination. The vaccine, however, is recommended in asymptomatic human immunodeficiency virus (HIV) patients. Although the vaccine is a live virus, transmission to susceptible individuals does not occur, and it can be given in households where pregnant women or immunocompromised persons reside. Subacute sclerosing panencephalitis is rare and usually milder than that caused by the actual measles virus. Arthralgias and, occasionally, arthritis are attributed to the rubella component in 1%–2% of children.

169. The answer is D. *(Neurology; neurofibromatosis)*
Neurofibromatosis (usually type I) generally has an autosomal dominant pattern of inheritance. Type II may present as bilateral acoustic neuromas (chromosome 22 as opposed to the chromosome 19 of type I). Six or more café au lait spots greater than 1.5 cm in diameter are diagnostic, and intracranial hamartomas are common, as well as hamartomas in other organs (e.g., kidneys, heart).

170. The answer is D. *(Pediatrics; Haemophilus influenzae type B)*
Haemophilus influenzae type B is the most common cause of epiglottitis. This bacteria can be recovered from the blood and the epiglottis. Although nontypable *H. influenzae* is a more common cause of otitis media, type B is sometimes responsible. Septic arthritis can be caused by *H. influenzae* B in the appropriate age-group. Orbital cellulitis is most commonly caused by *H. influenzae* B in children younger than 5 years of age. Neonatal meningitis is most commonly caused by group B streptococcus, *Escherichia coli*, and *Listeria monocytogenes*. The majority of *H. influenzae* infections occur between 6 months and 5 years of age.

171. The answer is D. *(Neurology; multiple sclerosis)*
Multiple sclerosis (MS) is a disorder of the white matter, and aphasia is clearly a cortical (gray matter) disorder. The aphasia and the right arm weakness best describe a patient with a transient stroke. Bilateral trigeminal neuralgia is strongly suggestive of MS. Bilateral intranuclear ophthalmoplegia suggests bilateral demyelinative lesions of the median longitudinal fasciculi. Magnetic resonance imaging (MRI) scans are very sensitive for MS, usually showing plaques in the white matter of the brain.

172. The answer is A. *(Pediatrics; specialized vaccines)*
Haemophilus influenzae B vaccine is indicated for the prevention of invasive diseases such as meningitis and epiglottitis. The majority of otitis media caused by *Haemophilus* is due to nontypable strains. Influenza vaccine is recommended for children at risk of serious pulmonary complications, such as children with congenital heart disease, severe asthma, bronchopulmonary dysplasia, cystic fibrosis, renal disease, diabetes, and sickle cell anemia. Pneumococcal vaccine is much more effective after 2 years of age. It is currently recommended that all newborns be immunized against hepatitis B virus (HBV). Newborns of HBV-antigen–positive mothers should also receive hepatitis

B immune globulin at birth, but it should be administered at a separate site from the vaccine.

173. The answer is A. *(Cardiology; role of low-density lipoprotein in coronary artery disease)*
Cholesterol and high-density lipoprotein (HDL) levels are the best screens for primary prevention of coronary artery disease when there is no history or evidence of the disease. Low-density lipoprotein (LDL) is the initial screen for secondary prevention when there is known disease and is also used to decide whether drug therapy is indicated.

LDL carries most of the cholesterol in the blood and is derived from very low-density lipoprotein (VLDL). Oxidized LDL is more atherogenic than native LDL. It is taken up by the scavenger pathway, via high-affinity LDL receptors on macrophages, to form foam cells that contribute to the formation of fatty streaks in the atherosclerotic process. Antioxidants (vitamins A, C, and E) are thought to neutralize oxidized LDL, thereby reducing atherogenicity. LDL is calculated as follows: LDL = (cholesterol − HDL) − (triglyceride II 5). Levels less than 130 mg/dl are normal; levels between 130 and 159 mg/dl indicate a borderline high risk; and a level equal to or greater than 160 mg/dl is medically significant.

The goal of therapy in primary prevention is to attain an LDL lower than 130 mg/dl. However, in secondary prevention, the goal is an LDL lower than 100 mg/dl, because these patients already have coronary artery disease.

174. The answer is E. *(Pediatrics; accidents)*
Any self-poisoning in a child older than 5 years should be considered self-inflicted or abuse. Suffocation is more common in the first year of life, sometimes in infants who sleep with their parents. One in three infants who use walkers will have an accidental fall, usually a fall down stairs. The majority of drownings occur in the 1- to 4-year age-group. Pool drownings are most common in children 1 to 3 years of age. Most of these children are unsupervised in a pool with no fence around it. Pedestrian injuries are most common in the 3- to 7-year age-group.

175. The answer is B. *(Cardiology; ejection fraction)*
The ejection fraction (EF) is the ratio of stroke volume (SV) to left ventricular end-diastolic volume (LVEDV). It is measured by echocardiography or radionuclide angiography. Because the normal SV is 80 ml and the LVEDV is 120 ml, the normal EF is 0.66 (80/120). The SV is increased by increasing preload ("the more it fills, the more it ejects"), decreasing afterload (impedance to ejection), or increasing contractility (the vigor of contraction) without increasing LVEDV. Contractility is increased by increasing sympathetic stimulation of the heart or by administering positive inotropic agents, such as digitalis and β-agonists. Contractility is decreased by negative inotropic agents, such as propranolol, heart failure, myocardial ischemia, myocardial fibrosis, and metabolic acidosis.

Patient A has a decreased EF, which would be expected in a ventricular aneurysm, because much of the myocardial tissue is replaced by noncontractile fibrous tissue. It could also be due to a myocardial infarction involving the left ventricle (decreased contractility), congestive cardiomyopathy (decreased contractility), hypertrophic cardiomyopathy (increased afterload), or severe aortic stenosis (increased afterload).

Patient B has a normal EF, as discussed previously. Increasing cardiac contractility increases the EF in a normal person; it is what occurs in a well-trained long-distance runner (see next paragraph). A β-blocker, such as propranolol, reduces the EF in a normal patient because it decreases contractility.

Patient C has an increased EF, representative of a long-distance runner. Well-trained athletes compared with untrained individuals have a lower resting heart rate, less increase in heart rate with exercise, a greater SV, and a greater EF. The increase in SV is due to an increase in contractility because of physiologic left ventricular hypertrophy (LVH). LVH increases the size and force of contraction of individual myocardial fibers.

176. The answer is A. *(Pediatrics; active versus passive immunization)*
Active immunization is the administration of a vaccine or toxoid which stimulates formation of

antibodies. Rabies vaccine provides active immunization. In passive immunization, preformed antibodies are given to confer temporary immunity. Immune globulin, Rh immune globulin, diphtheria antitoxin, and crotalin antivenin are all examples of agents used for passive immunization.

177. The answer is E. *(Laboratory medicine; laboratory values in geriatric patients)*
A mild glucose intolerance is normal in the elderly because of the increase in adipose tissue, which decreases the number of insulin receptors available for glucose. Alkaline phosphatase is increased in the elderly because of an increase in degenerative arthritis. Reactive bone formation occurs at the margins of the joints (osteophytes) in response to wear and tear of the articular cartilage. An increase in autoantibodies with age is secondary to a decrease in CD8 T-suppressor cells. The creatinine clearance decreases as age increases, primarily as a result of a decrease in the glomerular filtration rate. The hemoglobin concentration in elderly men is in the range of the hemoglobin concentration in adult women (12–16 g/dl). This decrease is due to a decrease in testosterone, which decreases the stimulation of erythropoietin, leading to a slight decrease in erythropoiesis in the bone marrow.

178. The answer is B. *(Pulmonology; pulmonary function studies in restrictive and obstructive lung disease)*
Pulmonary function studies are very important in differentiating restrictive from obstructive lung diseases. Restrictive diseases, (e.g., sarcoidosis) show decreased compliance of the lungs (difficulty in expansion) because of interstitial fibrosis but increased elasticity (good recoil once they are expanded). Obstructive diseases (e.g., emphysema) have increased compliance (ease of expansion) but decreased elasticity (poor recoil) because of destruction of elastic tissue in the supporting structures. Therefore, on expiration, air becomes trapped in the lungs behind the collapsed distal airways that lack elastic tissue support.

Spirometry is used to determine volumes (e.g., tidal volume) and capacities (two or more volumes; e.g., total lung capacity) in the lung as well as measurements of flow rate of air out of the lungs (e.g., forced expiratory volume in 1 second [FEV_1]). In restrictive lung disease, the poor compliance affects all volumes and capacities equally; therefore, they are all decreased. In obstructive lung disease, the inability to eliminate all of the air on expiration increases the residual volume (air left in the lung after maximal expiration). This increase in air increases the total lung capacity (sum of all of the lung volumes) and expands the chest cavity to produce an increased anteroposterior diameter (barrel chest) and flattened diaphragms. Limited expansion of the rigid chest wall accompanied by an ever-expanding residual volume eventually decreases the other lung volumes and capacities such as tidal volume (volume of air entering or leaving the lungs in quiet inspiration or expiration, respectively) and vital capacity (maximal amount of air exhaled from the lungs after full inspiration).

Regarding flow studies, an FEV_1 refers to the amount of air that is forcibly expelled in 1 second after maximal inspiration. Normally, a person expels 4 L of air in 1 second. The forced vital capacity (FVC) is the total amount of air expelled after maximal inspiration. Normally, the FVC is 5 L. When expressed as a ratio, the FEV_1/FVC is 80% (4 L/5 L). In both restrictive and obstructive lung disease, the FEV_1 is decreased, but the magnitude of the decrease is less in restrictive (e.g., 3 L) than in obstructive lung disease (e.g., 2 L), because of the greater problem in expelling air in the latter disease. In restrictive lung disease, the FEV_1 and the FVC are almost identical, because the increased elasticity in the lungs quickly expresses air out of the lung in 1 second. Therefore, the FEV_1/FVC ratio is increased (e.g., 3 L/3 L = 100%). In obstructive lung disease, however, the FVC is usually 3 L or less; therefore, the ratio of FEV_1/FVC is usually decreased (e.g., 2 L/3 L = 66%). The $Paco_2$ is usually increased in obstructive lung disease (respiratory acidosis), because CO_2 remains behind in the lung on expiration. In restrictive disease, the $Paco_2$ is either normal or decreased, because the patient must breathe more frequently for adequate ventilation of lungs that do not expand well on inspiration. A comparison of restrictive and obstructive lung disease follows.

	Obstructive	Restrictive
Total lung capacity	Increased	Decreased
Residual volume	Increased	Decreased
Tidal volume	Decreased	Decreased
Vital capacity	Decreased	Decreased
FEV_1	Decreased (++)	Decreased (+)
FVC	Decreased (+++)	Decreased (+)
FEV_1/FVC	Decreased	Increased
$PaCO_2$	Increased	Normal to decreased

+ indicates degree of magnitude.

179. The answer is E. *(Pediatrics; stages of child development)*

Babbling and cooing occur by 2 months of age. The social smile also is present by this time. Lifting the head and chest occurs by 3 months of age. A 2-month-old infant can use the eyes well enough to follow an object through 180 degrees. Rolling over from the prone to supine position usually does not occur until 4 to 6 months of age.

180. The answer is E. *(Emergency medicine; poisons and their antidotes)*

Methanol is an alcohol that is found in paint strippers and fluid for automobile windshield wipers. It is metabolized into formic acid, which irritates the optic nerve to produce optic neuritis and the potential for permanent blindness. Addition of formic acid to the extracellular fluid compartment also produces an increased anion gap metabolic acidosis. Because methanol competes with ethanol for alcohol dehydrogenase, ethanol infusion is used as an antidote until hemodialysis is performed.

Gold poisoning is most commonly seen in the setting of treatment for rheumatoid arthritis. Acute tubular necrosis, central necrosis of the liver, membranous glomerulonephritis, and hematologic changes including agranulocytosis, pancytopenia (aplastic anemia), and thrombocytopenia are potential complications. Dimercaprol is a gold chelating agent.

Organophosphates are irreversible cholinesterase inhibitors that are found in insecticides. They are readily absorbed through the skin, respiratory tract, and gastrointestinal tract. The accumulation of acetylcholine in the nerve endings stimulates muscarinic receptors to produce increased lacri-

mation, salivation, and sweating as well as bronchospasm, miotic pupils, bradycardia, and fecal incontinence. Acetylcholine accumulation at nicotinic receptors produces muscle weakness, the potential for tachycardia rather than bradycardia, paralysis, and muscle fasciculations. Measurement of serum or red blood cell cholinesterase levels is useful in documenting acute intoxication. Pralidoxime competitively inhibits the binding of organophosphates to acetylcholinesterase and is given to the majority of patients with significant intoxication. Atropine is useful for the muscarinic effects. Respiratory depression is the usual cause of death.

β-adrenergic blockers, like propranolol, compete with catecholamines for $β_1$ and $β_2$ receptor sites. $β_1$ receptors normally increase inotropism and rate in the heart, whereas the $β_2$ receptors are responsible for vasodilatation, bronchodilation, and stimulation of glycogenolysis. Therefore, β-receptor blockade could result in bradycardia, hypotension, convulsions, bronchoconstriction, and hypoglycemia. Profound myocardial depression is the most common cause of death. Because glucagon increases intracellular cyclic adenosine monophosphate (cAMP) by a different mechanism than that of β receptors, it is useful in treating the hypotension with β blockade. It also stimulates glycogenolysis and gluconeogenesis to raise the glucose level. Atropine or isoproterenol is used for treating advanced atrioventricular block.

Tricyclic antidepressants, like amitriptyline, are anticholinergics. Major effects include coma with shock and metabolic acidosis, respiratory depression, agitation or delirium, neuromuscular irritability and seizures, hyperpyrexia, bowel and bladder paralysis, and various cardiac abnormalities including arrhythmias and toxic cardiomyopathies. Atropine, which itself is an anticholinergic agent, is contraindicated. Lidocaine, propranolol, or phenytoin is useful for the cardiac abnormalities. Sodium bicarbonate is useful for treating the metabolic acidosis up to a pH of 7.2.

181–182. The answers are: 181-C, 182-A. *(Psychiatry; mood disorders)*

Nortriptyline exemplifies an antidepressant with a "therapeutic window." Dosages that achieve a blood level of 50–100 ng/ml are associated with good patient responses. Increasing the dosage diminishes the response. This therapeutic window has not been demonstrated for other tricyclic antidepressants.

Lithium has a threshold for response at a dosage that produces a blood level of approximately 1.0 mEq/L. Lower doses are ineffective. Higher doses do not appreciably increase the degree of response, but are associated with more untoward effects. Graph B represents a graded response, as might be seen with antipsychotic medication. Graph D represents a lack of response. Graph E represents a negative response to a medication.

183–184. The answers are: 183-B, 184-C.
(Hematology; polycythemia)
Polycythemia refers to an increase in red blood cell (RDC) mass, which, in an adult, is any hematocrit greater than 55%. The differential of polycythemia is based on whether there is an absolute increase in RBC mass or whether it is a relative increase related to a decrease in plasma volume contracting around a normal RBC mass. Next, it must be decided whether it is appropriate, owing to the stimulus of hypoxemia; or inappropriate from ectopic secretion or autonomous production of RBCs in the bone marrow.

An arterial blood gas is the first step in the workup of any polycythemia state and immediately characterizes the polycythemia as appropriate or inappropriate. RBC mass and plasma volume are also useful, because they define whether the polycythemia is absolute or relative. Erythropoietin levels are increased only if the polycythemia is appropriate or ectopically secreted. A low oxygen saturation, increased RBC mass, normal plasma volume, and increased erythropoietin indicate an appropriate polycythemia, because the oxygen saturation is decreased. It is

also absolute, because the RBC mass is increased. The normal plasma volume and increased erythropoietin levels are expected when hypoxemia is the cause of the secondary polycythemia. Hypoxemia is associated with chronic obstructive pulmonary disease (COPD), restrictive lung diseases, cyanotic congenital heart disease, and high-altitude residence, to name a few.

A normal oxygen saturation, normal RBC mass, decreased plasma volume, and normal erythropoietin indicate an inappropriate polycythemia, because the oxygen saturation is normal. It is relative because the RBC mass is normal. This combination is characteristic of dehydration and stress polycythemia. Both are associated with hemoconcentration secondary to a reduction in plasma volume. Stress polycythemia is typically seen in obese, male hypertensives.

Polycythemia rubra vera is a myeloproliferative disease with unregulated production of RBCs, leukocytes, and platelets in the marrow. The oxygen saturation is normal; RBC mass and plasma volume are both increased; and the erythropoietin is decreased.

Renal adenocarcinoma and other disorders characterized by increased production of erythropoietin (e.g., hepatocellular carcinoma, cerebellar hemangioblastoma, uterine leiomyomas, renal cysts) have normal oxygen saturations, increased RBC mass, normal plasma volumes, and increased erythropoietin levels.

Another subset of polycythemia is smoker's polycythemia. In this disorder, the carbon monoxide in smoke causes tissue hypoxia and the release of erythropoietin; other components in smoke, for unexplained reasons, decrease plasma volume. They have variable oxygen saturations.

The following chart summarizes the different types of polycythemia and the expected laboratory findings.

Condition	RBC mass	Plasma volume	Sao$_2$	Erythropoietin
Polycythemia rubra vera	I	I	N	D
Hypoxemia (COPD)	I	N	D	I
Ectopic erythropoietin	I	N	N	I
Smoker's polycythemia	I	D	V	I
Stress polycythemia	N	D	N	N
Dehydration	N	D	N	N

I = increased; D = decreased; N = normal; V = variable Sao$_2$ = oxygen saturation in arterial blood gas.

185–187. The answers are: 185-E, 186-D, 187-A. *(Pharmacology; cardiac drugs)*
Guanethidine is an effective antihypertensive agent that initially decreases cardiac output, but with chronic use lowers peripheral resistance. Its actions on sympathetic neurons depend on its uptake into nerve terminals via the norepinephrine transporter. Tricyclic antidepressants, which inhibit the uptake of guanethidine, may decrease its antihypertensive actions. The major adverse effects of the drug are postural hypotension and increased gastrointestinal motility.

Hydralazine relaxes arteriolar smooth muscle, thereby decreasing systemic vascular resistance. Tachyphylaxis occurs, so the drug is usually used in combination with other agents in the treatment of hypertension. A syndrome that includes arthralgia, myalgia, fever, and skin rashes may occur at high doses, chiefly in patients who slowly acetylate the drug.

Nifedipine appears to block the L-type calcium channels in vascular smooth muscle at concentrations below those required for significant cardiac effects. Therefore, unlike verapamil and diltiazem, it is not useful in the treatment of supraventricular tachycardias. All calcium channel blockers exert negative inotropic actions that are potentially deleterious in patients with heart failure.

188–189. The answers are: 188-D, 189-A. *(Psychiatry; substance abuse)*
Approximately 4% of young adults have used cocaine in the last month. This number has decreased steadily since the mid-1980s. However, the use of crack cocaine has become endemic in some areas, where it starts at an earlier age.

Approximately 28% of young adults smoke tobacco regularly. This percentage has held constant for a few years. There is evidence to suggest that the number of young adult smokers has started to rise again. In contrast, tobacco use in the overall population continues to decline.

190–191. The answers are: 190-B, 191-A. *(Pharmacology; anesthesia and analgesia)*
With inhalational anesthetics, the rate of onset of anesthesia depends on the physicochemical properties of the compound, which are reflected in its blood:gas partition coefficient. Anesthetics with high partition coefficients have slow rates of onset. In practice, the rate of onset of anesthetic action can be accelerated by increasing anesthetic concentration in the inspired air and by increasing the ventilation rate.

Minimal alveolar concentration (MAC) value of an inhalational anesthetic is defined as the concentration (expressed as percentage of the alveolar gas mixture) that results in immobility in 50% of a patient population exposed to a noxious stimulus. It is a measure of anesthetic potency and represents a single point on a dose/response curve. A MAC value greater than 100% for drug A shows that it is the least effective anesthetic of those listed. If inhaled at a concentration of 80%, less than half of a patient population is immobilized. Thus, if used alone, such a compound is unlikely, on theoretical grounds, to provide an anesthetic state that is adequate for most surgical procedures.

192–195. The answers are: 192-F, 193-B, 194-E, 195-A. *(Nephrology; urinary casts in nephrotic syndrome, acute glomerulonephritis, acute pyelonephritis, and end-stage renal disease)*
Urinary casts are a mold of the renal tubules. They consist of a mixture of protein, with or without cells or cellular debris that is present in the renal tubules as a result of a normal process or disease. Their presence in the urine indicates pathological processes that are occurring in the kidneys rather than in the lower urinary tract.

Children who present with generalized edema (anasarca) associated with a 24-hour urine protein greater than 3.5 g have the nephrotic syndrome. Minimal change disease (nil disease, lipoid nephrosis) is the most common cause of the nephrotic syndrome in children. The syndrome results from the loss of polyanions (negative charge) in the glomerular basement membrane, with massive loss of albumin in the urine. Hypoalbuminemia reduces the plasma oncotic pressure, resulting in generalized, pitting edema. In addition, the hypoalbuminemia stimulates liver production of excess cholesterol, resulting in hypercholesterolemia. Some of the cholesterol is lost in the urine where it produces lipiduria, fatty casts, and oval fat bodies (renal tubular cells or macrophages with cholesterol).

The white blood cell (WBC) cast distinguishes acute pyelonephritis from acute cystitis. Acute pyelonephritis is an acute tubulointerstitial disease most commonly secondary to ascending infection (usually *Escherichia coli*) from the bladder. Acute inflammation results in the presence of neutrophils that form microabscesses in the kidney and in the renal tubules. Lower urinary tract infections like acute cystitis have neutrophils in the urine (pyuria), but do not have casts, which are formed only in the kidney.

Waxy casts are acellular casts that represent the progressive degeneration of a cellular cast. The progression is thought to occur as follows: cellular cast [leukocytes, red blood cells (RBCs), renal tubular cells] → coarsely granular cast → finely granular cast → waxy cast. They are highly refractile and have sharp borders, unlike a hyaline cast, which has soft features and round borders. Waxy casts are a marker for end-stage chronic renal disease.

RBC casts are a marker for glomerulonephritis, which is divided into the nephritic and nephrotic types (discussed previously). The nephritic type is commonly seen in poststreptococcal glomerulonephritis, as in this patient recovering from scarlet fever, and in renal involvement in systemic lupus erythematosus (SLE), to name two. RBC casts, hematuria (smoky urine), and mild to moderate proteinuria are the hallmarks of the nephritic syndrome.

Renal tubular casts are associated with acute tubular necrosis secondary to ischemic or nephrotoxic damage. They are partially responsible for the oliguria associated with acute tubular necrosis.

Hyaline casts are the most common overall cast. When present in small numbers, they have the least clinical significance of all casts. Formed from the protein gel in the renal tubule, these casts are called Tamm-Horsfall mucoprotein. One hyaline cast per low-power field is commonly seen in normal urine. However, increased numbers are associated with any condition accompanied by proteinuria (e.g., fever, exercise, renal disease).

196–197. The answers are: 196-C, 197-B.
(Pharmacology; cardiac drugs)
Minoxidil acts to open potassium channels in smooth muscle membranes and, like hydralazine,

dilates arterioles but not veins. It should be used in combination with a β blocker and a loop diuretic because reflex sympathetic stimulation leads to tachycardia and fluid retention. Topical use may stimulate hair growth in baldness.

Why not hydrochlorothiazide? Used as single-drug therapy, thiazides are mild antihypertensives that cause diuresis and vasodilation (especially indapamide). The hypotensive action of angiotensin converting enzyme (ACE) inhibitors such as captopril occurs via inhibition of the peptidyl dipeptidase, which converts angiotensin I to angiotensin II and which also hydrolyzes bradykinin, a potent vasodilator. This action is decreased by nonsteroidal anti-inflammatory drugs (NSAIDs), which appear to block bradykinin-mediated vasodilation through inhibition of prostaglandin synthesis. Blood counts and urinalyses are advised during the first months of treatment with ACE inhibitors, because bone marrow suppression and nephrotoxicity may occur.

198–200. The answers are: 198-D, 199-I, 200-F.
(Hematology; lead poisoning, autoimmune hemolytic anemia, folate deficiency)
Anemias are quickly separated on the basis of mean corpuscular volume (MCV) into microcytic (MCV < 80 μm^3), normocytic (MCV 80–100 μm^3), and macrocytic (MCV > 100 μm^3). Microcytic anemias include iron deficiency, anemia of chronic disease, α- and β-thalassemia, and sideroblastic anemias (e.g., lead poisoning). The most common macrocytic anemias are B_{12} and folate deficiencies. Normocytic anemias are subdivided into those with corrected reticulocyte counts of less than 2% (aplastic anemia, renal disease, blood loss for less than 1 week) and those with corrected reticulocyte counts of greater than 3% (hemolytic anemias, blood loss for more than 1 week).

The reticulocyte count represents the bone marrow response to an anemia, which is called effective erythropoiesis. Next to the complete blood count (CBC), the reticulocyte count is the most important laboratory test to perform in the workup of anemia. It must be corrected for the degree of anemia by the following formula: patient hematocrit/45 × reticulocyte count. For example, a patient with a reticulocyte count of 9% and a hematocrit of 15% has a corrected reticulocyte count of 3% (15/45 × 9% = 3%). A corrected reticulocyte count of less than 2% indicates a poor marrow response to the anemia (ineffective erythropoiesis), whereas a corrected count of greater than 3% portends a good marrow response to the anemia (effective erythropoiesis). It takes at least 1 week before the marrow responds to anemia with an appropriate reticulocyte count. Therefore, patients with an acute bleed or those who are being treated for known deficiencies (e.g., iron deficiency) will not have an elevated count until at least 5 to 7 days of treatment have passed.

Lead poisoning is most commonly seen in children who have exposure to toys that contain lead in the paint. There is often a history of pica, or the child may have an unusual craving for eating such things as dirt. In adults, inhalation is the most important route of exposure, usually from burning car batteries. Lead concentrates in the skeleton where it deposits in the epiphyses to produce densities that are visible on x-ray.

Lead interferes with heme synthesis by inhibiting two major enzymes—aminolevulinic acid dehydrase (ALA dehydrase) and ferrochelatase. The latter enzyme catalyzes the reaction that joins iron to protoporphyrin to form heme. This reaction underscores the use of the red blood cell (RBC) protoporphyrin level as a screen for lead poisoning because it is elevated in the majority of cases. ALA dehydrase catalyzes the reaction between δ-aminolevulinic acid (ALA) and porphobilinogen. In lead poisoning, inactivation of this enzyme results in an increase of ALA in the urine. Lead also inactivates nucleotidase, which breaks down RNA in RBCs. Inactivation of this enzyme is responsible for the coarse basophilic stippling in RBCs, which is an extremely good marker of lead poisoning in the setting of a microcytic anemia. Lead also injures the RBC membrane, producing a mild hemolytic component to the anemia, as evidenced by the increase in corrected reticulocyte count in the patient. The anemia is microcytic; because whenever hemoglobin synthesis is decreased because of inadequate iron supplies (iron deficiency, anemia of chronic disease), decreased production of heme (lead poisoning), or decreased production of globin chains (the thal-assemias), extra mitotic divisions in the marrow result in the production of microcytes.

Clinical findings include demyelination in the central and peripheral nervous systems (CNS and PNS) [e.g., wrist and foot drop] and encephalopathy caused by increased vessel permeability, producing cerebral edema. Severe, colicky abdominal pain is also noted. When excreted in the kidney, lead produces a nephrotoxic tubular necrosis. A lead line on the gums is frequently observed. Treatment for lead poisoning involves the use of dimercaprol and edetate calcium disodium.

Patients with autoimmune diseases [e.g., systemic lupus erythematosus (SLE)] are prone to developing other autoimmune diseases. Therefore, in the setting of a patient with known SLE, the presence of anemia with an elevated corrected reticulocyte count is most likely an autoimmune hemolytic anemia (AIHA). The gold standard test for AIHA is the Coombs' test, which detects the presence of immunoglobulin G (IgG), C3, or both on the surface of RBCs (direct Coombs') or the presence of IgG antibodies against RBC antigens in the serum (indirect Coombs').

AIHA is subdivided into cold (30%) or warm (70%) type. Cold AIHA is characterized by the presence of IgM and C3. IgM reacts best at cold temperatures (cold agglutinin) and is a potent stimulator of the classic complement pathway. Rarely, the blood bank can identify the exact type of IgM antibody that is causing the hemolysis (e.g., anti-I, anti-i). Most of the time, they are nonspecific cold agglutinins. Hemolysis is either intravascular or extravascular depending on how far the complement system is activated. If activation stops at C3, the macrophages in the spleen and liver will phagocytize and destroy the cells extravascularly. If the complement system is activated all the way through C9, then intravascular hemolysis occurs. Cold AIHA is seen in diseases like *Mycoplasma pneumoniae* infections (anti-I), infectious mononucleosis (anti-i), malignant lymphomas, and chronic lymphocytic leukemia. Alkylating agents are the mainstay of therapy.

Patients with SLE account for the majority of those with warm AIHA (40%–50%), which is characterized by the presence of IgG antibodies with or without C3. Splenomegaly is commonly associated with the disease and is often responsible for the immunologic destruction of leukocytes and platelets as well, as illustrated in this patient. Extravascular destruction of RBCs is the rule. Damage to the RBCs inflicted by the macrophages frequently results in the presence of spherocytes in the peripheral blood, which could be confused with congenital spherocytosis except for the presence of a positive direct Coombs' in autoimmune hemolysis. The marked reticulocytosis frequently produces macrocytic indices, as exemplified by the increased MCV in this patient. Other causes of warm AIHA include drugs (approximately 20%), chronic lymphocytic leukemia, Hodgkin's disease, viral infections, and other collagen vascular diseases. Treatment is extremely difficult and, depending on how the patient responds, progresses in the following manner: corticosteroids to splenectomy to immunosuppressive therapy.

Macrocytic anemias associated with macroovalocytes and hypersegmented neutrophils are due to either B_{12} or folate deficiency. Folate deficiency is the most common of the two and is most commonly associated with improper dietary intake in alcoholics. The patient represented in this case exhibits end-stage alcoholic liver disease, which is manifested by the presence of hepatosplenomegaly and ascites. Spider angiomata and gynecomastia indicate the buildup of estrogen, because it cannot be metabolized by a damaged liver. Splenomegaly is secondary to portal hypertension. The enlarged spleen frequently traps leukocytes and platelets in the sinusoids, with their eventual destruction, as noted in this patient. This condition is called hypersplenism. B_{12} is found primarily in animal products, whereas folate is present in both animal and plant products. The liver has at least a 5-year supply of B_{12} as opposed to only a 3- to 4-month supply of folate, so folate deficiency develops quite rapidly when the dietary intake is decreased. B_{12} deficiency is associated with decreased intake (pure vegetarian) or decreased absorption. Examples include pernicious anemia, with a lack of intrinsic factor; bacterial overgrowth in the small bowel from diverticular disease or motility problems; and terminal ileal disease, where the receptors for intrinsic factor are located for absorption of B_{12}. Folate deficiency is associated with decreased intake (malnutrition, alcoholism), decreased absorption (malabsorption syndromes), increased use (pregnancy and lactation, disseminated cancer), and impaired use (methotrexate and trimethoprim inhibiting dihydrofolate reductase).

Clinically, patients present with the same gastrointestinal manifestations, such as glossitis and hematologic findings (discussed later). However, a neurologic disease called subacute combined degeneration is unique to B_{12} deficiency. This demyelinating disease is characterized by involvement of the posterior columns and lateral corticospinal tracts, peripheral nerves, and cerebrum itself. The findings include numbness and paresthesias of the extremities (earliest sign), hyporeflexia, vibratory loss, ataxia, and dementia. Folate therapy is able to correct all of the clinical signs, symptoms, and laboratory abnormalities of B_{12} deficiency except the neurologic findings; therefore, the distinction between the two diseases is important.

Because B_{12} and folate are necessary for DNA synthesis, their absence results in enlarged, immature nuclei in all the nucleated cells in the body. The hematopoietic cells in the marrow are called megaloblastic, therefore the term megaloblastic anemia. A classic marrow cell that typifies megaloblastic change is the giant-band neutrophil. Because all of the hematopoietic cells are abnormal, the majority are destroyed in the marrow by the macrophages. Therefore, patients present with severe anemia, leukopenia, and thrombocytopenia (pancytopenia).

Serum B_{12} is decreased in patients with B_{12} deficiency. The Schilling test is useful in localizing the B_{12} deficiency to deficient intrinsic factor (pernicious anemia), bacterial overgrowth, or small bowel disease. The serum and RBC folate are useful in diagnosing folate deficiency. The RBC folate has the greater specificity because it represents the storage state of folate in the body. Bone marrow aspirates are usually not indicated.

B_{12} deficiency is treated with parenteral B_{12} injections. Folate deficiency is treated with oral replacement therapy.

Test II

QUESTIONS

DIRECTIONS: Each of the numbered items or incomplete statements in this section is followed by answers or by completions of the statement. Select the ONE lettered answer or completion that is BEST in each case.

1. Two days after surgical repair of a femoral head fracture, a normotensive 65-year-old woman develops a third heart sound, distention of the jugular neck veins, bibasilar rales, and dependent pitting edema. These signs most likely represent

(A) endotoxic shock
(B) cardiogenic shock
(C) volume overload
(D) fat embolism syndrome

2. A 23-year-old woman presents with recurrent history of epistaxis and menorrhagia that is exacerbated whenever she takes aspirin. Her father and paternal aunt also have bleeding tendencies. Laboratory studies show a normal prothrombin time (PT), prolonged activated partial thromboplastin time (aPTT), prolonged bleeding time, and a normal platelet count. The most likely diagnosis in this patient is

(A) disseminated intravascular coagulation
(B) von Willebrand's disease
(C) a qualitative platelet defect due to aspirin
(D) hemophilia A
(E) factor VII deficiency

3. A 7-year-old boy wakes up in the night with his right face twitching and with speech arrest. He is able to run to his parents' room, where the attack stops within 1 minute. His electroencephalogram (EEG) is completely normal except for a prominent spike focus that emerges over the left central area during sleep. What is the most likely explanation for this occurrence?

(A) Childhood absence epilepsy
(B) Left temporal lobe tumor
(C) Benign rolandic epilepsy
(D) Sleep terrors
(E) Hypsarrhythmia

4. A 35-year-old woman who has delivered her third child is 7 days post emergency cesarean section under general anesthesia for active phase arrest. She has persistent spiking fevers despite broad-spectrum antibiotic coverage of both aerobes and anaerobes for the past 6 days. Pelvic examination and ultrasound show no abnormal pelvic masses. Which treatment modality would be most appropriate?

(A) Exploratory laparotomy
(B) Intravenous heparin
(C) Antifungal antibiotics
(D) Uterine curettage
(E) Pelvic examination under anesthesia

5. Bladder rupture is most commonly associated with

(A) urinary tract obstruction
(B) previous radiation therapy to the pelvis
(C) pelvic fracture
(D) blunt trauma with a full bladder

6. Which statement about the epidemiology of bipolar disorder is true?

(A) It has a lifetime incidence of between 5% and 10%
(B) It is more common in women than in men
(C) It usually is first clinically evident between age 20 and 30
(D) It is more common in higher socioeconomic groups
(E) It occurs more frequently in Amish populations

7. A newborn infant has excessive drooling along with coughing and choking with feeding. Cyanosis is present and is unrelieved by crying. Bilateral pulmonary rales are present. There is abdominal distention with tympany on percussion. The most likely diagnosis is

(A) choanal atresia
(B) respiratory distress syndrome
(C) Zenker's diverticulum
(D) a tracheoesophageal fistula
(E) duodenal atresia

8. A 29-year-old woman who has had three miscarriages and three abortions is in her thirteenth week of pregnancy. Her mother took diethylstilbestrol (DES) while this 29 year old was in utero. On examination her cervix is 0.5 cm long; before 20 weeks' gestation, she has lost three consecutive normally formed fetuses. The best treatment modality would be

(A) cervical cerclage
(B) oral terbutaline
(C) progesterone suppositories
(D) human chorionic gonadotropin (hCG) injections
(E) human menopausal gonadotropin (hMG) injections

9. A 65-year-old man is in the coronary care unit with an acute anterior myocardial infarction of 4 days' duration. He now experiences substernal chest pain similar in intensity to his initial pain. Positive physical findings include a third heart sound and bibasilar rales. Pertinent negative findings include the absence of a murmur and friction rub. Laboratory studies reveal the presence of creatine kinase (CK) isoenzyme MB and a lactate dehydrogenase (LDH) isoenzyme study with an LDH_1/LDH_2 flip. This patient most likely has

(A) recurrent angina
(B) Dressler's syndrome
(C) reinfarction
(D) a ruptured posteromedial papillary muscle
(E) a pulmonary embolism

10. Given the standardized 2 × 2 table below, which option reflects the study group in a retrospective investigative design?

	Disease Present (D+)	Disease Absent (D−)	Totals
Exposed (E+)	a	b	a + b
Nonexposed (E−)	c	d	c + d
Totals	a + c	b + d	

(A) a + c
(B) b + d
(C) c + b
(D) a + b
(E) c + d

11. A significant risk factor for breast cancer in women is

(A) a history of using birth control pills
(B) a high-fiber, low-fat diet
(C) late menarche
(D) early menopause
(E) a history of endometrial carcinoma

12. If a man with hemophilia A marries a female carrier for hemophilia A, what percentage of their sons will have hemophilia A?

(A) 0
(B) 25
(C) 50
(D) 75
(E) 100

13. A 45-year-old woman with polyhydramnios delivers a male infant with Down syndrome. A few hours after birth, the infant begins to vomit bile-stained fluid. An x-ray of the chest and abdomen reveals a "double bubble" sign. The most likely diagnosis is

(A) congenital pyloric stenosis
(B) duodenal atresia
(C) an intussusception
(D) a diaphragmatic hernia
(E) a perforated viscus

14. Which statement about the pathophysiology of schizophrenia is most accurate?

(A) Findings include increased thickness of the corpus callosum
(B) Findings include increased activity in the prefrontal cortex
(C) Findings include decreased cerebral asymmetry
(D) Findings include decreased size of lateral ventricles
(E) Abnormalities of dopaminergic transmission are pathognomonic

15. A patient with myasthenia gravis who has been well controlled with pyridostigmine for 2 years comes to the emergency room complaining of progressive weakening during the last 24 hours. He has trouble swallowing and suffers from double vision. The patient has had "flu" for the past week. What is the immediate course of action?

(A) Increase the dose of pyridostigmine
(B) Replace pyridostigmine with physostigmine
(C) Give a small dose of edrophonium
(D) Lower the dose of pyridostigmine
(E) Administer succinylcholine

16. A 33-year-old woman with a total thyroidectomy for a papillary carcinoma of the thyroid is noted to have both carpal spasm when her blood pressure is taken and facial muscle contraction with tapping over the facial nerve. Which set of laboratory data would most closely represent the expected findings in this patient? $\downarrow Ca^{2+}$

	Serum calcium	Serum phosphorus	Serum parathormone (PTH)	
(A)	Increased	Decreased	Increased	1° Hyper PTH
(B)	Increased	Decreased	Decreased	Malignancy ↑ Ca²⁺
(C)	Decreased	Increased	Decreased	HYPO PTH
(D)	Decreased	Decreased	Increased	Malabsorp vit D
(E)	Decreased	Increased	Increased	Renal Failure

17. A 15-year-old girl presents with sudden onset of abdominal pain. Physical examination reveals a tender mass in the left adnexa. A pregnancy test is negative. An x-ray exhibits a mass lesion of the left ovary, with focal areas of calcification. The most likely diagnosis is

(A) follicular cyst
(B) mucinous cystadenoma
(C) cystic teratoma
(D) Brenner's tumor
(E) serous cystadenoma

18. A 52-year-old woman has a 3-cm movable, firm, nontender mass in the right parotid that has been present for the last 6 years. No adenopathy is present. This mass most likely represents

(A) adenoid cystic carcinoma
(B) Warthin's tumor
(C) pleomorphic adenoma (mixed tumor)
(D) mucoepidermoid carcinoma

19. Given the standardized 2 × 2 table below, which option reflects the study group in a prospective investigative design?

	Disease Present (D+)	Disease Absent (D−)	Totals
Exposed (E+)	a	b	$a + b$
Nonexposed (E−)	c	d	$c + d$
Totals	$a + c$	$b + d$	

(A) $a + c$
(B) $b + d$
(C) $c + b$
(D) $a + b$
(E) $c + d$

20. The most feared complication of benign intracranial hypertension (pseudotumor cerebri) is

(A) visual loss
(B) sixth nerve palsy
(C) herniation syndrome
(D) migraine headache

21. Which feature is most useful in differentiating false labor from true labor?

(A) Character of pain
(B) Progressive descent of fetus to birth canal
(C) Uterine contractions
(D) Bloody show
(E) Effacement and cervical dilation

22. A 65-year-old man presents to the emergency room with sudden onset of left retroperitoneal pain. Physical examination reveals hypotension and a pulsatile mass in the abdomen. The pathogenesis of this patient's disease is most closely related to

(A) hypertension
(B) atherosclerosis
(C) elastic tissue fragmentation
(D) immune complex–mediated inflammation
(E) vasculitis secondary to syphilis

23. A heterozygote with neurofibromatosis marries a normal person. What is the possibility that they will have a child with neurofibromatosis?

(A) 0%
(B) 25%
(C) 50%
(D) 75%
(E) 100%

24. Which of the statements about the epidemiology of schizophrenia is most accurate?

(A) The risk is higher in families with certain patterns of interpersonal communication
(B) The risk of developing schizophrenia varies with the season of birth
(C) The concordance rate in identical twins approaches 100%
(D) The course is almost always characterized by progressive deterioration
(E) The lifetime incidence is between 0.1% and 0.5%

25. A 52-year-old woman with type II diabetes mellitus presents with altered mental status to the emergency room. She is taking 250 mg of chlorpropamide daily. Physical examination is unremarkable. Her skin turgor is normal. Laboratory studies indicate the following values: serum sodium concentration of 120 mEq/L (normal is 135–147 mEq/L), serum potassium concentration of 3.2 mEq/L (normal is 3.5–5.0 mEq/L), serum chloride concentration of 90 mEq/L (normal is 95–105 mEq/L), serum bicarbonate concentration of 21 mEq/L (normal is 22–28 mEq/L), serum glucose concentration of 140 mg/dl (normal is 70–110 mg/dl), and serum blood urea nitrogen (BUN) concentration of 5 mg/dl (normal is 7–18 mg/dl). Random urine sodium level is 80 mEq/L (normally > 20 mEq/L indicates increased loss, < 20 mEq/L indicates increased reabsorption). In the management of this patient, the physician would

(A) restrict both water and sodium from her diet
(B) restrict only sodium from her diet
(C) restrict only water from her diet
(D) add sodium to her diet
(E) increase her water intake

26. A 66-year-old woman with ascites presents with left-sided pleural effusion containing clumps of malignant cells with glandular configuration. Her Pap smear is atrophic. The most likely diagnosis in this patient is

(A) metastatic endometrial carcinoma
(B) advanced cervical malignancy
(C) ovarian carcinoma
(D) metastatic uterine leiomyosarcoma
(E) Krukenberg's tumor

27. A 65-year-old man with known diverticulosis presents with fever and severe, diffuse abdominal pain. Abdominal examination reveals generalized rebound tenderness, absent bowel sounds, and guarding. The pathogenesis of this patient's findings relates to

(A) perforation
(B) obstruction
(C) intra-abdominal bleeding
(D) ischemic bowel disease

28. Two carriers for cystic fibrosis marry. What is the chance that they will have a child with cystic fibrosis?

(A) 0%
(B) 25%
(C) 50%
(D) 75%
(E) 100%

29. Which characteristic most accurately describes somatization disorder?

(A) Lack of association with drug abuse
(B) No real association with neuromotor and sexual dysfunction
(C) Frequent presentation in the fifth decade
(D) Greater occurrence in men
(E) Association with family histories of alcoholism and antisocial behavior

30. A 65-year-old man presents with complaints of heartburn, belching, and epigastric pain, which is aggravated when drinking coffee or eating fatty foods. Physical examination is unremarkable. Endoscopy shows erosive ulceration at the gastroesophageal junction. The primary mechanism for this patient's complaint is

(A) decreased acid production in the stomach

(B) increased gastric emptying

(C) increased esophageal peristalsis

(D) inappropriate relaxation of the lower esophageal sphincter (LES)

31. The measurement corresponding to the obstetric conjugate is the distance from the middle of the sacral promontory to the

(A) superior surface of the pubis

(B) ischial tuberosity

(C) inferior surface of the pubis

(D) ischial spines

(E) closest point of the pubis

32. If the data set is 2,5,7,8,8, which option gives the correct mean, median, and mode in the correct order?

(A) 7,8,6

(B) 8,7,5

(C) 7,6,8

(D) 5,7,8

(E) 6,7,8

33. A 75-year-old woman has massive lower gastrointestinal bleeding requiring blood transfusion. Which of the following sets of diseases would be the most likely causes of the bleeding?

(A) Colon cancer, volvulus

(B) Intussusception, ischemic bowel disease

(C) Diverticulosis, angiodysplasia

(D) Meckel's diverticulum, solitary rectal cancer

(E) Ulcerative colitis, anal fissure

34. The complaint of a 30-year-old patient is the sudden onset of a severe headache so intense that she had lost consciousness. She has a moderate diffuse headache, sensitivity to light, and a stiff neck. A noncontrasted head computed tomography (CT) scan is read by the emergency room physician as "probably normal for age." The next step should be

(A) admission to the hospital with hourly neurologic checks

(B) narcotics for pain

(C) spinal tap

(D) intravenous antibiotics (ceftriaxone)

(E) electroencephalography (EEG)

35. What is body dysmorphia?

(A) A somatic delusional syndrome

(B) An effect of hallucinogen intoxication

(C) A "depressive equivalent"

(D) A characteristic set of behaviors resulting from abnormalities in physical appearance

(E) A preoccupation with an imagined (or minor) defect in appearance

36. A patient with the last name Smith, who is O negative, is transfused with a unit of A-positive blood ordered for a different person, whose last name is also Smith. The patient develops fever, hypotension, chills, and severe backache. Blood is noted to ooze out of multiple venipuncture sites as well. The next step in the management of this patient is to

(A) administer isotonic saline to maintain adequate tissue perfusion
(B) stop infusing the unit of blood
(C) give an intravenous dose of a loop diuretic
(D) administer antipyretics
(E) give an intravenous dose of mannitol to begin osmotic diuresis

37. Which of the following modalities for treating hepatic encephalopathy is most effective in reducing serum ammonia levels?

(A) Lactulose
(B) Antibiotic sterilization of the bowel
(C) Reduced protein intake
(D) Loop diuretic

38. Which statement about alcohol dependence is most accurate?

(A) Sons of alcoholic fathers at risk for alcoholism seem to have a greater tolerance for the neuromotor effects of alcohol
(B) Socially appropriate drinking is a more practical goal of treatment than is total abstinence
(C) There do not appear to be subtypes of alcohol dependence
(D) The highest prevalence of alcohol abuse occurs in the fourth decade
(E) The risk for alcohol dependence is about equal in all ethnic backgrounds when economic variables are controlled

39. Which laboratory parameter maintains its normal reference range in both pregnant and non-pregnant states?

(A) Creatinine clearance
(B) Blood urea nitrogen (BUN)
(C) Hemoglobin
(D) Serum glutamic oxaloacetic transaminase (SGOT)
(E) Alkaline phosphatase (ALP)

40. What is the incidence of sickle cell disease in the population if the carrier rate for sickle cell trait is 1/12?

(A) 1/144
(B) 1/288
(C) 1/576
(D) 1/1936
(E) 1/3600

41. A 66-year-old man develops a fever 6 days following biliary tract surgery. This is most likely due to

(A) resorption of blood from the peritoneum
(B) endotoxic shock
(C) atelectasis
(D) a wound infection

42. A 25-year-old woman who is 13 weeks pregnant with her first child presents with vaginal bleeding, a blood pressure of 160/95, 3+ proteinuria, and a fundus measurable at the umbilicus. Which diagnosis is most likely to explain these findings?

(A) Gestational diabetes
(B) Twin pregnancy
(C) Fetal anencephaly
(D) Inevitable abortion
(E) Molar pregnancy

43. Which statement about cocaine dependence is true?

(A) Concurrent alcohol abuse is rare

(B) It is often associated with opiate abuse

(C) Its overall prevalence is decreasing among high-school students

(D) Cocaine intake is usually continuous over many months

(E) Cocaine abuse is uncommon in patients with preexisting schizophrenia

44. A 30-year-old, female nonsmoker presents with bilateral puffiness and swelling of the fingers and joint pains. Cold exposure and stress cause episodes of blanching or cyanosis of the fingers. She is not on any medications. The mechanism for this patient's disease is most likely the result of

(A) vasospasm and thickening of the digital arteries

(B) hyperviscosity due to an increase in immunoglobulin M (IgM) antibodies

(C) an immune complex vasculitis

(D) thrombosis of the digital vessels

45. A laboratory test has a reference mean value of 20 mg/dl and a standard deviation of 2. The range in which 95% of repeated laboratory determinations would be expected to fall is

(A) 20 to 22

(B) 18 to 22

(C) 16 to 24

(D) 14 to 26

(E) 19 to 21

46. A 48-year-old woman requiring systemic total parenteral nutrition has sudden onset of dyspnea following insertion of a central venous catheter into the subclavian vein. This is most likely caused by

(A) air embolism

(B) pneumonia

(C) ipsilateral pneumothorax

(D) a cardiac arrhythmia

47. A patient with a long-standing history of epilepsy sees the physician in the office after he has his first seizure in 3 years. His phenytoin level is 11 mg/dl (therapeutic range 10–20 mg/dl), and he is compliant with his regimen of 300 mg/day. What is the best therapeutic maneuver?

(A) Repeat an electroencephalogram (EEG)

(B) Raise the phenytoin dosage

(C) Add phenobarbital

(D) Substitute carbamazepine

(E) Perform an imaging study (computed tomography [CT] or magnetic resonance imaging [MRI]) to rule out tumor

48. Which statement about intrapartum electronic fetal monitoring is true?

(A) A normal fetal heart rate tracing ensures a healthy, normal newborn

(B) A normal fetal baseline heart rate can vary from 120 to 170 beats/min

(C) Variable decelerations most commonly indicate placental insufficiency

(D) Normal Apgar score and cord pH value frequently occur with abnormal patterns

(E) Early decelerations require prompt intervention

49. Which congenital disease includes saber shins, rhagades, snuffles, pneumonia alba, and hepar lobatum?

(A) Cytomegalovirus (CMV) infection
(B) Rubella
(C) Toxoplasmosis
(D) Syphilis
(E) Herpes infection

50. A 25-year-old recently married woman has a blood pressure of 145/95 after multiple readings on two separate visits. She is a one-pack/day smoker. There is no family history of hypertension. Physical examination is unremarkable. She is using triphasic oral contraception. The most likely diagnosis of this woman's hypertension is

(A) essential hypertension
(B) Turner's syndrome
(C) renal artery fibromuscular hyperplasia
(D) pheochromocytoma
(E) iatrogenic etiology

51. Which statement about opiate dependence is true?

(A) It is a fairly common sequel to opiate use for acute pain management
(B) It usually lasts for less than a decade
(C) Deviant social behavior is rare in addicts with ready access to opiates
(D) It commonly induces an organic delusional syndrome
(E) Addicted individuals tend to be isolated and lonely

52. Digoxin, an inotropic agent with a low therapeutic index, is frequently monitored in patients by measurements of drug levels in the plasma. The usual therapeutic plasma concentration range is 0.5 to 2 ng/ml. However, drug measurements are not advised during the first 6 hours following any dose because digoxin exhibits

(A) an elimination half-life greater than 6 days
(B) a low volume of distribution
(C) high plasma protein binding
(D) a slow rate of distribution
(E) extensive first-pass metabolism

53. A 75-year-old woman presents with colicky midabdominal pain, with nausea and vomiting. An abdominal x-ray shows distention of the small bowel, a radiopaque mass in the distal small bowel, and air in the biliary tree. The patient most likely has

(A) acute pancreatitis
(B) gallstone ileus
(C) acute appendicitis
(D) acute pylephlebitis
(E) a small bowel infarction

54. The condition that can cause a low maternal serum alpha-fetoprotein (MSAFP) level is

(A) spina bifida
(B) anencephaly
(C) Turner's syndrome
(D) Down syndrome
(E) omphalocele

55. Using the following code (IRE = incidence rate among exposed; IRN = incidence rate among nonexposed), which formula is used to calculate attributable risk?

(A) IRE + IRN
(B) IRE − IRN
(C) IRN − IRE
(D) IRN + IRE

56. A 35-year-old fireman with second-degree burns involving 15% of his body surface and third-degree burns involving 20% of his body surface develops fever. Biopsy of one of the wound sites and culture would most likely reveal which of the following organisms?

(A) *Staphylococcus aureus*
(B) *Pseudomonas aeruginosa*
(C) *Candida albicans*
(D) Group A streptococcus

57. Headache associated with a brain tumor is most common in which clinical setting?

(A) Upon awakening in the morning
(B) After eating breakfast
(C) After eating lunch
(D) After eating dinner

58. A 3-year-old child presents with a 3-day history of fever, conjunctivitis, swelling and peeling of the hands and feet, and cervical adenopathy. Laboratory findings include an absolute neutrophilic leukocytosis and left shift, thrombocytosis, and an elevated erythrocyte sedimentation rate. The most likely diagnosis is

(A) Still's disease
(B) scarlet fever
(C) acute rheumatic fever
(D) periarteritis nodosa
(E) Kawasaki disease

59. Autism is strongly associated with a history of

(A) emotionally unavailable parents
(B) childhood sexual abuse
(C) intrauterine rubella
(D) maternal cocaine abuse
(E) early childhood lead exposure

60. A 55-year-old woman presents with a breast mass in the left upper outer quadrant that is movable and nontender on palpation. A needle aspiration of the mass is negative for cyst fluid. The next step in the management of this patient is to

(A) perform a fine-needle aspiration of the mass with cytologic evaluation
(B) repeat the needle aspiration in 6 months
(C) schedule the patient for a modified radical mastectomy
(D) order a mammogram to define whether the mass is malignant or benign

61. In spite of taking sublingual nitroglycerin, a patient has frequent attacks of angina. Some of these attacks begin while he is asleep and others when he is exercising. The logical approach to prophylactic therapy in this patient is

(A) transdermal nitroglycerin patch changed to a fresh one every 24 hours
(B) nifedipine chronically with sublingual nitroglycerin as needed for attacks
(C) propranolol chronically with sublingual nitroglycerin as needed for attacks
(D) transdermal and sublingual nitroglycerin as needed for attacks
(E) propranolol chronically and oral verapamil as needed for acute attacks

62. Which congenital anomaly is the most common?

(A) Spina bifida occulta
(B) Hypospadias
(C) Phocomelia
(D) Cleft palate
(E) Club feet

63. A 22-year-old Asian woman presents for a routine physical examination and a cervical Pap smear. Her menstrual history and physical examination are unremarkable. A stool guaiac is negative. A hemogram shows a hemoglobin of 11 g/dl (normal is 12–16 g/dl), a red blood cell (RBC) count of 5.8 million cells/μl (normal is 3.5–5.5 million cells/μl), a mean corpuscular volume (MCV) of 70 μm³ (normal is 80–100 μm³), a normal RBC distribution width (RDW—10 +/– 5), and normal leukocyte and platelet counts. The mild anemia in this patient is most likely related to

(A) absent iron stores in the bone marrow
(B) iron blockade in the macrophages
(C) hemolysis of RBCs in the spleen
(D) decreased globin chain synthesis
(E) decreased heme synthesis

64. Childhood sexual abuse has been most often reported by patients with

(A) multiple personality disorder
(B) hypochondriasis
(C) major depression
(D) antisocial personality disorder
(E) autism

65. The difference in mean diastolic blood pressure among 150 subjects in a low-salt diet group and 150 subjects in a no-added-salt group is 10 mm Hg, a difference significant at a P value of less than 0.05. Which statement about the two groups is true?

(A) The blood pressure difference is clinically significant
(B) The chance that an individual would benefit from a low-salt diet is less than 0.05
(C) If the low-salt diet is effective in lowering blood pressure, the probability of the reported finding is less than 0.05
(D) If the low-salt diet is ineffective in lowering blood pressure, the probability of the reported finding is less than 0.05
(E) Increasing the number of subjects would tend to change the P value from significant to nonsignificant

66. A 62-year-old woman with a history of diabetes and hypertension presents to the emergency room with the right eye deviated outward and an obvious ptosis. The pupils are normal size. She has a slight headache. The most likely diagnosis is

(A) cavernous sinus thrombosis
(B) superior oblique palsy
(C) posterior cerebral artery aneurysm with third nerve impingement
(D) vasculopathic (noncompressive) third nerve palsy
(E) intranuclear ophthalmoplegia

67. A 23-year-old sexually active woman presents with fever, pain, and effusion in her left knee, as well as scattered erythematous papular lesions on the fingers, toes, and extremities. The most likely diagnosis is

(A) secondary syphilis
(B) disseminated lymphogranuloma venereum
(C) disseminated gonococcemia
(D) Reiter's syndrome
(E) hepatitis B serum sickness

68. The chromosome defect associated with autism is

(A) fragile X syndrome
(B) cri du chat syndrome (deletion of short arm of 5)
(C) Turner's syndrome (XO)
(D) Klinefelter's syndrome (XXY)
(E) trisomy 21

69. Which characteristic primarily determines the prognosis in patients with tetralogy of Fallot?

(A) Degree of pulmonic stenosis
(B) Overriding aorta
(C) Level of hypoxemia at birth
(D) Size of the ventricular septal defect
(E) Degree of right ventricular hypertrophy

70. Bloody nipple discharge in a 35-year-old woman without a palpable breast mass is most likely caused by

(A) intraductal papillomatosis
(B) a breast abscess
(C) an intraductal papilloma
(D) an infiltrating ductal carcinoma
(E) fibrocystic change

71. A 23-year-old woman with prolonged premature rupture of the membranes at 30 weeks' gestation undergoes a cesarean section for breech presentation. She develops lower abdominal pain and spiking fevers on the third postoperative day. She is placed on broad-spectrum intravenous aerobic and anaerobic antibiotic coverage for 72 hours, but her fever does not respond. The patient is placed on intravenous heparin, with resolution of the fever within 48 hours. The most likely diagnosis is

(A) tubo-ovarian abscess
(B) septic pelvic thrombophlebitis
(C) retained placenta
(D) acute endometritis
(E) acute pyelonephritis

Questions 72–73

A 12-year-old boy has a 5-year history of episodes of severe bronchospasm that have resulted in repeated hospitalizations. He has been using an inhaler by day and long-acting theophylline at night. He comes to the emergency room with severe respiratory distress, cyanosis, and tachycardia. The examination is consistent with severe bronchoconstriction and shows no other complicating factors.

72. Which statement about treatment is accurate?

(A) A β-adrenoceptor agonist is likely to exacerbate his symptoms
(B) Parenteral corticosteroids should not be given until the bronchospasm is relieved
(C) The present problem is due to excessive use of the inhaler
(D) Cromolyn by aerosol should be given until the bronchospasm is relieved
(E) Prophylactic corticosteroid therapy after recovery from this episode should be considered

73. Which statement about the drugs discussed in the previous question is correct?

(A) The β_2-agonist drugs now used in asthma have no cardiac actions
(B) Cromolyn blocks the airway smooth muscle contraction that occurs in response to vagal stimulation
(C) The use of glucocorticoids by aerosol appears to be as effective as oral prednisone in prophylaxis
(D) Tolerance develops in terms of the bronchodilating actions of methylxanthines
(E) Chronic use of inhaled glucocorticoids increases bronchial reactivity

74. A mother says that her teenage daughter has developed peculiar eating habits. She has been secretly inducing vomiting as a form of weight control. The daughter will not confirm this behavior. Which physical findings best support the mother's contention?

(A) Erosion of tooth enamel and abraded fingers
(B) Pharyngeal discharge and cheilosis
(C) Superficial wrist lacerations
(D) Esophageal tears and bruises
(E) Hoarseness

75. A 24-year-old woman presents with acute onset of localized areas of erythema and vesicle formation where she has pierced ears. She states that these findings correlate with the purchase of new earrings that she has been wearing for the last 2 days. The mechanism responsible for this reaction most closely resembles

(A) an urticarial reaction associated with type I hypersensitivity
(B) a localized Arthus reaction
(C) a positive purified protein derivative (PPD) skin reaction
(D) antibody-dependent cytotoxicity
(E) an immune complex reaction

76. A 31-year-old woman is 6 days post emergency cesarean for active phase arrest. She has persistent fever to 103° F despite 72 hours of appropriate antibiotic therapy covering both aerobes and anaerobes. She has normal lochial flow. The next step in management is to rule out the diagnosis of

(A) septic pelvic thrombophlebitis
(B) acute pelvic inflammatory disease (PID)
(C) retained placenta
(D) blood in the peritoneal cavity
(E) pelvic abscess

77. Laboratory parameters to change first after acute hemorrhage include

(A) arterial pH, P_{O_2}, and P_{CO_2}
(B) hemoglobin and hematocrit
(C) central venous pressure
(D) oxygen saturation

78. Which histologic finding is most characteristic of the endometrium of a 13-year-old girl whose menarche began 1 year ago and who has been bleeding irregularly for the past 3 months?

(A) Serrated endometrial glands with inspissated secretions *ovulation*
(B) Tubular endometrial glands with many mitoses *proliferative*
(C) Back-to-back endometrial glands with prominent nuclei *CA*
(D) Decidual reaction forming around endometrial arterioles *Pregnancy*
(E) Hyperchromatism and loss of cellular polarity *CA*

79. In recent literature, family dynamics during childhood are often given a causal role in

(A) autism
(B) panic disorder
(C) bipolar disorder type II
(D) melancholic depression
(E) anorexia nervosa

80. Differential cyanosis is a feature of which congenital heart disease?

(A) Ventricular septal defect
(B) Infantile coarctation of the aorta
(C) Patent ductus arteriosus with coarctation
(D) Corrected transposition of the great vessels
(E) Atrial septal defect

81. A 27-year-old woman in the thirty-second week of pregnancy with her first child presents with a blood pressure of 160/110, 3+ proteinuria, confusion, and retinal hemorrhages. Which medication would be indicated in the treatment of this patient?

(A) Ritodrine
(B) Magnesium sulfate
(C) Terbutaline
(D) Progesterone
(E) Indomethacin

82. A patient presents with increased anxiety and depression following a recent marital separation. This situation is an adjustment disorder if

(A) the patient has a history of difficulty in adjusting to new situations and is often anxious and depressed
(B) the patient has a pattern of anxiolytic medication abuse
(C) the patient's reaction is not part of a pattern of overreaction to stress
(D) the patient and spouse are engaged in a symbiotic relationship
(E) the stressor is beyond the range of normal human experience

83. A 55-year-old alcoholic with chronic pancreatitis and steatorrhea is best treated by

(A) total pancreatectomy
(B) broad-spectrum antibiotic therapy
(C) a gluten-free diet
(D) oral pancreatic enzymes before, during, and after meals

84. A 68-year-old woman with congestive heart failure and normal blood pressure has been taking captopril and hydrochlorothiazide for 5 years. Which statement is accurate?

(A) Although this regimen may be effective, it is much more hazardous than other methods used in heart failure

(B) Captopril is used in heart failure because it acts on the heart to increase cardiac force and reduce heart size

(C) In heart failure, thiazide doses should be lower than would be required for maximal diuresis because maximal cardiac benefits occur at lower doses

(D) Digoxin could not be added to this regimen because captopril sensitizes the system to digitalis toxicity

(E) This regimen can reduce both preload and afterload and has been shown to increase the life span of patients with congestive heart failure

85. Below is shown the antigenic makeup of a woman, man, and their child.

Mother	Child	Father
XXXX	XXOO	OOOO

Which graft combination will be accepted by the recipient?

	Graft donor	**Graft recipient**
(A)	Mother	Child
(B)	Mother	Father
(C)	Father	Mother
(D)	Child	Mother
(E)	Child	Father

86. Twin gestation increases a woman's risk for

(A) urinary tract infection
(B) pregnancy-induced hypertension
(C) gestational diabetes
(D) low maternal serum alpha-fetoprotein (MSAFP)
(E) vaginal moniliasis

87. Which spinal fluid profile fits an otherwise healthy patient with aseptic (viral) meningitis?

(A) Glucose 50, protein 85, white blood cells (WBCs) 22 (95% lymphocytes)
(B) Glucose 15, protein 115, WBCs 4200 (99% polys)
(C) Glucose 68, protein 40, WBCs 2 (100% lymphocytes)
(D) Glucose 22, protein 100, WBCs 55 (85% lymphocytes)
(E) Glucose 68, protein 10, WBCs 0

88. A 42-year-old woman describes continual and, in her opinion, irrational worry that she has been contaminated with industrial chemicals in her workplace. She says that she is showering longer and longer every night to remove these chemicals. Which neurotransmitter system is implicated in such symptoms?

(A) Acetylcholine
(B) γ-Aminobutyric acid (GABA)
(C) Serotonin
(D) Dopamine
(E) Norepinephrine

89. Third-space fluid loss is most commonly associated with

(A) bacterial peritonitis
(B) severe vomiting
(C) severe diarrhea
(D) acute appendicitis
(E) acute cholecystitis

90. A 65-year-old woman has a protrusion from her anterior vagina. She has a long history of urinary stress incontinence. The most likely diagnosis is

(A) cystocele
(B) urethral diverticulum
(C) embryonal rhabdomyosarcoma
(D) rectocele
(E) enterocele

91. An 8-month-old infant presents with fever, runny nose, cough, nasal flaring, and hyperexpansion of the chest. Expiratory wheezes are present. The most likely diagnosis is

(A) croup
(B) bronchiolitis
(C) asthma
(D) acute epiglottitis
(E) cystic fibrosis

92. An 8-year-old boy becomes terrified whenever his parents leave the house. He also avoids going to school in order to remain with his mother. Which anxiety disorder is a sequel to these symptoms?

(A) Obsessive-compulsive personality disorder
(B) Somatoform pain disorder
(C) Dysthymia
(D) Panic disorder
(E) Schizophrenia

93. The percentage of all health care costs incurred by the elderly in the United States is

(A) 30%
(B) 40%
(C) 50%
(D) 60%
(E) 70%

94. A 23-year-old married woman comes to the office after recent exposure to a person with active hepatitis A. She has a long history of recurrent sinopulmonary infections and bronchial asthma. In addition, after her last pregnancy she received a blood transfusion for severe postpartum hemorrhage. After receiving an intramuscular dose of immune serum globulin as prophylaxis against hepatitis A, she develops an anaphylactic reaction. This patient most likely has

(A) a hemolytic transfusion reaction
(B) immunoglobulin A (IgA) deficiency with anti-IgA antibodies
(C) contaminated immune serum globulin
(D) a type IV hypersensitivity reaction against a protein in the immune serum globulin

95. Which technique is the most specific for assessing fetal lung maturity?

(A) Lecithin/sphingomyelin ratio greater than 2
(B) Presence of vernix in amniotic fluid
(C) Ossification of distal femoral epiphyses
(D) Ferning pattern on a glass slide
(E) Increased amniotic fluid creatinine

96. Compression of a mass on the anterior thigh of a 45-year-old man with high-output cardiac failure results in slowing of the pulse rate. A continuous machinery murmur is heard on auscultation. The origin of this lesion is most closely associated with

(A) penetrating injury
(B) blunt trauma
(C) previous femoral artery bypass
(D) a mycotic aneurysm
(E) a congenital malformation

97. A child with cystic fibrosis has pneumonia secondary to *Staphylococcus aureus*. The child suddenly develops increased respiratory distress, decreased breath sounds in the left chest, and tracheal deviation to the right. The child most likely has

(A) empyema
(B) a pleural effusion
(C) a ruptured tension pneumatocyst
(D) adult respiratory distress syndrome
(E) a pulmonary infarction

98. The presumptive sign of pregnancy is

(A) mapping of fetal outline by palpation
(B) ballottement of the fetus
(C) softening of uterine isthmus
(D) palpation of uterine contractions
(E) purplish red vaginal mucosa (Chadwick's sign)

99. The leading cause of death in men 25 to 44 years old in the United States is

(A) accidents
(B) suicide
(C) homicide
(D) acquired immune deficiency syndrome (AIDS)
(E) cancer

100. A 23-year-old college student goes to Mexico on his spring break. Two days into the vacation he develops low-grade fever associated with nausea, vomiting, diarrhea with mucus and blood, and abdominal cramps. The mechanism most likely responsible for this patient's diarrhea is

(A) enterotoxin stimulation of cyclic adenosine monophosphate (cAMP)
(B) invasion of the bowel wall by a bacteria
(C) enterotoxic damage to the bowel mucosa
(D) acquired disaccharidase deficiency combined with the osmotic effect of undigested carbohydrates

101. Seizures occur during withdrawal from

(A) heroin
(B) benzodiazepines
(C) cocaine
(D) LSD
(E) marijuana

102. The patient is a 10-year-old boy whose school performance has decreased over 2 months. He has a headache, gait ataxia, and double vision, all progressing with time. The immediate test of choice is

(A) computed tomography (CT) scan of the brain
(B) electroencephalogram (EEG)
(C) urine drug screen
(D) urine for amino acid screen
(E) magnetic resonance imaging (MRI)

103. A 26-year-old woman presents with increased facial hair, a deep voice, and clitoromegaly on physical examination. A mass is palpated in the left ovary. She most likely has a

(A) granulosa-theca cell tumor
(B) Brenner's tumor
(C) Sertoli-Leydig cell tumor
(D) fibroma
(E) dysgerminoma

104. Measles-mumps-rubella (MMR) vaccine is first administered at which age?

(A) 2 Months
(B) 4 Months
(C) 6 Months
(D) 12 Months
(E) 15 Months

105. A solitary nodule in the thyroid is expected to have the greatest chance of being malignant if it is

(A) a cold nodule on an iodine 131 (^{131}I) scan in a woman
(B) cystic on fine-needle aspiration
(C) in a patient with previous irradiation of the neck
(D) associated with hyperthyroidism
(E) in a patient with Hashimoto's thyroiditis

106. A 25-year-old man is very upset with his coworkers and describes fantasies of driving to work and "beating them up." The most ominous sign that he may take action is

(A) a lack of anxiety
(B) the presence of temporal lobe epilepsy
(C) a history of violence
(D) the presence of persecutory delusions
(E) a history of alcohol abuse

107. A 20-year-old college student who is not sexually active states that she has not had a period for the last 5 months. Her menarche was at 12 years of age. She feels that she is at least 25 pounds overweight. She is 5′ 6″ and weighs 102 pounds. She has normal secondary sex characteristics, and the pelvic examination is normal. Serum prolactin, estradiol, and human chorionic gonadotropin (hCG) studies are normal. The most likely diagnosis is

(A) Turner's syndrome
(B) hypogonadotropic hypogonadism
(C) polycystic ovary disease
(D) Asherman's syndrome
(E) anorexia nervosa

108. The leading causes of death in the United States across age-groups in descending order are

(A) cancer, heart disease, stroke
(B) heart disease, cancer, stroke
(C) acquired immune deficiency syndrome (AIDS), heart disease, cancer
(D) heart disease, AIDS, cancer
(E) cancer, stroke, heart disease

109. Which nutritional supplement is recommended in a normal pregnancy in the United States?

(A) Folate and vitamin C
(B) Vitamin C and D
(C) B complex and folate
(D) Iron and folate
(E) Vitamin B_{12} and folate

110. A 48-year-old woman with a parathyroid adenoma and a pheochromocytoma has a mass in the thyroid gland. The best screening test for this thyroid mass is

(A) an iodine 131 (^{131}I) scan
(B) measurement of the serum thyroid-stimulating hormone level (TSH)
(C) measurement of the serum thyroxine (T_4) level
(D) serum calcitonin screening

111. Which disorder is the most common cause of neonatal hypoglycemia in premature infants or in those who are small for gestational age?

(A) Leucine sensitivity
(B) Nesidioblastosis
(C) Inadequate fat and glycogen stores
(D) Immature pituitary–hypothalamic axis
(E) Mother with diabetes

112. Both delirium and chronic undifferentiated schizophrenia are associated with

(A) gross cognitive impairment
(B) elaborate delusions
(C) a prolonged clinical course
(D) hallucinations
(E) severe memory problems

113. The highest percentage of deaths in adolescents results from

(A) suicide
(B) homicide
(C) drug overdose
(D) automobile accidents
(E) cancer

114. Which condition would be expected to show decreased cardiac output?

(A) Early endotoxic shock
(B) Severe anemia
(C) Aortic regurgitation
(D) Hypertrophic cardiomyopathy
(E) Thyrotoxicosis

115. Dementia is distinguished from delirium by

(A) memory impairment
(B) poor prognosis
(C) presence of structural central nervous system (CNS) disease
(D) prolonged clinical course
(E) cognitive impairment

116. A 19-year-old sexually active woman presents with a desquamating rash involving her palms and soles, diarrhea, fever, hypotension, headache, myalgias, and red eyes. Her last menstrual period was 4 days ago. The most likely diagnosis is

(A) viral influenza
(B) Rocky Mountain spotted fever
(C) Kawasaki's disease
(D) scarlet fever
(E) toxic shock syndrome (TSS)

117. An example of a delusion of reference would be

(A) a belief that others are monitoring the person's thoughts through listening devices in the walls
(B) formication
(C) a belief that one has a special mission to save the world
(D) the feeling that a voice is singing in the wind
(E) a belief that a street address is a secret message describing the end of the universe

118. Newborns of mothers with systemic lupus erythematosus (SLE) have an increased risk for which disorder?

(A) Complete heart block
(B) Coarctation of the aorta
(C) Open neural tube defects
(D) Microcephaly
(E) Polycystic kidney disease

119. The most common malignancy of the female genital tract is

(A) vulvar squamous carcinoma
(B) vaginal squamous carcinoma
(C) cervical squamous carcinoma
(D) endometrial adenocarcinoma
(E) ovarian carcinoma

120. A homeless 30-year-old man dressed in tattered clothes is brought into the emergency room by police after he was found haranguing passersby. Which additional finding is most suggestive of psychosis?

(A) Hyper-religiosity and ascetic living habits
(B) Rumination about the meaninglessness of material things
(C) A belief that his thoughts are controlled via secret television messages
(D) Disorientation to time and place
(E) An unfounded suspicion that others are plotting against the government

121. Which fetal anomaly is associated with parvovirus infection in the mother?

(A) Chorioretinitis
(B) Hydrops fetalis
(C) Rhagades
(D) Microcephaly
(E) Hutchinson's teeth

122. A 58-year-old woman presents with a rapidly enlarging, painful breast mass. The overlying skin exhibits edema, warmth, and erythema. There is nonpainful adenopathy in the ipsilateral axilla. The most likely diagnosis is

(A) breast cancer with plugging of the dermal lymphatics by tumor
(B) Paget's disease of the breast
(C) cystosarcoma phyllodes
(D) erysipelas due to group A streptococci

123. A 22-year-old woman who is pregnant with her second child presents for her first prenatal visit in her eighth week of pregnancy. On pelvic examination, the physician palpates a 5-cm left adnexal mass. A pelvic sonogram shows it to be cystic. Which prognosis is most likely for this adnexal mass?

(A) It is benign and will gradually enlarge
(B) It is benign and will remain the same size
(C) It is benign and will spontaneously regress
(D) It is malignant but will remain encapsulated
(E) It is malignant and will metastasize

124. Flight of ideas describes

(A) the sudden disappearance of thoughts from consciousness
(B) catatonic excitement
(C) illogical thought processes
(D) rapid shifting from one thought to another
(E) increased imaginary abilities

125. Although a 75-year-old patient goes to bed each night at 11 P.M. and wakes up at 7 A.M., he feels sleepy all day. His wife reports that he snores loudly and sleeps fitfully. This patient's condition is most likely to be

(A) narcolepsy
(B) sleep–wake schedule disorder
(C) insomnia
(D) Kleine-Levin syndrome
(E) sleep apnea

126. A 42-year-old woman on ampicillin for acute cystitis presents with sudden onset of fever, oliguria, and a generalized skin rash. Laboratory findings include eosinophilia, moderate proteinuria, and eosinophiluria. The mechanism for this patient's findings is

(A) the development of immune complex glomerulonephritis
(B) a drug-induced hypersensitivity reaction
(C) progression of acute cystitis into acute pyelonephritis
(D) development of endotoxic shock

127. Which diameter of the female pelvis normally has the smallest measurement?

(A) True conjugate
(B) Obstetric conjugate
(C) Bispinous
(D) Diagonal conjugate
(E) Posterior sagittal

128. The most common cause of death in children between 1 and 12 months of age is

(A) an accident
(B) sepsis
(C) sudden infant death syndrome (SIDS)
(D) a congenital defect
(E) acute leukemia

129. The cerebrospinal fluid (CSF) finding most associated with successful suicide is

(A) low levels of serotonin
(B) increased protein
(C) high levels of norepinephrine
(D) low glucose

130. The most common malignancy in children is

(A) Ewing's sarcoma
(B) acute lymphocytic leukemia
(C) Wilms' tumor
(D) neuroblastoma
(E) cerebellar astrocytoma

131. A 52-year-old woman has biopsy evidence of an in-situ lobular carcinoma in the right breast. In managing this patient the physician also should be concerned about

(A) a high incidence of negative estrogen- and progesterone-receptor assays in these tumors
(B) the aggressive natural history of these tumors
(C) the increased likelihood of breast cancer occurring in the contralateral breast
(D) the high incidence of chest wall involvement by this tumor

132. Which pair of antibody tests has the highest combined specificity for diagnosing systemic lupus erythematosus (SLE)?

(A) Anti-SSA (Ro) and semi-Sm (Smith)
(B) Anti-ds (double stranded) DNA and anti-Sm
(C) Anti-SSB (La) and anti-ds DNA
(D) Anticentromere and antiribonucleoprotein
(E) Antimitochondrial and antihistone

133. A term indicating an abnormal fetal attitude is

(A) occipitoposterior position
(B) frank breech presentation
(C) oblique fetal lie
(D) sacrum anterior
(E) brow presentation

134. A girl in second grade shows the intellectual ability of a sixth grader. What is the intelligence quotient (IQ) category of this child?

(A) Low average
(B) Average
(C) High average
(D) Superior
(E) Very superior

135. Which feature is most characteristic of the orgasmic phase of the female sexual response cycle?

(A) Vascular transudation with vaginal lubrication
(B) Proximal vaginal "tenting" and expansion
(C) Reflex clonic levator sling contractions
(D) Erythematous rash over chest and neck
(E) Vascular engorgement of pelvic viscera

136. A 55-year-old man presents to the emergency room with massive hematemesis. Physical examination reveals abdominal distention, shifting dullness on percussion of the abdomen, and spider angiomata over the face and upper chest. An emergency endoscopic examination reveals blood rapidly filling the distal esophagus. The hematemesis is most likely due to

(A) pyloric obstruction
(B) ruptured esophageal varices
(C) a gastric ulcer
(D) esophageal carcinoma

Questions 137–140

A 3-year-old boy with growth retardation has a long history of recurrent pneumonia and chronic diarrhea. His mother states that he has six to eight foul-smelling stools per day. Physical examination reveals a low-grade fever, scattered rhonchi over both lung fields, crepitant rales at the left lung base and dullness on percussion, mild hepatomegaly, and slight pitting edema of the lower legs. Preliminary laboratory data are as follows:

Hemoglobin	7.5 g/dl
WBC count	18,000 cells/mm³, with neutrophilic leukocytosis and 15% bands; occasional hypersegmented neutrophils
Mean corpuscular volume	90 μm³
Red blood cells	Dimorphic population with both microcytic and macrocytic cells
Serum albumin	2.5 g/dl
Serum calcium	7.0 mg/dl
Serum phosphorus	4.0 mg/dl
Serum sodium	138 mEq/L
Serum chloride	112 mEq/L
Serum potassium	3.2 mEq/L
Serum bicarbonate	18 mEq/L
Serum alkaline phosphatase	300 U/L
Serum SGOT	115 U/L
Serum SGPT	125 U/L
Total bilirubin	0.9 mg/dl
Urine pH	5
Urine dipstick protein	Negative
Chest x-ray	Left lower lobe consolidation; generalized osteopenia

137. The most appropriate step in arriving at the primary diagnosis would be to order

(A) a plasma growth hormone assay
(B) a complete skeletal survey
(C) a sweat chloride test
(D) endoscopy of the upper gastrointestinal tract
(E) acute viral serologies

138. Which additional laboratory test would be LEAST indicated at this stage in the patient's workup?

(A) Serum iron, total iron-binding capacity, percent saturation
(B) Serum B$_{12}$ and folate levels
(C) Bone marrow aspiration and biopsy
(D) Quantitative stool for fat
(E) Sputum for Gram stain, culture, and sensitivity

139. The primary disease most likely responsible for this patient's clinical findings is

(A) celiac disease
(B) chronic granulomatous disease (CGD) of childhood
(C) Bruton's agammaglobulinemia
(D) cystic fibrosis
(E) nephrotic syndrome

140. All of the following secondary diagnoses are present in this patient EXCEPT

(A) combined iron and folate deficiency
(B) left lower lobe pneumonia
(C) malabsorption
(D) viral hepatitis
(E) vitamin-D deficiency

141. A 23-year-old woman in her first trimester of pregnancy is diagnosed as having deep venous thrombosis in her right lower extremity. The most appropriate therapy would be

(A) coumarin
(B) heparin
(C) aspirin
(D) dipyridamole
(E) streptokinase

142. A 28-year-old female secretary has the onset of insomnia, irritability, increased psychomotor activity, and impulsivity. This combination suggests

(A) psychosis
(B) antisocial traits
(C) mania
(D) anxiety
(E) depression

143. If convulsions follow after administering a diphtheria–tetanus–pertussis (DTP) vaccine, which procedure is recommended for future immunizations?

(A) Leave out the diphtheria component of the vaccine, and give pertussis and tetanus on the next immunization
(B) Leave out the tetanus component of the vaccine, and give diphtheria and pertussis on the next immunization
(C) Leave out the tetanus and pertussis components of the vaccine, and give diphtheria toxoid alone on the next immunization
(D) Leave out the pertussis component of the vaccine, and give diphtheria–tetanus toxoid on the next immunization
(E) Give DTP again on the next immunization

144. A 65-year-old man dies within 24 hours of a carotid endarterectomy. The most likely cause of death is

(A) an embolic stroke
(B) pulmonary embolism
(C) air embolism
(D) acute myocardial infarction

145. The labor and delivery nurse calls the physician to see a 20-year-old woman because of excessive vaginal bleeding 1 hour after spontaneous vaginal delivery of a 4400-g male infant (her third child). The duration of her labor was 7 hours, and she received oxytocin augmentation for the last 2 hours. The most likely explanation for her postpartum hemorrhage is

(A) retained placental tissue
(B) genital tract trauma
(C) uterine atony
(D) uterine inversion
(E) coagulation disorder

Questions 146–148

A 42-year-old obese woman, who does not smoke, presents with diastolic hypertension and menstrual irregularities. Pertinent findings on physical examination show a full, plethoric-appearing face, increased facial hair, predominantly truncal obesity with purple stria around the abdomen, and scattered ecchymoses over the entire body. Laboratory studies indicate a hemoglobin of 18 g/dl (normal is 12–16 g/dl), a white blood cell (WBC) count of 18,000 cells/μl (4500–11,000 cells/μl are normal), and a normal platelet count. The leukocyte differential shows an absolute neutrophilic leukocytosis and absolute lymphopenia and eosinopenia. The chest x-ray is normal.

146. Which screening test would be most useful in the initial workup of this patient?

(A) Rapid-sequence intravenous pyelography
(B) Plasma cortisol at 8 A.M. and 4 P.M.
(C) Clonidine suppression test
(D) Bone marrow aspiration and biopsy
(E) Low-dose dexamethasone suppression test

147. Which laboratory test result would be expected in this patient?

(A) Normal red blood cell (RBC) mass
(B) Normal 24-hour urine for 17-ketosteroids
(C) Hypoglycemia
(D) Increased 24-hour urine for free cortisol
(E) Normal 24-hour urine for 17-hydroxycorti-
      costeroids

148. The most likely diagnosis is

(A) obesity with cushingoid features
(B) pheochromocytoma
(C) fibromuscular hyperplasia of the renal artery
(D) polycythemia rubra vera
(E) Cushing's syndrome

149. A 25-year-old man being evaluated for social withdrawal states that he has no friends, is not really interested in other people, and does not feel particularly lonely. A mental status examination reveals no peculiar thought processes. The most likely personality diagnosis is

(A) schizotypal personality disorder
(B) paranoid personality disorder
(C) narcissistic personality disorder
(D) avoidant personality disorder
(E) schizoid personality disorder

150. The most accurate way to rule out an individual accused of having raped a woman is

(A) DNA typing of specimens from the victim and alleged rapist
(B) ABO studies of material from the rape victim
(C) polygraph, or lie detector, test
(D) absence of sperm in the victim's vagina
(E) absence of prostatic acid phosphatase in the victim's vagina

151. A 42-year-old patient with peptic ulcer disease associated with a basal acid output of 60 mEq/hr (normal is < 5 mEq/hr) and a serum gastrin level of 1000 pg/ml (normal is < 300 pg/ml) most likely has

(A) Ménétrier's hypertrophic gastritis
(B) a gastric adenocarcinoma
(C) a glucagonoma
(D) a malignant islet cell tumor

152. A 5-month-old nonimmunized child presents with a 2-week history of paroxysmal coughing that usually follows expiration, fever, vomiting, and rhinorrhea. Physical examination reveals bilateral otitis media and conjunctival hemorrhages. Scattered inspiratory rales are present bilaterally. The complete blood count (CBC) shows a white blood cell (WBC) count of 45,000 cells/mm³, 95% of which represent lymphocytes. The most likely diagnosis is

(A) acute lymphoblastic leukemia
(B) infectious lymphocytosis
(C) whooping cough
(D) bronchiolitis
(E) respiratory syncytial viral pneumonitis

153. The benzodiazepine associated with severe withdrawal is

(A) clorazepate
(B) alprazolam
(C) clonazepam
(D) lorazepam
(E) diazepam

154. The gold standard for working up a patient for suspected endometriosis is

(A) history
(B) laparoscopy
(C) pelvic examination
(D) hysterosalpingogram (HSG)
(E) culdocentesis during menses

155. Which of the following pretransplantation tests is most important in preventing a hyperacute rejection of a kidney?

(A) ABO and lymphocyte crossmatch compatibility with the donor
(B) Proper matching of the HLA-A, B, and C loci of the recipient with the donor
(C) Proper matching of the HLA-D loci of the recipient with the donor
(D) Results of testing for the graft-versus-host reaction

156. A 55-year-old stroke patient cannot copy a simple drawing. Which area of the brain is most likely to be affected?

(A) Nondominant frontal lobe
(B) Nondominant temporal lobe
(C) Nondominant parietal lobe
(D) Dominant temporal lobe
(E) Dominant frontal lobe

157. A 4-month old infant is brought to the emergency room with the sudden onset of lethargy, poor feeding, constipation, generalized hypotonia and weakness, and ophthalmoplegia. The child is afebrile. The mother sweetens the milk with honey. The most likely diagnosis is

(A) gray syndrome
(B) hypothyroidism
(C) Werdnig-Hoffmann's disease
(D) infant botulism
(E) hypomagnesemia

DIRECTIONS: Each of the numbered items or incomplete statements in this section is negatively phrased, as indicated by a capitalized word such as NOT, LEAST, or EXCEPT. Select the ONE lettered answer or completion that is BEST in each case.

158. All of the following statements concerning retinopathy of prematurity are correct EXCEPT

(A) it may or may not be associated with increased delivery of oxygen to the lungs
(B) it may be prevented with vitamin E therapy
(C) it usually involves both eyes
(D) greater than 90% of cases spontaneously arrest and show regression of retinal changes
(E) the disease begins at the periphery of the retina and moves centrally

159. A 65-year-old man has moderately severe, drug-resistant diastolic hypertension of 5 years' duration. A renal arteriogram shows narrowing of the left renal artery orifice. Rapid-sequence intravenous pyelography shows delayed filling of the left kidney. Physical examination reveals hypertensive retinopathy, diminished pulses in both lower extremities, and a bruit in the epigastric area. Which finding would NOT be expected?

(A) Hypokalemia and metabolic acidosis
(B) An exaggerated increase in plasma renin activity over the baseline after giving captopril
(C) Increased plasma aldosterone
(D) Increased plasma renin activity from the right renal vein
(E) Severe atherosclerosis of the left renal artery

160. The Arnold-Chiari syndrome includes all of the following deformities EXCEPT

(A) platybasia
(B) communicating hydrocephalus
(C) elongation of the medulla oblongata
(D) meningocele
(E) absence of the cerebellar vermis

161. Which finding is NOT characteristic of hyperemesis gravidarum?

(A) Hypokalemia
(B) Weight loss
(C) Ketonemia
(D) Nausea and vomiting
(E) Metabolic acidosis

162. All of the following statements about schizophrenia are true EXCEPT

(A) genetic predisposition has been established
(B) there is evidence that early use of antipsychotic medication alters the course of the illness
(C) there is a progressive downhill course
(D) there is no clear pattern of predisposing family dynamics
(E) changes in eye-tracking task performance have been regularly noted

163. The following water deprivation test involves three patients with polyuria and a normal control. Their maximal urine osmolality (U_{osm}) and plasma osmolality (P_{osm}) after prolonged water deprivation are recorded in addition to the effect of an intramuscular injection of vasopressin (antidiuretic hormone [ADH]) on U_{osm}.

Patients	Maximal P_{osm} (mmol/kg)	Maximal U_{osm} (mmol/kg)	U_{osm} postvasopressin (mmol/kg)
Control	290	760	780
Patient A	305	160	400
Patient B	310	125	150
Patient C	290	690	710

All of the following statements about these results are true EXCEPT

(A) patient A could be a person who suffered head injury in the past and now presents with polydipsia and polyuria
(B) patient B could be a patient who has primary polydipsia
(C) U_{osm} in patient C shows an appropriate response to administration of vasopressin
(D) U_{osm} in patient B does not respond appropriately after administration of vasopressin

164. All of the following conditions indicate psychosis EXCEPT

(A) referential delusions
(B) severe anxiety
(C) visual hallucinations
(D) loose associations
(E) auditory hallucinations

165. An ultrasound performed on a 31-year-old woman at 25 weeks' gestation reveals a twin gestation with two placentas, two sacs, and same-gender fetuses. Which statement about this pregnancy is NOT true?

(A) Risk of maternal anemia is increased over a single gestation
(B) The embryologic development of the twins must be dizygotic
(C) Umbilical cord entanglement is a rare occurrence
(D) Preterm delivery is a significant possibility
(E) The septum between the two fetuses has four layers

166. All of the following statements about prevalence and predictive value are correct EXCEPT

(A) as the prevalence for a disease decreases, the predictive value (PV) of a positive test result decreases
(B) as the prevalence for a disease increases, the PV of a negative test result increases
(C) prevalence does not affect the sensitivity and the specificity of a test
(D) when the result of a test with 100% specificity is normal, it can be either a true-negative or a false-negative
(E) when the result of a test with 100% sensitivity is normal, it is more likely to be a true-negative rather than a false-negative test result

167. All of the following symptoms are characteristic of a major depressive episode EXCEPT

(A) dysphoria
(B) sleep difficulty
(C) psychomotor agitation or retardation
(D) worry
(E) worsening of symptoms in the evening

168. All of the following syndromes characterized by deafness are associated with the correct abnormality EXCEPT

(A) leopard syndrome—pulmonary stenosis
(B) Pendred's syndrome—hypothyroidism
(C) Usher's syndrome—retinitis pigmentosa
(D) Alport's syndrome—nephrotic syndrome
(E) Waardenburg's syndrome—white forelock

169. All of the following orthopedic disorder–most common age-group relationships are accurate EXCEPT

(A) Osgood-Schlatter disease—girl 6 months to 2 years old
(B) subluxation of the radial head—1 to 4 years old
(C) Legg-Calvé-Perthes disease—boy 3 to 10 years old
(D) slipped capital femoral epiphysis—obese boy 9 to 15 years old
(E) idiopathic scoliosis—girl 10 to 16 years old

170. Tests with very high sensitivity are necessary in all of the following clinical disorders EXCEPT

(A) phenylketonuria
(B) hypothyroidism
(C) pheochromocytoma
(D) multiple sclerosis
(E) venereal disease

171. Which statement about fetal pulmonary maturity is NOT true?

(A) Type II pneumonocytes produce pulmonary surfactant
(B) Surfactant decreases alveolar surface tension
(C) The most important components of surfactant are phospholipids
(D) The most important surfactant phospholipid is lecithin
(E) An immature lecithin/sphingomyelin (L/S) ratio has a low false-negative rate

172. All of the following drug-overdose–therapy relationships are accurate EXCEPT

(A) salicylate poisoning—acetazolamide plus an alkaline urine
(B) iron poisoning—parenteral ethylenediamine-tetraacetic acid (EDTA)
(C) organophosphate poisoning—atropine plus pralidoxime
(D) methanol poisoning—ethanol
(E) acetaminophen poisoning—acetylcysteine

173. The major differences between heparin and warfarin include all of the following EXCEPT

	Variable	Heparin	Warfarin
(A)	molecular size	large	small
(B)	in vitro action	yes	no
(C)	route	injection	oral
(D)	duration	short	long
(E)	antagonist	vitamin K	protamine

174. A 29-year-old woman who is 40 weeks' pregnant is admitted to the labor room. She is 3-cm dilated and is having regular contractions. She dilates to 5 cm over the next 3 hours but has remained without cervical change for the past 2 hours. She had been up the previous night with contractions and asks how long she must continue with her labor. Which action would NOT be part of appropriate management?

(A) Perform a cesarean delivery for cephalopelvic disproportion
(B) Assess the intensity and frequency of her uterine contractions
(C) Rupture membranes and place an intrauterine pressure catheter
(D) Consider administration of intravenous oxytocin
(E) Perform pelvimetry to determine pelvic adequacy

175. Which condition is least likely to be responsible for newborn jaundice in the first 24 hours of life?

(A) Cytomegalovirus (CMV) hepatitis
(B) Neonatal sepsis
(C) ABO incompatibility
(D) Normal premature infant
(E) Rh hemolytic disease of the newborn

176. Resistance to methotrexate (MTX) in tumor cells can involve all of the following EXCEPT

(A) decreased activity of hypoxanthine–guanine phosphoribosyltransferase (HGPRT)
(B) increased expression of the multidrug-resistant (MDR) 1 gene
(C) change in sensitivity of dihydrofolate (DHF) reductase
(D) increases in a cell-surface glycoprotein
(E) increased synthesis of DHF reductase (DHFR)

177. Examples of lysosomal storage diseases include all of the following EXCEPT

(A) Tay-Sachs disease
(B) Gaucher's disease
(C) Niemann-Pick disease
(D) Hurler syndrome
(E) von Gierke's disease

178. Pruritus is likely to be associated with all of the following conditions EXCEPT

(A) carcinoid syndrome
(B) polycythemia rubra vera
(C) primary biliary cirrhosis
(D) atopic dermatitis
(E) uremia

179. Characteristics of galactosemia include all of the following EXCEPT

(A) deficiency of galactose-1-phosphate uridyl-transferase
(B) cataracts due to osmotic damage
(C) aminoaciduria
(D) liver disease
(E) hyperglycemia

180. Features of Klinefelter's syndrome include all of the following EXCEPT

(A) mental retardation
(B) presence of a Barr body
(C) gynecomastia
(D) azoospermia
(E) absent Leydig cells

181. All of the following statements concerning phenylketonuria (PKU) are true EXCEPT

(A) phenylalanine hydroxylase is deficient
(B) children have a musty smell because they have abnormal metabolites of phenylalanine
(C) cord blood should be used to screen for the disease
(D) early institution of phenylalanine-free diets prevents severe mental retardation
(E) mothers with PKU should be on a phenylalanine-free diet before they get pregnant to prevent problems with pregnancy

182. All of the following disease–gold standards for diagnostic relationships are true EXCEPT

(A) primary syphilis—rapid plasma reagin (RPR) or Venereal Disease Research Laboratories (VDRL)
(B) acute myocardial infarction—creatine kinase isoenzymes (CK-MB)
(C) deep venous thrombosis of the legs—venography
(D) cholelithiasis—ultrasound
(E) pulmonary embolus—pulmonary angiography

183. All of the following conditions are associated with a high amniotic-fluid level of alpha-fetoprotein (AFP) EXCEPT

(A) omphalocele
(B) anencephaly
(C) open neural tube defects
(D) Down syndrome
(E) twin gestation

184. A 46-year-old female alcoholic with a long history of chronic pancreatitis presents with weight loss and a 3-month history of frequent, greasy stools. Physical examination shows pitting edema of the lower extremities; mild, tender hepatomegaly; and scattered ecchymoses in areas of trauma. An ultrasound examination of the pancreas shows calcifications. Endoscopic biopsy in multiple locations of the small bowel is normal. The laboratory findings on the patient would be expected to include all of the following EXCEPT

(A) prolonged prothrombin time
(B) increased quantitative stool for fat
(C) abnormal D-xylose test
(D) hypoalbuminemia
(E) hypocalcemia

185. All of the following characteristics of postmature (postterm) infants are correct EXCEPT

(A) birth after 42 weeks' gestation
(B) large for gestational age
(C) absence of lanugo
(D) increased risk for meconium aspiration
(E) lethargic behavior

DIRECTIONS: Each set of matching questions in this section consists of a list of four to twenty-six lettered options (some of which may be in figures) followed by several numbered items. For each numbered item, select the ONE lettered option that is most closely associated with it. To avoid spending too much time on matching sets with large numbers of options, it is generally advisable to begin each set by reading the list of options. Then, for each item in the set, try to generate the correct answer and locate it in the option list, rather than evaluating each option individually. Each lettered option may be selected once, more than once, or not at all.

Questions 186–188

For each disease, select the serum protein electrophoresis pattern that most closely approximates the expected relationship.

186. Patient with sarcoidosis

187. Patient with alcoholic cirrhosis

188. Nonsmoking patient with panacinar emphysema involving the lower lobes

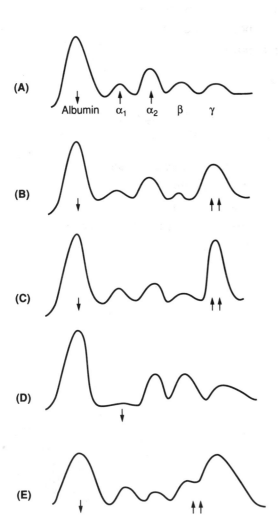

Questions 189–190

Match each drug with the related graph.

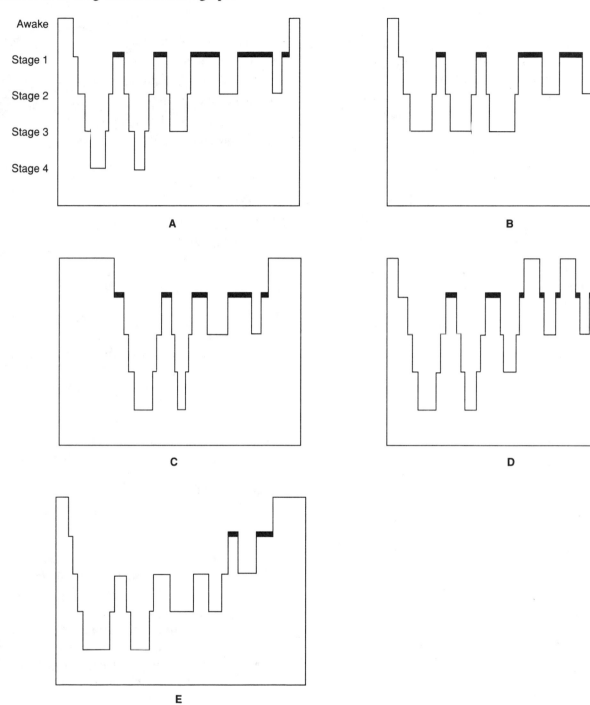

189. Diazepam

190. Benzodiazepine rebound

Questions 191–193

A 26-year-old African–American man presents with fever, chills, low-back pain, dysuria, and urinary frequency. Rectal examination reveals a tender prostate, the prostate massage specimen contains *Escherichia coli* (>100,000/ml), and bladder aspiration also shows many bacteria. The patient has no past history of urinary tract infections; and apart from the present situation, he has no health problems. He mentions that several years earlier he was given penicillin for a "sore throat" and developed a "bad skin rash." While in southeast Asia he had malaria, and one of the drugs given to him caused an acute hemolysis. Subsequently, the laboratory indicates that the *E. coli* is susceptible to gentamicin and tobramycin, most cephalosporins, the fluoroquinolones, and trimethoprim–sulfamethoxazole (TMP–SMZ), but it is penicillinase producing. This condition appears to be acute bacterial prostatitis with accompanying bladder infection. Since the man is otherwise healthy, his problem can be treated on an outpatient basis.

For each of the following descriptions, select the associated drug.

(A) Cefaclor
(B) Ciprofloxacin
(C) Gentamicin
(D) Ampicillin–sulbactam
(E) TMP–SMZ

191. Drug most likely to cause an allergic reaction in this patient

192. Drug most likely to cause hemolysis in this patient

193. Most appropriate drug to use for treatment of this man

Questions 194–195

Match each patient with the associated anxiety disorder.

(A) Acute stress disorder
(B) Agoraphobia
(C) Attention-deficit disorder
(D) Avoidant disorder of childhood
(E) Generalized anxiety disorder
(F) Obsessive–compulsive disorder
(G) Overanxious disorder of childhood
(H) Panic disorder
(I) Posttraumatic stress disorder
(J) Separation anxiety disorder
(K) Social phobia
(L) Specific phobia
(M) Substance-induced anxiety disorder

194. The parents of a 4-year-old boy seek marital therapy because they have grown steadily apart since the birth of their only child. They state that they never do things together anymore. It has been years since they left their child and went out to dinner with friends or took a vacation. They have little romantic life. They tried to leave their son with a baby-sitter several times, but the child became so upset that they cancelled the outing. The child sleeps in their bed every night. Occasionally they have tried putting him in his own bed, but he cries or crawls into their bed later.

195. A 35-year-old single male librarian seeks therapy because he is lonely and unhappy. He describes a solitary life spent cataloging books all day, then remaining alone at night and on weekends. He declines all invitations to dinners or get-togethers because he feels anxious around people. He says that he has tried to meet others but gets so uncomfortable that he goes home quickly.

Questions 196–198

For each of the following descriptions, select the most appropriate drug.

(A) Doxorubicin
(B) Cyclophosphamide
(C) Tamoxifen
(D) Vincristine
(E) Asparaginase

196. Pre- and posthydration are important for preventing hemorrhagic cystitis caused by this drug

197. Measurements of cardiac ejection fraction represent a noninvasive technique for monitoring declines in myocardial function that may occur with use of this drug

198. Used in the treatment of lymphoid malignancies, the major problem with this agent is the high incidence of hypersensitivity reactions

Questions 199–200

Match each patient with the associated defense mechanism.

(A) Blocking
(B) Denial
(C) Displacement
(D) Dissociation
(E) Distortion
(F) Intellectualization
(G) Projection
(H) Rationalization
(I) Reaction formation
(J) Regression
(K) Repression
(L) Sublimation
(M) Undoing

199. A political figure is engaged in a televised debate and comes under increasing pressure from his opponent. As his anxiety mounts, he begins to accuse his opponent of interrupting him, attacks his character, and finally throws down his papers and stalks offstage angrily.

200. An angry man murders his wife and disposes of her body. Initially, he is not a suspect; in fact, he receives much sympathy from others over his wife's disappearance. However, he becomes convinced that others suspect him and are watching him closely in order to gain evidence that will expose him. He even believes that his friends are taking a perverse pleasure in watching his anxiety build.

ANSWER KEY

1-C	31-E	61-B	91-B	121-B
2-B	32-E	62-B	92-D	122-A
3-C	33-C	63-D	93-A	123-C
4-B	34-C	64-A	94-B	124-D
5-D	35-E	65-D	95-A	125-E
6-C	36-B	66-D	96-A	126-B
7-D	37-C	67-C	97-C	127-E
8-A	38-A	68-A	98-E	128-C
9-C	39-D	69-A	99-D	129-A
10-A	40-C	70-C	100-A	130-B
11-E	41-D	71-B	101-B	131-C
12-C	42-E	72-E	102-E	132-B
13-B	43-C	73-C	103-C	133-E
14-C	44-A	74-A	104-E	134-E
15-C	45-C	75-C	105-C	135-C
16-C	46-C	76-E	106-C	136-B
17-C	47-B	77-C	107-E	137-C
18-C	48-D	78-B	108-B	138-C
19-D	49-D	79-E	109-D	139-D
20-A	50-E	80-C	110-D	140-D
21-E	51-B	81-B	111-C	141-B
22-B	52-D	82-C	112-D	142-C
23-C	53-B	83-D	113-D	143-D
24-B	54-D	84-E	114-D	144-D
25-C	55-B	85-A	115-D	145-C
26-C	56-B	86-B	116-E	146-E
27-A	57-A	87-A	117-E	147-D
28-B	58-E	88-C	118-A	148-E
29-E	59-C	89-A	119-D	149-E
30-D	60-A	90-A	120-C	150-A

151-D	161-E	171-E	181-C	191-D
152-C	162-C	172-B	182-A	192-E
153-B	163-B	173-E	183-D	193-B
154-B	164-B	174-A	184-C	194-J
155-A	165-B	175-D	185-E	195-K
156-C	166-B	176-A	186-B	196-B
157-D	167-E	177-E	187-E	197-A
158-C	168-D	178-A	188-D	198-E
159-D	169-A	179-E	189-B	199-J
160-E	170-D	180-E	190-C	200-G

ANSWERS AND EXPLANATIONS

1. The answer is C. *(General surgery; volume overload)*
The patient has volume overload most likely secondary to overzealous fluid and electrolyte therapy during and after surgery. A third heart sound is the first cardiac sign of left or right heart failure. Distention of the jugular veins and pitting edema reflect right heart failure, the most common cause of which is left heart failure. Loop diuretics as well as restriction of both water and salt intake would be helpful in removing the excess fluid. Endotoxic shock and cardiogenic shock are both unlikely, since the patient is normotensive and shows signs of right heart failure. Right heart failure is not a feature of the fat embolism syndrome.

2. The answer is B. *(Hematology; von Willebrand's disease)*
Classic von Willebrand's disease is an autosomal dominant disease characterized by a platelet adhesion defect (the most prominent manifestation) as well as a coagulation defect involving factor VIII (mild disease). Platelet defects most commonly manifest with epistaxis, mucosal bleeding, menorrhagia, excessive bleeding from scratches and cuts, and petechial lesions. Depending on the level of factor deficiency, coagulation defects present with late rebleeding of a wound, because patients cannot form a stable clot, or bleeding into potential spaces (e.g., joints).

Normally, the factor VIII molecule is divided into von Willebrand's factor (platelet adhesion factor), VIII antigen (inert carrier protein), and VIII coagulant (VIII:C), which is located in the intrinsic coagulation system. In classic von Willebrand's disease, the patients are deficient in all of these factors.

Von Willebrand's factor is synthesized by endothelial cells and megakaryocytes, the latter releasing the factor into the plasma as multimers of varying size. When vessels are injured, as manifested by a prolonged bleeding time, the exposed von Willebrand's factor in the damaged endothelium binds with von Willebrand's factor receptors on the surface of platelets, resulting in platelet adhesion. Adhesion stimulates formation of thromboxane A_2 (TXA_2) in the platelet, with subsequent platelet release of adenosine diphosphate (ADP) and thrombin. This adhesion produces platelet aggregation and formation of a temporary hemostatic plug, which ends the bleeding time. Therefore, deficiency of von Willebrand's factor prevents formation of this hemostatic plug, which produces laboratory evidence of a prolonged bleeding time or clinical evidence of excessive bleeding from scratches or cuts. Von Willebrand's factor is measured by a rocket technique or by ristocetin aggregation studies. Platelets lacking either von Willebrand's factor or its receptor are unable to aggregate in the presence of ristocetin, whereas the platelets of normal people with von Willebrand's factor or the receptor do aggregate.

Aspirin inactivates platelet cyclooxygenase and subsequent formation of TXA_2. It would be expected to exacerbate this patient's bleeding tendency, because both platelet adhesion and aggregation are defective.

The prothrombin time (PT) is a test of the extrinsic coagulation system, which is composed of factor VII. The activated partial thromboplastin time (aPTT) is a test of the intrinsic system, which consists of factors XII, XI, IX, and VIII. Both systems converge on factor X, which is at the head of the final common pathway and consist of X, V, II (prothrombin), and I (fibrinogen). Fibrinogen is converted by thrombin into fibrin, which forms a stable clot. The PT evaluates the extrinsic system (VII) down to the formation of a clot (VII, X, V, II, I → clot), whereas the aPTT evaluates the intrinsic system (XII, XI, IX, VIII) down to the formation of a clot (X, V, II, I → clot).

A platelet count is a quantitative measurement of platelets, but it provides no information about platelet function, for example, the bleeding time or platelet aggregation studies.

With this brief description of hemostasis, a patient with classic von Willebrand's disease would be expected to have a normal platelet count; a prolonged bleeding time, which would be exacerbated by the patient taking aspirin; a normal PT, because it does not include VIII coagulant; and a prolonged aPTT, because it includes VIII coagulant in the intrinsic system.

Disseminated intravascular coagulation refers to the formation of thrombi in the microcirculation, because inciting agents such as infection or malignancy activate the coagulation system. Clotting factors such as fibrinogen, factor V, factor VIII, and platelets are consumed in the clots. The fibrinolytic system is secondarily activated, therefore causing the release of plasmin, which breaks down intravascular clots into fibrin or fibrinogen degradation products that can be measured in blood. Laboratory studies in disseminated intravascular coagulation reveal a thrombocytopenia, prolonged PT and aPTT, prolonged bleeding time (thrombocytopenia), decreased plasma fibrinogen, and increased degradation products.

Qualitative platelet defects are most commonly due to aspirin. Aspirin prolongs the bleeding time, but has no effect on the coagulation tests.

Hemophilia A is a sex-linked recessive disease, with a deficiency of VIII coagulant leading to a prolonged aPTT. Since von Willebrand's factor is present, there is no platelet defect, so the bleeding time is normal.

Factor VII deficiency prolongs the PT because VII is in the extrinsic system. It does not affect the aPTT or bleeding time. Factor VII deficiency is also autosomal recessive, which would not fit this patient's family history because both parents must be carriers for the disease.

3. The answer is C. (*Pediatrics; benign rolandic epilepsy*)
Benign rolandic epilepsy (benign partial epilepsy of childhood) occurs in the school-age population and usually emerges during drowsiness or sleep. It is a benign condition that is eventually outgrown. Any anticonvulsant can manage the seizures; or it is legitimate not to treat if the events are isolated or rare, because they generally do not interrupt the day's activities. Childhood absence epilepsy would not present with focal manifestations and preserved alertness. A left temporal lobe tumor cannot be excluded but is less likely given the clinical presentation and would generally show persistent slowing on the left during an electroencephalogram (EEG). Sleep terrors, a parasomnia, occur during non–rapid eye movement (REM) sleep only and would not show an EEG abnormality. Hypsarrhythmia would present in a much younger age-group and be associated with developmental delay and flexor spasms.

4. The answer is B. (*Obstetrics; puerperal sepsis*)
The most likely diagnosis is septic pelvic thrombophlebitis, which is best treated with intravenous heparin. With a normal pelvic examination and ultrasound as described in this case, exploratory laparotomy, uterine curettage, and pelvic examination under anesthesia would not contribute to management. Unless the patient is immunosuppressed, antifungal antibiotics would be unnecessary.

5. The answer is D. (*General surgery; rupture of the bladder*)
Blunt trauma with a full bladder is the most common cause of bladder rupture. Pelvic fracture is associated with rupture of the bladder in approximately 15% of cases. Additional sources of bladder injury include puncture of the bladder during pelvic surgery or injury by cystoscopy. Previous irradiation to the bladder and urinary tract obstruction would not be expected to result in bladder rupture.

Intraperitoneal injury results in the release of urine and blood into the peritoneum, with subsequent peritonitis. Extraperitoneal injury results in a mass developing in the pelvis, which can eventuate in a pelvic abscess. Hematuria and suprapubic pain commonly occur along with suprapubic tenderness and guarding. Hemorrhagic shock may occur from loss of blood into the peritoneum. Cystography should precede excretory urography. If urethral trauma is suspected, retrograde urethrography should be performed before catheterization is attempted. Extraperitoneal extravasation should be drained, the bladder decompressed with a suprapubic or urethral catheter, and antibiotics given to avoid formation of a pelvic abscess. Intraperitoneal extravasation is treated with celiotomy, bladder closure, and bladder catheter drainage.

6. The answer is C. *(Psychiatry; bipolar disorder)*
Bipolar disorder is usually first evident in the third decade, but many exceptions exist. Its incidence is between 0.5% and 2%, and it is equally common in both sexes. There is no relationship to socioeconomic status. Amish populations have been the subject of heritability studies on bipolar disorder.

7. The answer is D. *(Pediatrics; tracheoesophageal fistula)*
Choking and cyanosis with feedings are the hallmarks of tracheoesophageal fistula. Rales can be heard and are caused by aspiration; abdominal distention results from swallowing air. A feeding tube fails to pass into the stomach. Choanal atresia presents as cyanosis relieved by crying. Cyanosis, grunting, and rales are seen in respiratory distress syndrome, but they are unrelated to feedings. Zenker's diverticulum does not appear in the newborn period. Biliary atresia is characterized by bilious vomiting.

8. The answer is A. *(Obstetrics; incompetent cervix)*
The most likely diagnosis is incompetent cervix in this diethylstilbestrol (DES) daughter with a foreshortened cervix. Terbutaline, progesterone, human chorionic gonadotropin (hCG), and human menopausal gonadotropin (hMG) are unlikely to provide the support needed to significantly prolong this pregnancy. Mechanical support of a cervical cerclage is the best treatment from this list.

9. The answer is C. *(Cardiology; acute myocardial infarction with reinfarction)*
Patients with an acute myocardial infarction who have reappearance of the CK isoenzyme MB after 3 days have reinfarction. After a myocardial infarction, the CK isoenzyme MB begins to rise within 4 to 8 hours, peaks in 24 hours, and disappears in 36 to 72 hours.

Lactate dehydrogenase (LDH) isoenzymes are composed of tetramers of H and M polypeptides to form five distinct isoenzymes that have different proportions in various tissues. Normally, the concentration of LDH_2 is greater than that of LDH_1, the concentration of LDH_1 is greater than that of LDH_3, and LDH_4 and LDH_5 concentrations are about equal. In order of decreasing concentration in tissue, LDH_2 is present in red blood cells (RBCs) and heart muscle, whereas LDH_1 is present in RBCs and heart muscle in reverse proportions. Therefore, myocardial damage results in an LDH_1/LDH_2 flip because LDH_1 has the higher concentration in cardiac muscle. The LDH_1/LDH_2 flip has a sensitivity of 80% and a specificity of 95%. It first is evident in 14 hours, peaks in 2 to 3 days, and disappears in 7 days; therefore, it is not very useful in documenting myocardial injury within the first 24 hours. Presence of an LDH_1/LDH_2 flip in this patient is expected on day 4 and does not contribute to the diagnosis of reinfarction.

Recurrent angina is ruled out by the reappearance of CK isoenzyme MB, which documents further injury. Dressler's syndrome is an autoimmune pericarditis that presents with fever, a pericardial friction rub, pleuritis, arthralgias, and neutrophilic leukocytosis in weeks to months following myocardial injury. It is not associated with the presence of CK isoenzyme MB. A posteromedial papillary muscle most commonly ruptures when the cardiac muscle is softest, and that occurs approximately day 4 to 7. The ruptured muscle would present with a murmur of mitral insufficiency. In addition, it is associated with thrombosis of the right coronary artery, which supplies the posterior part of the heart rather than being associated with the left anterior descending coronary artery, which would be responsible for the anterior myocardial infarction in this patient. A pulmonary embolus does not produce an increase in CK isoenzyme MB.

10. The answer is A. *(Biostatistics; retrospective investigative designs)*
In retrospective designs, the investigator first identifies a study group of individuals in whom a disease is present, then selects a control group of individuals free of the disease, and then notes to what extent each of the two groups was exposed to the proposed disease agent. The study group consists of those who have a disease ($a + c$), and the control group consists of those free of disease ($b + d$).

11. The answer is E. *(General surgery; breast cancer)*
Breast cancer is the most common cancer in adult women and the second most common cause of death. It occurs in approximately one in nine women in the United States. Predisposing factors for breast cancer include

- a family history of a first-degree relative with breast cancer or mother with breast cancer
- previous history of contralateral breast cancer
- early menarche and late menopause, both of which expose women longer to estrogen
- a low-fiber, high-fat diet
- nulliparity, which leaves women exposed to more estrogen without the benefit of the 9 months of progesterone
- a history of endometrial carcinoma, which is also an estrogen-induced cancer
- increasing age (the most common cause of a breast mass in women over 50 years of age)

Birth control pills do not predispose women to breast cancer. The progestins in the pill have an opposing effect on estrogen.

12. The answer is C. *(Biostatistics; risk of hemophilia A)*
Hemophilia A is transmitted as a sex-linked recessive trait. For an affected man to have a son, he must provide the Y chromosome and therefore cannot transmit the defective chromosome to his own son. The son, therefore, has a 50% chance of receiving the chromosome from his carrier mother, who is heterozygous.

13. The answer is B. *(Pediatrics; duodenal atresia)*
Although biliary atresia is more common than duodenal atresia in Down syndrome, duodenal atresia is often associated and appears in the first day of life as bilious vomiting after feedings. X-ray typically shows the double bubble; treatment is surgical. Pyloric stenosis appears at 3 to 4 weeks of age with nonbilious vomiting. A diaphragmatic hernia presents at birth, with respiratory distress and a scaphoid abdomen. Bowel sounds can be auscultated in the chest, and x-ray reveals abdominal contents in the thorax. A perforated viscus will show free air in the abdomen on x-ray.

14. The answer is C. *(Psychiatry; schizophrenia)*
Sophisticated studies of cerebral morphology and biochemistry in schizophrenia have yielded some fairly consistent findings, including decreased cerebral asymmetry. Also of note are a decreased size of the corpus callosum, decreased activity in the prefrontal cortex, and increased size of lateral ventricles. Although several abnormalities of dopamine metabolism have been reported, none are pathognomonic.

15. The answer is C. *(Pharmacology; autonomic drugs)*
The patient may have cholinergic crisis from taking an overdose of pyridostigmine or myasthenic crisis from not taking an adequate dose. Infections may alter drug requirement in myasthenics; and since gastrointestinal upsets are common in "flu," the physician cannot reliably use changes in bowel activity to aid in diagnosis. A small dose of edrophonium should be given, followed by careful observation of whether muscle strength improves (indicative of an inadequate dose of pyridostigmine) or worsens (indicative of an excessive dose). In the latter case, the worsening effect is quite brief, lasting only a few minutes. Physostigmine, a tertiary amine that exerts marked central effects, is not used in myasthenia gravis. Succinylcholine causes skeletal muscle paralysis.

16. The answer is C. *(Endocrinology; hypoparathyroidism)*
Hypoparathyroidism is most commonly caused by a total thyroidectomy. Because parathormone (PTH) normally increases calcium reabsorption in the kidney and decreases the reabsorption of phosphate, patients develop hypocalcemia, hyperphosphatemia, and decreased PTH. Hypocalcemia results in clinical evidence of tetany, such as carpal spasm after pumping up a blood pressure cuff (Trousseau's sign) and facial muscle contractions after tapping on the facial nerve (Chvostek's sign).

Hypercalcemia, hypophosphatemia, and increased PTH (choice A) are present in primary hyperparathyroidism, which is most commonly (85%) due to a benign parathyroid adenoma. It is the most common cause of hypercalcemia in the ambulatory population.

Hypercalcemia, hypophosphatemia, and decreased PTH (choice B) are characteristic of malignancy-induced hypercalcemia. This condition is most commonly due to secretion of a PTH-like peptide that acts on the kidney. The result is increased calcium reabsorption (hypercalcemia) and decreased phosphorus reabsorption (hypophosphatemia), but the hypercalcemia suppresses the patient's own PTH production. Other mechanisms for hypercalcemia in malignancy relate to the secretion of osteoclast-activating factor or prostaglandins.

Hypocalcemia, hypophosphatemia, and increased PTH (choice D) are seen in malabsorption of vitamin D due to celiac disease or other gastrointestinal diseases. Vitamin D normally increases the reabsorption of both calcium and phosphorus from the gut and kidneys. Therefore, deficiency results in hypocalcemia and hypophosphatemia, the former serving as a potent stimulus for PTH synthesis and secondary hyperparathyroidism.

Hypocalcemia, hyperphosphatemia, and increased PTH (choice E) are seen in renal failure. Since PTH normally increases the synthesis of the hydroxylating enzyme located in the renal tubules and is responsible for the second hydroxylation step of vitamin D, renal disease results in hypovitaminosis D, with a subsequent hypocalcemia and secondary hyperparathyroidism. The kidney is also the excretion route for phosphate; therefore, renal failure results in retention of phosphate. This constellation of findings is also seen in pseudohypoparathyroidism, which is a genetic disease that is associated with a resistance of the target tissue to PTH. Therefore, hypocalcemia and hyperphosphatemia are present; but, unlike primary hypoparathyroidism, the PTH is usually increased.

17. The answer is C. *(Gynecology; benign ovarian tumor)*
The human ovary can develop a wide variety of tumors, the majority of which are benign. These tumors can be functional, inflammatory, metaplastic, or neoplastic. Follicular cyst, mucinous cystadenoma, serous cystadenoma, cystic teratoma, and Brenner's tumor are all ovarian tumors. However, only cystic teratomas are characterized by frequent calcification.

18. The answer is C. *(Ear, nose, and throat; mixed parotid tumor)*
The patient has a mixed tumor (pleomorphic adenoma). This is the most common type of salivary gland tumor, and the parotid is the most common location. The ratio of benign to malignant salivary gland tumors is highest in the parotid and lowest in the minor salivary glands. Seventh-nerve palsy suggests the possibility of malignancy. A mixed tumor must be removed with a rim of normal parotid tissue around it; otherwise, it will recur. Adenoid cystic carcinomas are the most common malignant tumor of minor salivary glands. They have a propensity for perineural invasion. Warthin's tumors are most commonly located in the parotid. They are rarely malignant. Mucoepidermoid carcinoma is the most common malignant tumor of the major salivary glands. The greater the squamous component, the worse the prognosis.

19. The answer is D. *(Biostatistics; prospective investigative design)*
In prospective designs, the investigator first identifies a study group of individuals who will be exposed to a proposed disease agent, then selects a control group of individuals who will not be

exposed to the agent, and then notes to what extent each of the two groups develops the disease. The study group consists of those who are exposed to the agent ($a + b$), and the control group consists of those who will not be exposed to the agent ($c + d$).

20. The answer is A. (Neurology; benign intracranial hypertension)

Despite the name, long-standing benign intracranial hypertension can cause progressive visual loss related to direct pressure on the optic nerve sheath and head. An early finding might be an enlarged blind spot on visual field testing. Sixth nerve palsy can be seen in benign intracranial hypertension but is a temporary condition generally reversible when the pressure is normalized. Herniation syndrome is extremely rare with benign intracranial hypertension and is usually a consequence of an unrecognized mass lesion in the posterior fossa. Migraine headaches are not associated with benign intracranial hypertension. Benign intracranial hypertension is often self-limited, but it usually needs to be treated with diuretics, spinal taps, steroids, or even cerebrospinal fluid shunting.

21. The answer is E. (Obstetrics; diagnosis of labor)

Distinguishing between true and false labor is a difficult task prospectively because many features are found in both. Character of pain, descent of fetus, regular contractions, and bloody show may occur in false labor. However, the combination of progressive effacement and cervical dilation is the key distinguishing feature of true labor.

22. The answer is B. (General surgery; ruptured abdominal aortic aneurysm)

The patient has the classic triad for a ruptured abdominal aortic aneurysm: an abrupt onset of back pain, hypotension, and a pulsatile mass in the abdomen.

An aneurysm is a localized dilatation of a vessel. It is usually caused by structural weakness in the wall of the vessel due to atherosclerosis. Abdominal aortic aneurysms are the most com-

mon type of aneurysm in the vascular system, located below the orifices of the renal arteries. The majority occur in men over 55 years of age, who are asymptomatic. Ultrasound is the most effective means of making the diagnosis of an aneurysm.

Rupture of the aneurysm is the most common complication. Risk factors for rupture include the size of the aneurysm (> 5 cm), hypertension, and the presence of chronic obstructive pulmonary disease.

Indications for surgery include any symptomatic aneurysm or any asymptomatic aneurysm larger than 5 cm, since rupture is inevitable with time, and mortality rates exceed 90%.

23. The answer is C. (Genetics; risk of neurofibromatosis)

Neurofibromatosis is transmitted as an autosomal dominant trait. Therefore, a normal person is homozygous recessive. Half of the offspring would be heterozygous and therefore affected. Half of the offspring would be homozygous recessive and normal.

24. The answer is B. (Psychiatry; schizophrenia)

For unknown reasons, the risk for developing schizophrenia is higher for individuals born in winter months in temperate regions. The disease course is variable. No particular family communication style appears to cause schizophrenia. The concordance rate in identical twins is between 50% and 80%. The lifetime incidence is close to 1%.

25. The answer is C. (Nephrology; inappropriate antidiuretic hormone syndrome induced by chlorpropamide)

The inappropriate release of antidiuretic hormone (ADH) can be secondary to factors that stimulate the release of ADH from the hypothalamus or increase the sensitivity of its action in the kidneys, or both, or neoplastic conditions that ectopically secrete excess amounts of ADH. Some of these factors include chlorpropamide or other drugs, such as cyclophosphamide, clofibrate, morphine, or carbamazepine; small cell carcinoma of the lung; or any central nervous system (CNS) disturbance such as infection, tumor, or stroke.

The excess release of ADH results in the reabsorption of electrolyte-free water from the collecting ducts of the kidneys. Because the serum sodium equals the ratio of total body sodium (TBNa) to total body water (TBW), an increase in TBW produces a dilutional hyponatremia as water is added to the extracellular fluid compartment ($\downarrow\downarrow$ serum sodium = TBNa/$\uparrow\uparrow$ TBW). This change lowers the plasma osmolality, which is primarily determined by the sodium concentration. According to the law of osmosis, water moves from the point of low solute concentration, in this case the extracellular fluid, to high solute concentration, which is the intracellular fluid compartment. This influx of water into the brain produces cerebral edema, which is responsible for the altered mental status in this patient.

TBNa, which is primarily located in the extracellular fluid compartment, is determined by physical examination. Normal TBNa is reflected by the presence of normal skin turgor, as evident in this patient. Decreased TBNa is clinically reflected by signs of dehydration, such as dry mucous membranes, no axillary sweat, tenting of the skin, and hypotension. Increased TBNa is manifested as pitting edema and effusions into body cavities.

Continued presence of ADH results in an increase in arterial blood volume, which increases peritubular hydrostatic pressure in the kidneys. This decreases the reabsorption of all solutes that are normally removed by the proximal tubule, such as sodium (60%–80%), urea, uric acid, potassium, and glucose, leading to an increase in urine osmolality. Furthermore, the increase in arterial blood volume decreases the release of renin and, ultimately, aldosterone; therefore, additional sodium is lost in the distal tubules (10%–20%). This loss in sodium is reflected by an increased level of random urine sodium, as evident in this patient. Finally, the dilutional effect of excess plasma water not only affects the sodium concentration but also affects other electrolytes, such as potassium, chloride, and bicarbonate. Serum urea and uric acid are decreased, because they are lost in the urine by the mechanism discussed previ-

ously. This situation produces a classic triad for diagnosing inappropriate ADH syndrome, mainly severe hyponatremia, low serum blood urea nitrogen (BUN), and low uric acid.

The best treatment for the syndrome of inappropriate ADH is water restriction. Use of hypertonic saline infusions to raise serum sodium is only a temporary measure, because the sodium is eventually excreted in the urine by the mechanism previously discussed. Demeclocycline is an ADH antagonist that is primarily used in patients with small cell carcinoma.

Second-generation sulfonylureas do not have the water-retention properties of chlorpropamide and should be used if inappropriate ADH syndrome becomes a problem.

26. The answer is C. *(Gynecology; ovarian cancer)*
Ovarian cancer is the fifth most common cancer among women in the United States. It accounts for 25% of all gynecologic malignancies. The key feature in identifying ovarian carcinoma is the presence of ascites. Ovarian cancer typically spreads by dissemination and implantation throughout the peritoneal cavity. Endometrial, cervical, and uterine cancer do not have this finding. Krukenberg's tumor is a malignancy arising from the stomach and metastasizing to the ovary.

27. The answer is A. *(General surgery; diverticulosis with perforation and peritonitis)*
The patient has peritonitis secondary to rupture of a diverticulum, which occurs if the diverticulum is located above the peritoneal reflection. In such cases, the mesentery often covers the diverticulum, thus producing a localized collection of pus between the leaves of the mesentery rather than diffuse peritonitis.

Diverticula are most commonly located in the sigmoid colon. They are secondary to herniation of bowel mucosa through areas of weakness where the vessels penetrate the bowel wall. Constipation due to a low-fiber–high-fat diet increases intraluminal pressure, thus augmenting diverticula formation.

Most patients are asymptomatic. Symptomatic patients present with left lower quadrant pain secondary to diverticulitis (similar to acute appendicitis, but on the left side rather than the right). Computed tomography (CT) is excellent in identifying diverticulitis. Water-soluble contrast material should be used if a barium enema is performed.

Complications other than diverticulitis include massive lower gastrointestinal bleeding, perforation, fistula formation (usually colovesical), and a pericolic abscess. Treatment modalities include a high-fiber diet; surgery, if peritonitis or bleeding is present; and pentazocine for analgesia.

28. The answer is B. *(Genetics; risk of cystic fibrosis)*
Cystic fibrosis is transmitted as an autosomal-recessive disease; therefore, carriers are heterozygous. Two carriers who marry have a 25% chance of having an affected child, a 50% chance of having an unaffected carrier, and a 25% chance of having an unaffected child who is not a carrier.

29. The answer is E. *(Psychiatry; somatization disorder)*
Women with somatization disorder often have a higher incidence of male relatives with alcoholism and antisocial personality disorder. Somatization disorder is associated with analgesic and sedative hypnotic abuse and often involves neuromotor and sexual dysfunction. It almost always begins before age 30.

30. The answer is D. *(Gastroenterology; gastroesophageal reflux disease)*
Gastroesophageal reflux disease (GERD) is a chronic, recurrent disorder characterized by heartburn, eructation (belching), and epigastric pain. Prevalence of GERD increases with age; it is found more commonly in older men than in older women. The primary mechanism is inappropriate relaxation of the lower esophageal sphincter (LES). This condition is exacerbated by agents that decrease LES pressure, such as chocolate, coffee, ethanol, fat, peppermint, anticholinergics, theophylline, diazepam, barbiturates, and calcium channel blockers. Secondary factors that predispose to GERD include the acid concentration of the refluxate; delayed acid clearance, which is associated with low-amplitude peristalsis and recumbency; and impaired gastric emptying, which aggravates reflux. The acid concentration of the refluxate is the most important factor in determining progression to reflux esophagitis. The gold standard for the diagnosis of GERD is 24-hour intraesophageal pH monitoring.

Approximately 80% of adults with bronchial asthma have GERD. This percentage appears to be independent of bronchodilator therapy. GERD can also precipitate an asthmatic attack by reflux vagal stimulation or aspiration.

Complications associated with GERD are reflux esophagitis, stricture formation, and Barrett's esophagus. Barrett's esophagus is a premalignant condition characterized by glandular metaplasia of the distal esophagus. The risk of developing adenocarcinoma is 2% to 10%.

The treatment of GERD involves reducing gastroesophageal reflux, neutralizing the acid reflux, enhancing esophageal clearance, and protecting the esophageal mucosa from ulceration. Diet modification, weight loss, postural therapy, restriction of alcohol, and cessation of smoking along with pharmacologic treatment are used, the last in a stepwise approach reflecting patient response. A recommended progression of drugs includes antacids and alginic acid → histamine$_2$ (H$_2$) receptor antagonists at conventional doses → H$_2$ receptor antagonists at high doses, omeprazole, or prokinetic agents (metoclopramide) → antireflux surgery.

Reflux is commonly seen in pregnancy and is attributed to impaired LES competence and increased abdominal pressure.

31. The answer is E. *(Obstetrics; pelvic diameters)*
The actual space available to the fetus in relation to the pelvic inlet is the obstetric conjugate. It is the measurement from the sacral promontory to the closest point on the convex posterior surface of the symphysis pubis. It determines whether the presenting fetal part can engage.

32. The answer is E. *(Biostatistics; mean, median, mode)*
The mean is the sum of all of the numbers (2+5+7+8+8) divided by the number of numerals (5), which equals 6 in this set. The median is the number equidistant in order from the lowest and highest values, which is 7 in this set. The mode is the most frequently occurring number, which is 8 in this set. Therefore, mean, median, and mode are 6, 7, and 8.

33. The answer is C. *(General surgery; massive lower gastrointestinal bleeding)*
Diverticulosis and angiodysplasia are the two most common causes for massive lower gastrointestinal bleeding in elderly patients. Diverticula are juxtaposed to penetrating branches in the wall of the colon, thus predisposing the patient to massive bleeding. Angiodysplasia is more common in elderly, rather than younger, patients. It is characterized by dilated submucosal vessels, commonly located in the cecum and right colon, that can empty into the colon. There is an association with aortic stenosis and von Willebrand's disease. Colonoscopy may identify the bleeding sites, but mesenteric angiography is the preferred method for localizing the bleeding sites prior to surgery.

A solitary rectal ulcer is a painful superficial ulcer of unknown cause. Although uncommon, they can cause massive lower gastrointestinal bleeding. Intussusception, cancer, volvulus, ischemic bowel disease, and ulcerative colitis are all associated with bleeding but are rarely associated with massive lower gastrointestinal bleeding. Meckel's diverticulum is located 2 feet from the ileocecal valve. It is a true diverticulum, representing persistence of the omphalomesenteric duct. It is the most common cause of upper gastrointestinal bleeding in a child.

34. The answer is C. *(Emergency medicine; subarachnoid hemorrhage)*
A spinal tap should be performed to look for the presence of blood in the cerebrospinal fluid (CSF) as a means to exclude a subarachnoid hemorrhage. At least several percent of computed tomography (CT) scans may be negative in an initial study; and if the clinical suspicion justifies it, a spinal tap, arteriography, or both should be undertaken to look for bleeding from an arteriovenous malformation or aneurysm. Admission to the hospital is appropriate, but the more vital step is to identify a potentially lethal condition. Narcotics for pain should be undertaken only when the cause of the pain is identified or the appropriate test is underway. Intravenous antibiotics are appropriate for suspected meningitis, but the acuteness of the event makes this inflammation unlikely, and the stiff neck is likely to be secondary to the irritative property of blood rather than infection. Finally, the electroencephalogram (EEG) is useful in identifying focal lesions or seizures but would be particularly unhelpful in a possible subarachnoid hemorrhage.

35. The answer is E. *(Psychiatry; body dysmorphia)*
Body dysmorphia is a pathologic preoccupation with an imagined (or very minor) defect in appearance. The body parts most often involved are the nose, breasts, and thighs. The increased availability and effectiveness of reconstructive surgery have made diagnosis of this disorder more important. Surgical intervention is often ineffective in resolving it.

36. The answer is B. *(Hematology; hemolytic transfusion reaction)*
The majority of hemolytic transfusion reactions are due to clerical error, such as giving the wrong blood to a patient with the same name, a mislabeled unit, or not checking the patient's blood bank identification tag with the identification number on the unit. Because the patient in question is blood group O, immunoglobulin M (IgM) antibodies against A and B antigens are already present. Anti-A IgM antibodies in the patient will attach to the donor A cells, activate the classic complement pathway, and cause massive intravascular hemolysis (a type II hypersensitivity reaction), with subsequent hypotension and ischemic acute tubular necrosis. Approximately 50% of patients develop disseminated intravascular coagulation, as in this patient, who had blood

oozing out of venipuncture sites from the consumption of clotting factors (fibrinogen, factor V, factor VIII, platelets).

The first step in management of a hemolytic transfusion reaction is to stop the transfusion. The unit and a sample of blood and urine should immediately be sent to the blood bank for a transfusion reaction workup. Pink-staining plasma and hemoglobin in the urine are presumptive evidence of intravascular hemolysis. Shock is treated with normal saline or a balanced salt solution (e.g., Ringer's lactate). If the urine output is not increasing with the intravenous fluids or if there is volume overload from congestive heart failure, intravenous furosemide is given. If the patient's volume status is stable, intravenous mannitol is used to maintain an osmotic diuresis to prevent acute tubular necrosis. Antipyretics are not indicated, because this reaction is not febrile.

The donor is Rh-positive (A-positive), and the patient is Rh-negative (O-negative); however, this is not important in the pathogenesis of this patient's hemolytic anemia. If the patient survives, anti-D antibodies may develop against the D-positive donor cells. Administration of D-positive donor cells in the future could precipitate an extravascular hemolytic anemia. The anti-D (IgG antibody)–coated D-positive red blood cells (RBCs) are recognized by the Fc receptors for IgG on macrophages in the spleen, with subsequent removal and destruction of the RBCs.

37. The answer is C. *(General surgery; treatment of hepatocellular failure)*
Hepatocelluar failure is most commonly caused by alcoholic cirrhosis and chronic active hepatitis. Hepatic encephalopathy, one of many complications associated with hepatocellular failure, is a potentially reversible metabolic disorder characterized by diffuse slowing of brain waves on electroencephalography (EEG), altered levels of consciousness, asterixis (inability to sustain posture), and reversal of the day–night sleep rhythm. Possible causes include increased levels of false neurotransmitters [octopamine, γ-aminobutyric acid (GABA)], reduced levels of branched-chain amino acids, increased levels of aromatic amino acids, and increased levels of serum ammonia.

The most effective way of reducing serum ammonia levels is by reducing protein intake. This decreases the amount of protein available for bacteria to break down into absorbable ammonia (NH_3). Lactulose is given orally. It is broken down by colonic bacteria into hydrogen ions. These bind with NH_3 to form ammonium (NH_4), which cannot be reabsorbed in the bowel mucosa. Neomycin eliminates the bacteria that produce the ammonia. A loop diuretic could potentially precipitate hepatic encephalopathy, since metabolic alkalosis and hypokalemia are common complications.

38. The answer is A. *(Psychiatry; alcohol abuse)*
Those sons of alcoholics who have a greater innate tolerance for alcohol seem more likely to later develop alcohol problems. Abstinence appears to be the only way that former alcoholics can maintain sobriety. There appear to be distinct subtypes of alcoholism. The highest prevalence of alcoholism occurs in the third decade of life. Some ethnic groups have remarkably high or low rates of alcoholism.

39. The answer is D. *(Obstetrics; maternal physiology)*
The normal ranges for many laboratory values change with pregnancy. Enhanced renal plasma flow and glomerular filtration rate increase creatinine clearance and lower blood urea nitrogen (BUN). Hemoglobin decreases with the dilution effect of expanded plasma volume. Alkaline phosphatase (ALP) increases because of the placental contribution. Of the options listed, only serum glutamic–oxaloacetic transaminase (SGOT) remains unchanged with pregnancy.

40. The answer is C. *(Genetics; incidence of sickle cell disease)*
Sickle cell disease is transmitted as an autosomal-recessive disease and follows simple mendelian genetics. Therefore, if the carrier rate is 1/12, the odds that two carriers will meet are $1/12 \times 1/12 = 1/144$. The odds that two carriers will have an affected child are 1/4. Therefore, the incidence is $1/144 \times 1/4 = 1/576$.

41. The answer is D. *(General surgery; wound infections)*
The patient most likely has a postoperative wound infection, which occurs in 2% to 5% of patients who have had biliary tract surgery. The infections are usually the result of contamination of the wound either during or after surgery. Although infections can occur within 1 day in a grossly contaminated wound, they generally occur 5 to 10 days postoperatively.

Operative wounds are classified as clean (no gross contamination), clean–contaminated (e.g., in gastric or biliary tract surgery), contaminated (e.g., in unprepared colon surgery), or dirty and infected (infection encountered during the surgery).

The risk for wound infection increases if the wound is located in the abdomen, the surgery lasts longer than 2 hours, or contamination of the wound is encountered during surgery. One of the key factors that predisposes to infection is decreased oxygen tension in the tissues.

Attention to careful surgical techniques (reduced trauma to tissue, less suture material, removal of foreign bodies) and prophylactic use of antibiotics in certain types of surgeries reduce the chance of infection. Cefazolin is the drug of choice for prophylaxis during surgery when both aerobes and anaerobes are a concern. Antibiotic prophylaxis is only given in selected clean or clean–contaminated procedures, since antibiotic use in contaminated and dirty wounds is considered therapeutic. A single preoperative dose should be administered intravenously at the time of induction of anesthesia. Additional doses may be given after surgery but are usually discontinued within 24 hours.

Treatment of wound infections involves opening the wound and allowing drainage. Antibiotics are reserved for invasive infections. Atelectasis is the most common cause of fever within 24 hours of surgery. Endotoxic shock would be an unlikely cause of this man's fever. Endotoxic shock would be accompanied by warm shock, due to vasodilatation of peripheral vessels. Resorption of blood is not associated with fever.

42. The answer is E. *(Obstetrics; gestational trophoblastic neoplasia)*
The findings are those of first trimester pre-eclampsia. This unusual finding is unique to molar pregnancy. It is not characteristic of gestational diabetes, twin pregnancy, fetal anencephaly, or inevitable abortion.

43. The answer is C. *(Psychiatry; cocaine abuse)*
Although cocaine use is decreasing among high-school students, its use is becoming endemic in certain subgroups. Concurrent abuse of alcohol is common, often in an attempt to decrease agitation and dysphoria. Concurrent use of opiates is rare but dangerous. The rate of cocaine abuse in patients with schizophrenia is significant. The pattern of abuse usually involves bingeing rather than continuous use.

44. The answer is A. *(Rheumatology; Raynaud's phenomenon in systemic and localized scleroderma)*
Both systemic sclerosis (85%) and localized scleroderma, known as the CREST syndrome (95%), commonly present with Raynaud's phenomenon, often antedating other manifestations of the disease by years. Cold temperatures and stress are stimuli that produce color changes of the fingers (sometimes toes), which first blanch, then become cyanotic, and then red. Vasospasm and thickened digital vessels are responsible for these changes. Immune complexes are not present in the vessels.

CREST syndrome is characterized by **c**alcinosis of the digits, **R**aynaud's phenomenon, **e**sophageal motility dysfunction, **s**clerodactyly of the fingers, and **t**elangiectasia over the digits and under the nails. The anticentromere antibody is positive in over 50% of cases.

Systemic sclerosis is a more generalized disorder of connective tissue, characterized by degenerative and inflammatory changes that result in the subsequent increase of collagen tissue deposition in various tissues. Tightening of the skin of the face and extremities is a universal finding. Esophageal motility problems, with dysphagia for solids and liquids, occur in 80% of patients. Other problems include arthritis (80%), renal involvement (60%—onion skinning of the vessels), pericardial effusions (20%–50%), pulmonary fibrosis with restrictive lung disease (35%), and renal crisis (15%), which is the most common cause of death. The antinuclear antibody test is positive in 70% to 90% of cases. The anti–Scl-70 antibody is specific for systemic sclerosis and is noted in 40% to 70% of cases. Penicillamine may improve long-term survival.

Other causes of Raynaud's phenomenon are thromboangiitis obliterans (Buerger's disease), which is an inflammatory vasculitis producing thrombosis of the digital vessels in male smokers; cryoglobulinemia with proteins that precipitate in cold temperatures; cold agglutinins with immunoglobulin M (IgM) antibodies that clump red blood cells (RBCs) in the digital vessels; and ergotamine poisoning.

45. The answer is C. *(Biostatistics; normal distribution)*
Assuming a normal distribution, the mean ± 2 standard deviations describes the range in which it can be expected that 95% of repeated observations or determinations would fall. In the scenario described (with a mean of 20 and a standard deviation of 2), the normal range would be 20 ± 4, or 16 to 24.

46. The answer is C. *(General surgery; spontaneous pneumothorax from subclavian vein catheterization)*
The patient has a pneumothorax as a complication of subclavian vein catheterization. The subclavian vein courses under the clavicle near the subclavian artery and the apex of the lung. The artery is superior and deep to the vein. With a percutaneous approach, the vein is entered first before accidentally puncturing the artery. A chest x-ray should be obtained immediately to check placement of the catheter and to detect a possible (usually small) pneumothorax, which may occur in 10% of cases. A sudden onset of dyspnea related to catheter placement would not be expected in air embolism, pneumonia, or cardiac arrhythmia.

47. The answer is B. *(Neurology; epilepsy)*
The patient had been doing well for 3 years on phenytoin monotherapy, and raising the dosage slightly is likely to take care of the small risk of additional seizures. Ordering another electroencephalogram (EEG) adds little to the long-term management, because the seizure disorder is already diagnosed. Adding phenobarbital is less preferable because of the sedative properties and the increased risk of side effects and interactions with anticonvulsant polypharmacy. Carbamazepine is another excellent anticonvulsant; but in a patient who has a single breakthrough seizure while in the low therapeutic range, substitution is less preferable than optimizing a proven medicine. Finally, an imaging study adds little to the management in a patient with long-standing epilepsy unless there are new neurologic deficits or additional breakthrough seizures not explained by low medication levels.

48. The answer is D. *(Obstetrics; intrapartum fetal assessment)*
Normal fetal heart rate patterns are reassuring but do not always mean a healthy baby. Normal baseline rate is 120 to 160 beats/min. Variable decelerations indicate cord compression. Early decelerations are usually benign and require no intervention. Normal Apgar score and cord pH value frequently occur with abnormal patterns.

49. The answer is D. *(Pediatrics; congenital syphilis)*
Manifestations of congenital syphilis are divided into early and late. Early manifestations present during the first 2 years of life and include fever, anemia, failure to thrive, a maculopapular rash, hepatomegaly, and snuffles. Late manifestations are skeletal in nature and include saber shins, saddle nose, Hutchinson's teeth, and rhagades (perioral fissures or cracks in the skin).

50. The answer is E. *(Gynecology; contraception)*
Oral contraceptives increase the release of renin precursors from the liver and can result in hypertension in a small percentage of women. Although essential hypertension, pheochromocy-

toma, and renal artery fibromuscular hyperplasia are possible explanations for this mild hypertension, the best working diagnosis is iatrogenic etiology as a result of oral contraception. Turner's syndrome is not related to hypertension.

51. The answer is B. *(Psychiatry; heroin abuse)*
Opiate dependence is surprisingly time-limited—usually approximately 7 years. Use of opiates for acute pain management rarely causes dependence. Deviant behavior seems to occur in opiate addicts even if opiates are readily available. Opiates do not produce an organic delusional syndrome. Opiate addiction is most commonly a group phenomenon.

52. The answer is D. *(Pharmacology; cardiac drugs)*
Chronic treatment with digitalis requires attention to pharmacokinetics because toxicity occurs when plasma levels of the drugs exceed the therapeutic range. Sensitive plasma digoxin assays are available at most medical centers and should be used when patient response is not as predicted from the dosing schedule. Digoxin has an oral bioavailability of greater than 70%, a volume of distribution of over 400 L, and an elimination half-life of 40 hours. Plasma protein binding is low (25%); nonetheless, digoxin is distributed to tissues very slowly, and measurements of blood levels are erratic for up to 6 hours following an oral dose.

53. The answer is B. *(Gastroenterology; gallstone ileus with small bowel obstruction)*
Gallstone ileus is mechanical obstruction of the bowel by a large gallstone lodged in the lumen. It is most commonly seen in elderly women who have a chronically inflamed gallbladder that adheres to the bowel and forms a cholecystenteric fistula with the small bowel or colon. Stones that produce mechanical obstruction are usually greater than 2.5 cm. They are frequently radiopaque, as in this case. Air in the biliary tree from the cholecystenteric fistula is seen in 40% of cases. Treatment involves immediate surgery to remove the stone. The fistula usually closes spontaneously. An elective cholecystectomy is per-

formed at a later date if symptoms of gallbladder disease persist.

Because the findings in this patient are those of obstruction, acute pancreatitis, acute appendicitis, small bowel infarction, and acute pylephlebitis (inflammation and thrombosis of the portal vein) are unlikely.

54. The answer is D. *(Obstetrics; fetal anomaly screening)*
Maternal serum alpha-fetoprotein (MSAFP) screening is routine in many states in the United States to identify pregnancies requiring special care. MSAFP levels tend to be lower with Down syndrome. AFP levels are increased in spina bifida, anencephaly, and omphalocele. Turner's syndrome is not associated with MSAFP abnormalities.

55. The answer is B. *(Biostatistics; attributable risk)*
Attributable risk expresses the amount of absolute risk for a particular condition or disease that can be assigned to a specific exposure. The risk is calculated by subtracting the disease incidence in the nonexposed group from the disease incidence in the exposed group; that is, IRE − IRN.

56. The answer is B. *(General surgery; infection in burns)*
Infection is the most common complication of burns. *Pseudomonas aeruginosa* is the organism most frequently involved and the most common cause of death in burn patients. *Staphylococcus aureus, Candida albicans* (usually involved in catheter-related sepsis), and group A streptococcus are less common offenders.

Burn patients who develop fever do not always have an infection. Thermal injury releases interleukin-1, which can produce fever by stimulating the hypothalamus to synthesize prostaglandins, which, in turn, stimulate the thermoregulatory center in the brain. This underscores the need to biopsy suspicious burn wounds for culture in order to ascertain whether infection is the cause of fever. Antibiotics are not recommended for prophylaxis in burn patients.

57. The answer is A. *(General surgery; brain tumor)*
Headache can be a presenting sign of increased intracranial pressure. When associated with a brain tumor, the headache typically occurs in the morning and improves with standing because venous flow away from the brain is enhanced. Vomiting usually relieves the headache, whereas sneezing and coughing can make it feel worse.

58. The answer is E. *(Pediatrics; Kawasaki disease)*
Mucocutaneous lymph node syndrome (MLNS, Kawasaki disease) is a febrile vasculitis of children. Criteria for diagnosis are fever of 5 days' duration and four of the following five conditions: bilateral nonpurulent conjunctivitis, changes of the mucosa of the oropharynx (dry, cracked lips, strawberry tongue), changes of the peripheral extremities (edema, erythema, peeling of hands and feet), a polymorphous rash, and cervical lymphadenopathy. Many experts believe that in the presence of classic features, the diagnosis can be made before 5 days of fever. MLNS occurs generally in children less than 5 years of age. Thrombocytosis appears in the second or third week. Leukocytosis, elevated C-reactive protein, and elevated erythrocyte sedimentation rate are common laboratory findings.

59. The answer is C. *(Psychiatry; developmental disorder)*
Intrauterine rubella has a strong association with autism. Other intrauterine and postnatal insults also increase the risk for autism, but the association is much less clear-cut. No data suggest that any type of parenting is more likely to produce autism.

60. The answer is A. *(General surgery; breast mass)*
The patient requires fine-needle aspiration with cytologic evaluation to establish the histologic diagnosis of the breast mass. The sensitivity of fine-needle aspiration in correctly diagnosing breast cancer is in the range of 95%. The age of the patient, the location of the mass (upper outer quadrant is the most common site for cancer), the nontender nature of the mass, and the fact that it is solid and not cystic suggest that it is malignant.

The combination of physical examination, mammography, and fine-needle aspiration is highly accurate in diagnosing breast cancer when all of the tests give the same result. The combination increases overall specificity, thus decreasing false-positive results. The purpose of mammography is to evaluate the breasts for clinically occult lesions. Mammography has a sensitivity approaching 90% in diagnosing breast cancer, with a false-positive rate of approximately 10%. It has a specificity approaching 85%, with a false-positive rate of approximately 15%. These percentages reflect the deficits in mammography in detecting breast cancer in general, and in distinguishing benign from malignant tumors. The sensitivity of correctly diagnosing breast cancer by physical examination is between 60% and 85%.

A suggested management plan of a palpable breast mass is to perform a fine-needle aspiration first. If the mass is cystic and the mammogram is negative, the patient should be observed. If the mass is cystic and the mammogram is positive, or if the mass persists, the fluid is bloody, or there are multiple recurrences, an outpatient biopsy is recommended. If the mass is solid, the fine-needle aspiration is negative or suspicious, and the mammogram is positive or negative, an outpatient biopsy is recommended. If the fine-needle aspiration is positive for malignancy and the mammogram is positive or negative, an intraoperative biopsy is performed with frozen section before the definitive surgery is performed.

61. The answer is B. *(Pharmacology; cardiac drugs)*
This patient appears to be suffering from variant angina rather than angina of effort. Nitrates and calcium channel blockers are more effective than β-blockers in variant angina. Sublingual nitroglycerin, which acts within 1 or 2 minutes, is the most common agent used for relief of acute attacks, but it is not suitable for maintenance therapy because of its short duration of action. The clinical efficacy of transdermal nitroglycerin patches for prophylaxis is limited by the development of tolerance. The slow onset of action of oral verapamil renders it unsuitable for management of acute anginal attacks.

62. The answer is B. *(Pediatrics; congenital anomaly; hypospadias)*
Hypospadias occurs in approximately 1/500 live births and has an incidence of 8.2/1000 male births. Clubfoot has an incidence of 1/1000 births. Cleft palate alone occurs in approximately 1/2500 births and 1/1000 if associated with cleft lip. Phocomelia can occur spontaneously but has decreased dramatically since the discovery of its association with the use of thalidomide during pregnancy. Spina bifida occurs with a frequency of 1/650.

63. The answer is D. *(Hematology; α thalassemia)*
Thalassemia is a common cause of a microcytic anemia, particularly in the Asian and black populations. It is a defect in globin chain synthesis resulting in decreased production of hemoglobin leading to a microcytic anemia.

The normal globin chains are alpha (α), beta (β), delta (δ), and gamma (γ). Hemoglobin A is the predominant hemoglobin in adults and accounts for 96% to 98% of the hemoglobin in red blood cells (RBCs). Hemoglobin A_2 and F are present in trace amounts (1.5%–3% and 0%–2%, respectively). Adult hemoglobin is a tetramer composed of two α and two β chains, hemoglobin A_2 has two α and two δ chains, and hemoglobin F consists of two α and two γ chains. The synthesis of α chains is controlled by four genes, and deletions in these genes result in varying severity of disease from mild (1–2 gene deletions) to severe (3–4 gene deletions). A slight decrease in α-chain production (1–2 gene deletions) automatically leads to a proportional decrease in hemoglobin A, A_2, and F. Since hemoglobin electrophoresis detects only abnormal hemoglobins or an increase in a hemoglobin, it is normal in mild α thalassemia. In severe forms of α thalassemia (3–4 gene deletions), four β chains combine to form a tetramer called hemoglobin H or four γ chains combine to form hemoglobin Barts. Because these hemoglobins are abnormal, they are detected in a hemoglobin electrophoresis.

In β thalassemia, the decrease in β chains results in a decrease in hemoglobin A. There is an increase in hemoglobins A_2 and F because α-, β-, δ-, and γ-chain syntheses are unaffected.

An unexplained finding in the thalassemias in general is a normal to increased RBC count in the presence of a reduced hemoglobin concentration and mean corpuscular volume (MCV). This has spawned a number of ratios that are useful in differentiating thalassemia from other microcytic anemias (e.g., iron deficiency and the anemia of inflammation). The Mentzer index is the ratio of MCV to RBC count. A value less than 13 is highly predictive for thalassemia, whereas values greater than 13 usually indicate iron deficiency or anemia of inflammation. In this patient, the ratio is 12 (70/5.8). The red cell distribution width, or RDW, is a measure of RBC shape. Abnormally shaped cells increase the RDW. When working through the differential diagnosis of a microcytic anemia, iron deficiency, anemia of inflammation, thalassemia, and sideroblastic anemias are the prime suspects. The RDW is most consistently abnormal in iron deficiency, whereas it is usually normal in all the other microcytic anemias.

Mild α thalassemia, or α thalassemia minor, is a diagnosis of exclusion. If the hemoglobin electrophoresis is normal previously and the listed findings for thalassemia are present, the diagnosis is α thalassemia minor. However, if the hemoglobin electrophoresis indicates an increase in hemoglobin A_2 and F, the patient has β thalassemia minor. Iron studies are normal in mild $\alpha\beta$ thalassemia and are not indicated in the initial workup of these patients. Severe forms of either disease (e.g., hemoglobin Bart's disease or β thalassemia major) are uncommon in the United States. There is no specific treatment for thalassemia.

Regarding the other mechanisms listed in the question, absent iron stores indicate iron deficiency. Iron blockade is associated with the anemia of inflammation. Hemolysis of RBCs is present only in very severe forms of thalassemia. Decreased heme synthesis characterizes the sideroblastic anemias, which could be due to lead poisoning, pyridoxine deficiency, and the toxic effect of alcohol, to name only a few.

64. The answer is A. *(Psychiatry; multiple personality disorder)*
Patients with multiple personality disorder report a much higher incidence of childhood sexual abuse than those individuals with an antisocial personality disorder, major depression, hypochondriasis, or autism. Childhood sexual abuse is also associated with borderline personality disorder. Adult violence is sometimes associated with a history of childhood physical abuse.

65. The answer is D. *(Biostatistics; probability)*
Clinical significance and statistical significance are different entities; therefore, option A is incorrect. Similarly, option B is incorrect because it alludes to clinical benefit, which cannot be determined by P value alone. Option C would be correct if the word "effective" were changed to "ineffective." Therefore, option D is correct. Option E is erroneous: If the number of subjects were increased (assuming that the means and the standard deviations of the groups remained the same), the P value would tend to be more, rather than less, significant.

66. The answer is D. *(Neurology; vasculopathic third nerve palsy)*
Vasculopathic third nerve palsy is the correct diagnosis because the third nerve deficit (rotation outward from medial rectus weakness and ptosis from levator palpebrae weakness) is associated with a normal pupillary size. A compressive lesion such as an aneurysm or a tumor would compress the dorsomedial portion of the third nerve and cause a dilated, unreactive pupil. This distinction is important because a third nerve lesion that is pupillary-sparing is generally nonemergent, whereas lesions that involve the pupil are best considered medical emergencies. Cavernous sinus thrombosis, although possible, is less likely because it would generally involve other cranial nerves as well. A superior oblique palsy (from fourth cranial nerve damage) is usually traumatic in cause and would not present with eyelid abnormality. Intranuclear ophthalmoplegia from interruption of the medial longitudinal fasciculus could be either vasculopathic or demyelinative in cause, but would have promi-

nent sixth nerve (abducent nerve) palsies and spared medial rectus function on convergence.

67. The answer is C. *(Gynecology; disseminated gonorrhea)*
Fever and skin rash can be manifestations of a number of the options listed. However, the presence of a joint effusion along with a fever and skin rash in a sexually active young woman is highly suggestive of disseminated gonococcemia. Aspiration of the effusion and Gram's staining of the fluid can confirm the diagnosis if intracellular gram-negative diplococci are found.

68. The answer is A. *(Psychiatry; developmental disorder)*
Fragile X syndrome has been associated with mental retardation and autistic symptoms. Turner's syndrome is associated with various cognitive, social, and behavioral problems. Klinefelter's syndrome is associated with cognitive and emotional difficulties. Trisomy 21 is associated with mental retardation and Alzheimer's disease.

69. The answer is A. *(Pediatrics; tetralogy of Fallot)*
Classic tetralogy of Fallot consists of pulmonic stenosis, overriding aorta, right ventricular hypertrophy, and ventricular septal defect. Fallot's tetralogy is the most common congenital heart disease with cyanosis, although cyanosis may not be present at birth. Typical chest x-ray shows a boot-shaped heart (coeur en sabot) with diminished pulmonary vascular markings. Patients are at higher risk for cerebral thromboses and brain abscess. Treatment is surgical. Prognosis depends on the degree of pulmonic stenosis, which determines the degrees of hypoxemia and right ventricular hypertrophy.

70. The answer is C. *(General surgery; bloody nipple discharge)*
Bloody nipple discharge in a woman under 50 years of age is most commonly caused by an intraductal papilloma located in the lactiferous duct. In most cases, a mass is not palpable. The involved duct is identified by applying pressure

circumferentially around the nipple to see which lactiferous duct is emptying blood. Cytology can be performed on this material. Intraductal papillomas can be multicentric (involve other ducts) or can involve the contralateral breast in 25% of cases. A segmental resection of the lactiferous duct is recommended.

A bloody nipple discharge in a woman older than 50 years of age is most commonly associated with malignancy. Any bloody discharge from a male nipple is usually due to malignancy. A subareolar abscess, most commonly due to *Staphylococcus aureus,* would produce a purulent nipple discharge. Intraductal papillomatosis refers to ductal hyperplasia in fibrocystic change.

A green–brown nipple discharge in a premenopausal woman just prior to menstruation is usually due to mammary duct ectasia (plasma cell mastitis). The material is debris that collects in dilated lactiferous ducts. The ducts are surrounded by a heavy plasma cell infiltrate. Milky discharge (galactorrhea) in a woman can be due to a prolactinoma in the anterior pituitary (the most common pituitary tumor), primary hypothyroidism [decreased thyroxine (T_4) causes an increase in thyrotropin-releasing hormone, which is a potent stimulator, or prolactin], and various drugs (e.g., birth control pills, chlorpromazine). Clear, serous, or milky discharges are frequently associated with birth control pills, particularly prior to the onset of menses.

71. The answer is B. (*Obstetrics; puerperal sepsis*)
Prolonged premature membrane rupture and emergency cesarean delivery are predisposing factors for puerperal sepsis. The response of this patient's fever to intravenous heparin, following a failed response to adequate parenteral antibiotic therapy, strongly suggests septic pelvic thrombophlebitis as the best diagnosis. Tubo-ovarian abscess usually requires drainage, and retained placenta requires tissue removal for a response to occur. Acute endometritis and pyelonephritis generally respond to appropriate broad-spectrum antibiotic coverage.

72–73. The answers are: 72-E, 73-C. (*Pharmacology; respiratory drugs*)
Parenteral glucocorticoids and β_2-selective adrenoceptor agonists by aerosol are appropriate for acute management in this situation. Maximal bronchodilation occurs within 30 minutes following metaproterenol or albuterol via aerosol. The clinical signs are not consistent with excessive use of the inhaler. Because the current prophylactic regimen appears to have limited efficacy, a course of glucocorticoids given on alternate days (to avoid pituitary suppression) may be appropriate. Cromolyn is not effective in reversing asthmatic bronchospasm.

No β_2-agonist drug in clinical use is completely selective, and cardiac effects may occur through β_1-receptor activation. Cromolyn does not exert its prophylactic effects in asthma through blockade of muscarinic receptors. Tolerance does not occur with methylxanthines, but their effectiveness is limited by dose-dependent seizures or cardiotoxicity. Lipid-soluble glucocorticoids, including beclomethasone and flunisolide, are as effective as oral prednisone, but cause less systemic toxicity. Unlike other prophylactic treatments, the glucocorticoids decrease bronchial reactivity with chronic use.

74. The answer is A. (*Psychiatry; eating disorder*)
Frequent self-induced vomiting can cause caries and erosion of tooth enamel owing to gastric acid. Fingers can be abraded by insertion of fingers into the pharynx and by resultant scratches from teeth. Esophageal tears from self-induced vomiting are rare.

75. The answer is C. (*Dermatology; contact dermatitis*)
Contact dermatitis is a common inflammatory disorder of skin that is associated with exposure to various antigens and irritating substances. Four types have been described—allergic contact dermatitis, irritant contact dermatitis, contact photodermatitis, and contact urticaria.

Allergic contact dermatitis, of which this case is an example, is a cell-mediated type IV hypersensitivity reaction. Three conditions must be present for this reaction to occur, namely, a genetic predisposition, absorption of sufficient antigen through the skin surface, and a competent immune system. Antigenic substances of low molecular weight penetrate the skin, are phagocytized by Langerhans' cells, and are then transported to regional lymph nodes, where they are presented to T lymphocytes. The T lymphocytes release cytokines that are responsible for the inflammatory response in the tissue. Antigenic substances include rhus (found in poison ivy and poison oak), nickel (earrings, hair dyes), potassium dichromate (household cleaners, leather, cement), formaldehyde (cosmetics, fabrics), ethylenediamine (dyes, medications), mercaptobenzothiazole (rubber products), and paraphenylenediamine (hair dyes, chemicals in photography).

Because allergic contact dermatitis is a type IV hypersensitivity reaction, the positive purified protein derivative (PPD) reaction, which involves the interaction of T cells and macrophages, most closely resembles the mechanism of inflammatory response in this patient. Irritant contact dermatitis is not a cell-mediated immune response. It is due to the local toxic effect of the chemical on the skin. Contact photodermatitis is similar to allergic contact dermatitis except that reaction depends on ultraviolet light. Contact urticaria is a wheal-and-flare reaction that may be secondary to a type I hypersensitivity (IgE-mediated) reaction or a nonimmunologic reaction. The clinical presentation of contact dermatitis, regardless of the mechanism, ranges from localized areas of erythema with vesicle formation to erythematous plaques of thickened skin in chronic disease. The treatment involves removal of the offending agent along with the use of wet compresses with Burow's solution in acute disease, followed by local application of steroid cream to suppress inflammation. Subacute or chronic cases should be treated with local steroid creams without the compresses. Extensive disease may require the use of systemic corticosteroid therapy.

In terms of the other mechanisms listed in the question, type I hypersensitivity involves the interaction of immunoglobulin E (IgE) antibodies developed against specific antigens and mast cells. Reexposure to the antigen causes mast cell degranulation, with the release of histamine and other chemical mediators that produce increased vessel permeability, swelling of tissue, and an inflammatory reaction.

An Arthus reaction is a localized immune complex disease (type III hypersensitivity), which activates the complement system to produce anaphylatoxins and chemotactic agents that cause the inflammatory reaction. An example of an Arthus reaction is farmer's lung, in which exposure to a thermophilic actinomycetes in the air results in a localized immune complex deposition in the alveoli with subsequent inflammation and hypersensitivity pneumonitis. Systemic immune complex diseases, like systemic lupus erythematosus (SLE) or serum sickness, are also associated with immune complex deposition in various tissues, like the joints, skin, and vessels in the skin and glomerulus.

Antibody-dependent, cell-mediated cytotoxicity (ADCC) is a variant of type II hypersensitivity. It involves the presence of antibody against a target tissue, which attracts killer cells, natural killer cells, or macrophages. These cells interact with the antibodies and destroy the target tissue. Warm autoimmune hemolytic anemia, with destruction of IgG antibody-coated red blood cells (RBCs) by macrophages in the spleen, is a classic example of an ADCC reaction.

76. The answer is E. (*Obstetrics; puerperal sepsis*) With puerperal fever, unresponsive to appropriate antibiotic therapy, it is imperative to rule out a pelvic abscess before instituting long-duration intravenous heparin for a presumptive diagnosis of septic pelvic thrombophlebitis. Acute pelvic inflammatory disease (PID) is unlikely with the antibiotic therapy she has had. A retained placenta is unlikely with normal lochial flow. Peritoneal blood does not cause persistent fever.

77. The answer is C. (*General surgery; laboratory parameters in acute hemorrhage*) Volume loss from hemorrhage is first detected by a drop in the central venous pressure or capillary wedge pressure in the lungs. The hemoglobin and hematocrit often remain normal for 1 to 3 days since an equal amount of plasma and red blood cells are lost and the vascular tree contracts around the reduced volume of blood. Plasma is the first to be restored as fluid moves from the interstitial space into the blood vessels. This uncovers the deficit in the red blood cells, resulting in a drop in the hemoglobin and hematocrit. Intravenous administration of isotonic saline uncovers this deficit faster. The reticulocyte count, which represents the marrow response to anemia, increases in 5 to 7 days after a hemorrhage. An increased count reflects effective erythropoiesis in the bone marrow, which will replace the deficit in red blood cells, in the peripheral blood.

Anemia does not alter the pH, oxygen partial pressure (P_{O_2}), or carbon dioxide partial pressure (P_{CO_2}) of blood. However, it does reduce the total amount of oxygen available to tissue, thus producing tissue hypoxia. The oxygen saturation, which represents the total number of binding sites on hemoglobin that are occupied by oxygen, is normal since there is normal oxygenation of hemoglobin in the pulmonary capillaries. The problem in anemia is a decrease in hemoglobin, which automatically lowers the total oxygen content of blood.

78. The answer is B. (*Gynecology; anovulation*)
The description of this young woman, in the beginning of her reproductive life, is characteristic of anovulation with unopposed estrogen. The expected finding would be a proliferative histologic picture (B) without evidence of ovulation (A), endometrial carcinoma (C and E), or pregnancy (D).

79. The answer is E. (*Psychiatry; eating disorder*)
Family dynamics are strongly implicated in the development of anorexia nervosa. Patients' mothers are often seen as overly controlling and fathers are seen as inhibited and compulsive. Food restriction and weight loss are postulated as attempts to regain some control and, perhaps, avoid sexual issues. Psychotherapeutic intervention often involves family therapy.

80. The answer is C. (*Pediatrics; differential cyanosis; heart diseases*)
Differential cyanosis is seen when blood shunts from right to left across a patent ductus arteriosus in the presence of a coarctation or interrupted aortic arch. The patient has blue lower extremities and pink upper torso and extremities. Other signs of patent ductus arteriosus include bounding pulses and a to-and-fro machinery murmur.

81. The answer is B. (*Obstetrics; severe preeclampsia*)
Hypertensive disorders of pregnancy are among the main causes of maternal mortality in the United States. This patient's condition is characteristic of severe preeclampsia. Appropriate management is stabilization, prevention of seizures using magnesium sulfate, and then prompt delivery. Ritodrine, terbutaline, and indomethacin are tocolytics and would be contraindicated in this patient. Progesterone administration has no demonstrable indication in severe preeclampsia.

82. The answer is C. (*Psychiatry; adjustment disorder*)
An adjustment disorder can be diagnosed only if the symptoms are not part of a longer term pattern of overreaction to stressors. Situations and stressors that cause adjustment disorder vary greatly from individual to individual; moreover, they are not necessarily catastrophic. The duration of an adjustment disorder is, by definition, quite brief. It resolves when the stressor goes away or the patient learns to live with it.

83. The answer is D. (*General surgery; treatment of steatorrhea in chronic pancreatitis*)
Chronic pancreatitis produces steatorrhea (increased fat in the stool) because of a deficiency of lipase. Undigested lipid and fat-soluble vitamins are lost in the stool. Oral pancreatic enzyme preparations high in lipase before, during, and after the meal, with concurrent administration of a histamine$_2$ (H_2) antagonist to block inactivation of the enzyme by acid, facilitates absorption of fats. In addition, the patient should be on a low-fat diet.

A broad-spectrum antibiotic would not enhance lipid absorption, since bacterial overgrowth is not part of the pathophysiology of chronic pancreatitis. Bacterial overgrowth produces bile salt deficiency, which leads to steatorrhea. A gluten-free diet is the therapy of choice for celiac disease, which is the most common cause of malabsorption. Total pancreatectomy is a treatment option in chronic pancreatitis if intractable pain is present that is not amenable to medical therapy.

84. The answer is E. *(Pharmacology; cardiac drugs)*
Angiotensin converting enzyme (ACE) inhibitors such as captopril are now considered first-line agents (along with diuretics and digitalis) in the management of chronic heart failure. Their efficacy is equal to that of digoxin, with a more favorable therapeutic index. Captopril has no direct actions on the heart, but decreases cardiac work via peripheral vasodilation. In some patients, ACE inhibitors have been used concomitantly with cardiac glycosides. Maximal cardiac benefits of thiazides in heart failure directly parallel maximal diuretic response (this is not true in terms of their beneficial effects in hypertension).

85. The answer is A. *(Clinical immunology; transplantation)*
The basic concept in transplantation is that the recipient of a graft will accept the donor graft if no foreign antigens are present or will reject the graft if foreign antigens are present.

In choice A, the mother, who is XXXX, is the donor; and the child, who is XXOO, is the recipient. There are no foreign antigens in the mother's graft; therefore, it is accepted. In the other choices, the donor graft contains antigens that are foreign to the recipient; therefore, they are rejected.

86. The answer is B. *(Obstetrics; multiple gestation)*
Twin gestation increases risk for a variety of maternal and fetal complications. Pregnancy-induced hypertension risks are increased with twins. Although urinary tract infection, diabetes, and

moniliasis are increased in pregnancy, they are not influenced by the number of fetuses. Multiple gestation increases rather than decreases maternal serum alpha-fetoprotein (MSAFP).

87. The answer is A. *(Neurology; viral meningitis)*
A slightly low or normal glucose with a slightly elevated protein and a modest lymphocytosis is common for aseptic meningitis, although variation is common. A bacterial meningitis would best fit the profile in choice B, as shown by a remarkable leukocytosis with a left shift and an elevated protein with a very low glucose. An atypical infection such as tuberculosis (TB) or cryptococcal meningitis could fit choice D, although organisms visible on smears or cultures would be necessary to cement the diagnosis. The description in choice C would best fit a normal spinal fluid profile. Choice E could be normal, although the very low cerebrospinal fluid (CSF) glucose also might be seen in patients with benign intracranial hypertension (pseudotumor cerebri).

88. The answer is C. *(Psychiatry; obsessive-compulsive disorder)*
This case is most suggestive of obsessive-compulsive disorder. Serotonin has been implicated in obsessive-compulsive disorder because many of the most effective medications are serotonin agonists. Other neurotransmitters have not been specifically linked to it.

89. The answer is A. *(General surgery; third-space fluid loss)*
Third-space fluid loss refers to extracellular fluid sequestered from the plasma compartment. It reduces functional extracellular fluid; therefore, the patient is hypovolemic. However, since it is isotonic fluid, the serum sodium concentration is usually normal.

Inflammation associated with bacterial or chemical (e.g., bile, amylase) peritonitis results in a widespread increase of bowel permeability to interstitial fluid containing protein and electrolytes. In general, it is estimated that 1 L of extracellular fluid is sequestered in each of the abdominal quadrants that are traumatized (surgery) or inflamed (peritonitis).

Other conditions associated with third-space fluid loss to a lesser degree are acute pancreatitis, bowel obstruction, severe burns, severe muscle injury, and generalized sepsis. Acute appendicitis and acute cholecystitis do not result in significant third-space fluid loss. Fluids lost by vomiting and diarrhea are not sequestered, so they are not considered third-space fluids. However, the result is significant hypovolemia.

Reabsorption of third-space fluid in the healing process can result in significant volume overload.

90. The answer is A. *(Gynecology; pelvic relaxation)*
Urinary stress incontinence develops when the proximal urethra drops below the pelvic floor because of pelvic relaxation defects. This condition is frequently associated with a cystocele, the bulging of the bladder into the upper anterior vaginal wall. A urethral diverticulum is diagnosed via urethroscopy. Rectocele is associated with bulging of the posterior vaginal wall. Enterocele is herniation of the pouch of Douglas into the upper posterior vaginal wall. Rhabdomyosarcoma is extremely rare.

91. The answer is B. *(Pediatrics; bronchiolitis)*
Bronchiolitis results from inflammatory obstruction of the smaller airways. The inflammation occurs during the first 2 years of life, with a peak incidence at 6 to 12 months of age. Bronchiolitis starts insidiously as an upper respiratory infection—but develops to include wheezy cough, dyspnea, and tachypnea. Physical examination reveals tachypnea, nasal flaring, rales, wheezes, and retractions. Patients start showing gradual improvement after 72 hours in uncomplicated cases. Asthma can easily be confused with bronchiolitis, but asthma usually includes a history of repeated attacks of wheezing and a family history of asthma. Croup is characterized by a brassy, barking cough. Epiglottitis occurs in older children and is associated with fever, severe respiratory distress, and drooling. Cystic fibrosis presents with recurrent pulmonary infections, failure to thrive, and malabsorption.

92. The answer is D. *(Psychiatry; panic disorder)*
This case is most suggestive of separation anxiety disorder. A history of this disorder is common in adult patients with panic disorder. Schizophrenia is sometimes associated with a history of emotional withdrawal during childhood.

93. The answer is A. *(Behavioral science; health care costs)*
The elderly incur 30% of all health care costs. This figure is expected to reach 50% by 2020.

94. The answer is B. *(Clinical immunology; IgA deficiency and anaphylactic shock with blood products)*
Immunoglobulin A (IgA) deficiency is the most common immunodeficiency. It occurs in 1 in 500 individuals. There is an intrinsic defect in the differentiation of B cells committed to synthesizing IgA. Both circulating and secretory IgA are deficient; therefore, these patients are subject to mucosal problems, such as recurrent sinopulmonary infections, allergies, and diarrhea secondary to *Giardia* and other organisms. There is also an increased incidence of autoimmune disease. In some patients, a selective deficiency of IgG2 and IgG4 subclasses predisposes them to bacterial infections.

Exposure to blood products containing IgA (through blood transfusion) often sensitizes these patients to IgA, and they develop antibodies against IgA. Reexposure to IgA causes an anaphylactic reaction. Patients should not receive blood products containing IgA. If transfusions are necessary, blood from IgA-deficient patients must be used.

A hemolytic transfusion reaction, contamination of the immune serum globulin, and a type IV hypersensitivity reaction are not associated with the administration of this product and would not explain the patient's history of sinopulmonary disease and asthma.

95. The answer is A. *(Obstetrics; fetal lung maturity assessment)*
Of the options listed, only the lecithin/sphingomyelin ratio is specific for fetal lung maturity.

Vernix suggests skin maturity, femoral epiphysis ossification suggests long bone maturity, elevated amniotic fluid creatinine suggests renal maturity, but none are specific for pulmonary function. Amniotic fluid ferning is present throughout pregnancy.

96. The answer is A. *(General surgery; arteriovenous fistula)*

The patient has an arteriovenous (AV) fistula, which is most commonly a result of a penetrating injury (e.g., knife wound). Other causes of AV fistulas include congenital causes, which can result in hemihypertrophy of an extremity; erosion of an arterial graft or aneurysm into a subjacent vein; and bone disease, such as Paget's disease of the bone, in which the remodeling of bone creates intramarrow AV communications.

A continuous machinery murmur is usually heard on auscultation of an AV fistula. Proximally, the arteries and veins are dilated. The distal pulse is usually diminished in amplitude. Compression of the mass results in slowing of the pulse rate. This is called Branham's sign. Since an AV fistula bypasses the microcirculation, there is an increase in venous return to the right heart, which results in a high-output failure.

Magnetic resonance imaging (MRI) and angiography are very useful in delineating these lesions. Heart failure in this patient is an indication for surgical removal or embolization of the lesion under radiographic control.

97. The answer is C. *(Pediatrics; ruptured tension pneumatocyst)*

Sudden deterioration of respiratory status should lead one to suspect pneumothorax. Clinically, decreased breath sounds are heard on the affected side. X-ray shows extrapulmonary air, with deviation of the trachea away from the affected side. *Staphylococcus aureus* frequently causes pneumatocyst, which can rupture and create a pneumothorax. Empyema and pleural effusions are also caused by *S. aureus,* but these effusions have a different radiologic appearance.

98. The answer is E. *(Obstetrics; diagnosis of pregnancy)*

Presumptive signs are primarily those associated with skin and mucous membrane changes, such as Chadwick's sign. Mapping of the fetal outline by palpation, ballottement of the fetus, softening of the uterine isthmus, and palpation of uterine contractions are probable signs of pregnancy and are related to detectable physical changes in the uterus.

99. The answer is D. *(Behavioral science; acquired immune deficiency syndrome)*

Acquired immune deficiency syndrome (AIDS) is the leading cause of death in men 25 to 44 years old in the United States. It is the third leading cause of death in black women and the sixth in white women (*New York Times,* 11/93).

100. The answer is A. *(Infectious disease; traveler's diarrhea)*

Traveler's diarrhea is caused by bacterial enteropathogens in at least 80% of cases; of these, enterotoxigenic *Escherichia coli* is responsible for 50% to 75% of cases. Enterotoxins elaborated by the organism stimulate cyclic adenosine monophosphate (cAMP), resulting in a secretory diarrhea similar in mechanism to cholera. No mucosal damage is associated with the enterotoxin. The majority of cases are due to ingestion of contaminated food and, to a lesser degree, contaminated water.

Traveler's diarrhea occurs in people who reside in an industrialized country and travel to a developing tropical or semitropical country. It is defined as the passage of at least three to ten unformed stools in 24 hours, associated with low-grade fever, nausea and vomiting, abdominal cramps, and urgent stools with or without mucus and with or without blood. In 10% of patients, the diarrhea lasts longer than 1 week.

Drugs that are useful for prophylaxis include doxycycline, trimethoprim–sulfamethoxazole combination, fluoroquinolones, and bismuth subsalicylate.

Other causes of traveler's diarrhea include *Shigella* species, *Campylobacter jejuni, Salmonella* species, and rotavirus. Species like

Shigella and *Campylobacter* invade the bowel mucosa to produce mucosal injury and an inflammatory diarrhea with production of an exudate.

Acquired disaccharidase deficiencies commonly occur as a secondary event in gastroenteritis resulting from the loss of brush-border enzymes (e.g., lactase). This inflammation could produce an osmotic diarrhea secondary to the osmotic effect of undigested carbohydrate in the bowel as well as the osmotic effect of fatty acids from the breakdown of carbohydrate by colonic bacteria.

Toxin-induced damage of the mucosa is operative in pseudomembranous colitis because of *Clostridium difficile* overgrowth in patients on antibiotics such as ampicillin or clindamycin.

101. The answer is B. *(Psychiatry; drug abuse)*
Seizures are associated with benzodiazepine withdrawal. Other symptoms of benzodiazepine withdrawal include anxiety, insomnia, and psychosis. Seizures are not associated with withdrawal from opiates, cocaine, LSD, or marijuana.

102. The answer is E. *(Neurology; magnetic resonance imaging)*
With progressive deficits related to the posterior fossa (cerebellum and brain stem), a space-occupying lesion such as a tumor (medulloblastoma, ependymoma, brain-stem glioma) should be immediately excluded. Because of the presence of bone in the posterior fossa, a magnetic resonance imaging (MRI) scan is more sensitive than a computed tomography (CT) scan. Because of the progressive rather than acute nature, an electroencephalogram (EEG) or drug screen would be less likely to be diagnostic, although it might be considered in an acute process. Aminoacidurias tend to present at an earlier age.

103. The answer is C. *(Gynecology; ovarian tumors)*
Endocrinologically functioning (not functional) ovarian tumors include the granulosa-theca cell tumor, which promotes feminizing signs and symptoms, and the Sertoli-Leydig cell tumor, which promotes virilizing signs and symptoms,

as in this patient. Brenner's tumor, fibroma, and dysgerminoma are not endocrinologically active.

104. The answer is E. *(Pediatrics; measles-mumps-rubella vaccine)*
The measles-mumps-rubella (MMR) vaccine is first given at 15 months of age. A repeat vaccination is currently recommended at entrance to school or at 10 to 12 years of age. Immunization earlier than 15 months of age is recommended if the child is traveling to endemic areas.

105. The answer is C. *(General surgery; thyroid nodules and malignancy)*
The majority (60%) of solitary nodules in the thyroid gland are not neoplastic and represent cysts or a goiter. Approximately 25% are follicular adenomas, and the remaining 15% are malignant. Factors that suggest malignancy in a solitary nodule are: a history of previous irradiation of the neck; any solitary nodule in a man or a child; a hard, irregular nodule with cervical lymphadenopathy, or one that is greater than 3 cm to 4 cm; serum thyroglobulin greater than 100 ng/dl; a family history of a medullary carcinoma of the thyroid suggesting multiple endocrine neoplasia (MEN) IIa or IIb syndrome.

In managing a solitary nodule, some clinicians begin with ultrasound to see if the nodule is cystic or solid, while others first perform fine-needle aspiration. If the fine-needle aspiration is positive for cancer, surgery is performed. If it is inconclusive, a thyroid scan is ordered. A cold nodule is treated by surgery; a hot nodule is observed. Hot nodules are rarely malignant.

106. The answer is C. *(Psychiatry; violence)*
A history of violence is the strongest predictor of future violence. Alcohol abuse and persecutory delusions are not as strongly associated with violence. Temporal lobe epilepsy is rarely associated with premeditated violence.

107. The answer is E. *(Gynecology; secondary amenorrhea)*
For this patient with secondary amenorrhea, the height/weight discordance suggests anorexia nervosa. Turner's syndrome is associated with short

stature and primary amenorrhea. Hypogonadotropic hypogonadism is associated with absence of secondary sexual development. Patients with polycystic ovary disease are usually overweight. Asherman's syndrome arises from intrauterine synechiae following overzealous curettage.

108. The answer is B. *(Behavioral science; leading causes of death)*
The leading causes of death in the United States across age-groups in descending order are heart disease, cancer, and stroke. Women are more likely to have strokes than men; men are more likely to die as a result of a heart attack. Increased smoking in women has resulted in increased cancer deaths for women.

109. The answer is D. *(Obstetrics; nutrition in pregnancy)*
Iron supplementation with folate is the best choice of the options listed. Although vitamin supplementation in pregnancy is ubiquitous, there is no evidence that the outcome of a normal pregnancy is enhanced with supplementation of vitamin C, B complex, or B_{12}. Bone marrow iron stores in women are half those in men. Iron deficiency anemia is eight times more common in women than in men worldwide.

110. The answer is D. *(General surgery; MEN IIa syndrome)*
A patient with a parathyroid adenoma, pheochromocytoma, and a mass in the thyroid most likely has a medullary carcinoma of the thyroid and the autosomal-dominant disease called multiple endocrine neoplasia (MEN) syndrome, type IIa. Medullary carcinomas of the thyroid derive from C cells, which synthesize calcitonin. Only 10% of cases are familial and associated with MEN IIa or IIb; for this type, serum calcitonin is the best screen. A provocative stimulation test using pentagastrin or calcium can be used on family members to identify those who are at risk for developing medullary carcinoma. The other 90% of cases are sporadic. Serum thyroid-stimulating hormone (TSH) and serum thyroxine (T_4) levels are normal in patients with medullary carcinoma. An

iodine 131 (^{131}I) scan would be of no additional value in working up the patient.

Patients are treated with a total thyroidectomy and neck dissection. Patients with the familial variant have a 50% 5-year survival rate. Those with MEN IIa have a better survival than those with MEN IIb (medullary carcinoma, pheochromocytoma, mucosal neuromas).

111. The answer is C. *(Pediatrics; neonatal hypoglycemia in premature infants)*
Premature and low–birth-weight infants have inadequate stores of fat and glycogen. Consequently, they are at high risk for hypoglycemia. Early, frequent feedings help avoid this problem. Infants of diabetic mothers tend to be macrosomic. Their hypoglycemia is caused by relative hyperinsulinism.

112. The answer is D. *(Psychiatry; psychosis)*
Hallucinations are common in both delirium and schizophrenia. Gross cognitive impairment and severe memory problems are much more common in delirium. Elaborate delusions and a prolonged clinical course are much more characteristic of schizophrenia.

113. The answer is D. *(Behavioral science; death in adolescents)*
Accidents are the most common cause of death in adolescents, and 75% of these accidents occur in automobiles. Suicide and homicide are the second and third leading causes of death in adolescents. Children 13 years of age and younger are most likely to die as a result of accidents, cancer, and congenital abnormalities.

114. The answer is D. *(Cardiology; high-output and low-output failure)*
The cardiac output equals stroke volume times heart rate. Stroke volume is determined by afterload (resistance that the heart must overcome), preload (stretch on the ventricles), state of inotropy (contractility) of the heart, and synchronous contraction of the ventricles.

In hypertrophic cardiomyopathy, there is usually an asymmetric hypertrophy of the ventricular septum, with increased thickness of the free left ventricular wall. This condition decreases the left ventricular volume. The anterior leaflet of the mitral valve is closely approximated to the asymmetric interventricular septum and is drawn against that structure by the negative pressures created behind the ejected stream of blood, thereby obstructing blood flow and decreasing the cardiac output. Positive inotropic agents such as digitalis or β-agonists are contraindicated, because the increased force of contraction causes the anterior leaflet to obstruct the opening even earlier. Negative inotropic agents, such as propranolol decrease the force of contraction and also increase preload, thereby enhancing the cardiac output.

Early endotoxic shock, severe anemia, and thyrotoxicosis are associated with a high-output failure. High-output failure is the outcome of any condition that increases blood volume, increases positive inotropism (thyrotoxicosis), increases blood flow (decreased blood viscosity as in anemia), or decreases peripheral vascular resistance, with subsequent increase in venous return to the heart (early endotoxic shock with arteriolar vasodilation). Aortic regurgitation increases preload in the left ventricle, because blood drips back into the left ventricle in diastole, thereby increasing the left ventricular end-diastolic pressure and stroke volume.

115. The answer is D. *(Psychiatry; cognitive disorders)*
Dementia differs from delirium in that it often has a lengthy course. Delirium, by contrast, develops rapidly and usually has a short course. Both delirium and dementia can present with memory impairment and cognitive impairment. For both syndromes, the prognosis and the presence of structural central nervous system (CNS) disease depend on the nature of the underlying cause.

116. The answer is E. *(Gynecology; toxic shock syndrome)*
Toxic shock syndrome (TSS) is a rare, potentially fatal, multisystem condition associated with strains of staphylococci-producing toxins, including an epidermal exfoliative toxin. It has

been reported in menstruating women who leave tampons in place for a prolonged period of time. The case presented is classic for TSS because of the desquamating rash that distinguishes it from the other options listed.

117. The answer is E. *(Psychiatry; psychosis)*
A delusion of reference involves the assignment of personal significance to neutral events. Such a delusion, along with delusions of persecution and jealousy, are often a component of paranoia. They are common in paranoid schizophrenia, organic delusional disorders, and delusional disorder.

118. The answer is A. *(Pediatrics; systemic lupus erythematosus)*
The most common cause of congenital complete heart block is autoimmune injury by maternal immunoglobulin G (IgG) antibodies in a mother with systemic lupus erythematosus (SLE). The exact mechanism of damage is unknown. Most infants have mothers with antibodies to Ro/SSA or La/SSB. The heart damage may be permanent.

119. The answer is D. *(Gynecology; endometrial cancer)*
Cancer of the endometrium is the most common gynecologic malignancy in the United States and occurs twice as frequently as cervical cancer. It is the fourth most common malignancy found in women after breast, colorectal, and lung cancer.

120. The answer is C. *(Psychiatry; psychosis)*
Psychosis is clinically identified by the presence of hallucinations, delusions, or illogical thinking with grossly disorganized behavior. Since a delusion is a patently false belief, it would include the belief that his thoughts are controlled by secret television messages.

121. The answer is B. *(Pediatrics; parvovirus infection in mother)*
Pregnant women infected by parvovirus may be asymptomatic or have nonspecific symptoms. Fetal infection occurs via transplacental passage of virus and can result in stillbirth and nonimmune hydrops fetalis. Parvovirus is not consid-

ered a teratogen and is not associated with a typical syndrome. Chorioretinitis and microcephaly are seen in congenital toxoplasmosis. Rhagades and Hutchinson's teeth are typical findings of congenital syphilis.

122. The answer is A. *(General surgery; inflammatory carcinoma)*
The patient has inflammatory carcinoma of the breast. This cancer is characterized by a painful breast mass, with the overlying skin exhibiting edema, warmth, and erythema due to plugging of the dermal lymphatics by the tumor. It is the most malignant type of breast cancer and accounts for less than 3% of all cases. Metastasis occurs early, and the prognosis is extremely poor. Approximately 75% of patients already have axillary node involvement at presentation. Modified radical mastectomy is rarely performed. Radiation, hormone therapy, and chemotherapy are the mainstays of treatment.

Paget's disease of the breast (1% of breast cancers), most common in elderly women, presents as a scaly, eczematous rash usually involving the nipple. Unlike extramammary Paget's disease involving the vulva, the breast variant is always associated with an underlying cancer, which extends up into and involves the epidermis.

Cystosarcoma phyllodes is the most common malignant stromal tumor of the breast. It produces massive breast enlargement. The stroma is hypercellular, but the epithelial elements are benign. Whether low or high grade in its appearance, it rarely metastasizes to the axillary nodes and is treated with simple mastectomy.

Erysipelas is a brawny cellulitis associated with group A streptococci. Although it can simulate inflammatory carcinoma, it responds rapidly to antibiotics.

123. The answer is C. *(Obstetrics; ovarian tumors in pregnancy)*
Adnexal disease can coexist with pregnancy. Neoplastic ovarian masses must be ruled out. However, for this patient, the most likely diagnosis is a corpus luteum cyst that will spontaneously involute. Malignant adnexal masses are rare in this age-group.

124. The answer is D. *(Psychiatry; depression)*
Flight of ideas refers to a rapid flow of thoughts, often unconnected or tenuously related to one another. This condition is commonly associated with pathologically accelerated psychomotor activity, such as is seen in the manic phase of bipolar disorder.

125. The answer is E. *(Behavioral science; sleep apnea)*
In sleep apnea, the person stops breathing for a time. Anoxia then awakens him during the night and he becomes chronically tired. The elderly are at higher risk for sleep apnea. In narcolepsy, a patient falls asleep suddenly during the daytime. In insomnia, the person has difficulty initiating or maintaining sleep. In sleep–wake schedule disorder, patients sleep at the wrong time. Kleine-Levin syndrome includes periods of hypersomnia and hyperphagia.

126. The answer is B. *(Nephrology; acute drug-induced tubulointerstitial disease)*
The constellation of findings in acute drug-induced tubulointerstitial disease includes fever, sudden onset of oliguria, proteinuria (sometimes in the nephrotic range), skin rash, eosinophilia, and eosinophiluria (eosinophils in the urinary sediment). Various types of hypersensitivity reactions have been implicated, including type I (IgE-mediated), type II (antibodies), and type IV (cytotoxic T cells). The disease is a reversible cause of renal failure, because withdrawal of the drug reverses the disease. Failure to recognize the disorder results in renal failure in 50% of cases. Methicillin is the prototypical drug causing the disease. Other associated drugs include ampicillin, penicillin, cephalosporins, thiazides, furosemide, and nonsteroidal anti-inflammatory drugs (NSAIDs). The value of glucocorticoids in the treatment of the disease has not been established.

Drug-induced immune-complex glomerulonephritis commonly presents as a nephrotic syndrome, usually membranous glomerulonephritis. Proteinuria is greater than 3.5 g/24 hours. Ampicillin is not associated with this type of renal disease.

Acute pyelonephritis developing from a lower urinary tract infection would be associated with costovertebral angle pain, white blood cell (WBC) casts and pus in the urine, and a neutrophilic leukocytosis rather than an eosinophilia.

Endotoxic shock, presumably arising from an *Escherichia coli* septicemia, is more likely to be associated with acute pyelonephritis than with acute cystitis. The clinical course would be associated with the development of warm shock, which is not evident in this patient.

127. The answer is E. *(Obstetrics; pelvic diameters)*
The diameters of the pelvic planes represent the amount of space available at each level. The posterior sagittal diameter is always less than 10 cm. The diameters of the true conjugate, obstetric conjugate, bispinous, and diagonal conjugate average more than 10 cm in length.

128. The answer is C. *(Pediatrics; sudden infant death syndrome)*
Sudden infant death syndrome (SIDS) is the most common cause of death in children in the first year of life. Cancer causes more deaths than any other disease in children between 1 and 15 years of age.

129. The answer is A. *(Psychiatry; suicide)*
Some studies have shown lower levels of serotonin and its metabolites in the cerebrospinal fluid (CSF) of suicide victims and suicide attempters. No other biochemical findings have been consistently found in such studies.

130. The answer is B. *(Pediatrics; malignancies in children)*
The most common malignancy in children is acute lymphocytic leukemia. Leukemias in general are the most common form of cancer in children, accounting for about one-third of all new cases. Brain tumors, the most common solid tumors, are second. Cerebellar astrocytomas are the most common of the posterior fossa tumors. Neuroblastomas comprise the most common tumor of the central nervous system (CNS). Bone tumors have an incidence of 5.6/million in white

children and 4.8/million in black children; osteosarcoma is the most common. Wilms' tumor accounts for almost all cases of renal cancer in children.

131. The answer is C. *(General surgery; lobular carcinoma of the breast)*
Lobular carcinoma is the most common malignancy of the terminal lobule. It accounts for 5% to 10% of all breast cancers and is frequently difficult to detect as a palpable mass on self-examination. Left untreated, lobular carcinoma in situ tends to become invasive in 20% to 30% of patients over a prolonged period of time (10 to 15 years). It is associated with a high degree of bilaterality in the same quadrant in the contralateral breast. The contralateral tumor can be another lobular cancer or a ductal cancer. The majority of in-situ lobular carcinomas are estrogen- and progesterone-receptor positive. Simultaneous bilateral breast cancer occurs in less than 1% of cases. The presence of a breast cancer in one breast places the patient at increased risk for cancer in the contralateral breast, which underscores the need for mammography of the contralateral breast at regular intervals.

132. The answer is B. *(Rheumatology; serum antibody tests in systemic lupus erythematosus)*
The serum antinuclear antibody (ANA) test is the gold-standard screening test to rule out systemic lupus erythematosus (SLE) and other collagen vascular diseases. The major groups of ANA are antibodies against DNA (both double- and single-stranded), histones and nonhistone proteins, and nucleolar antigens. The ANA provides a titer of the antibody as well as a pattern on immunofluorescence. The patterns include diffuse (homogeneous), speckled, rim (peripheral), and nucleolar. Some patterns are specific for certain diseases. For example, a rim pattern is usually associated with anti–double-stranded (ds) DNA, which is very specific for SLE with renal involvement. A nucleolar pattern is specific for progressive systemic sclerosis.

The two most specific antibodies (least number of false-positives) for SLE are anti-ds DNA (98%) and anti-Sm (Smith) [100%]. Anti-SSA

(Ro) and anti-SSB (La) are positive in Sjögren's syndrome in 70% to 95% and 60% to 90%, respectively. The presence of anti-SSA (Ro) in a pregnant woman with SLE has a high association with complete heart block in newborns. Anticentromere antibodies are present in 90% of patients with the CREST syndrome. Antimitochondrial antibodies are noted in more than 90% of cases of primary biliary cirrhosis. Antihistone antibodies are present in more than 95% of patients with drug-induced SLE (most commonly due to procainamide). Antiribonucleoproteins are seen in more than 95% of patients with mixed connective tissue disease.

133. The answer is E. *(Obstetrics; malpresentation)*
Malpresentation of the fetus in labor can result in abnormal labor patterns or difficult delivery. The attitude of the fetus is the degree of extension or flexion of the fetal head. Occipitoposterior position, frank breech presentation, oblique fetal lie, and sacrum anterior do not describe fetal attitude. Brow presentation is really a misnomer because it does not describe true presentation but rather the orientation of the head midway between full flexion and full extension.

134. The answer is E. *(Pediatrics; intelligence quotient)*
A child in second grade is approximately 8 years old. If she shows the intellectual ability of a 12 year old (sixth grader), her intelligence quotient (IQ) (using the IQ formula of mental age/chronological age × 100) is approximately 150. Intelligence quotients greater than 130 are in the very superior category. With respect to IQ scores, low average is 80–89, average is 90–109, high average is 110–119, and superior is 120–129.

135. The answer is C. *(Gynecology; human sexual response)*
The orgasmic phase of the female sexual response cycle is mediated through the sympathetic nervous system and is characterized by genital musculature contractions. Vascular transudation with vaginal lubrication, proximal vaginal tenting and expansion, erythematous rash over chest and neck, and vascular engorgement of the pelvic viscera all occur in the excitement phase and are mediated by the parasympathetic nervous system.

136. The answer is B. *(General surgery; esophageal varices secondary to portal hypertension)*
The patient has portal hypertension complicated by hematemesis secondary to ruptured esophageal varices. The most common cause of portal hypertension is alcoholic cirrhosis. Approximately 50% of the deaths in cirrhosis are due to ruptured varices.

Bleeding varices cannot be diagnosed on the clinical presentation alone and require an emergency endoscopy to localize the source of bleeding. Most experts agree that emergency endoscopy with cautery of the bleeding varices is the most important step in management. Ice water lavage and balloon tamponade with a Sengstaken-Blakemore tube are not commonly used now. An intravenous vasopressin drip is used in some cases. On rare occasions, an emergency end-to-side portacaval shunt is performed to decompress the varices. Sclerotherapy is effective in obliterating the vessels once the bleeding is controlled.

Pyloric obstruction secondary to duodenal ulcer disease can be associated with gastric ulcers and bleeding, but it does not fit the clinical presentation of this patient. Although hematemesis is most frequently associated with peptic ulcer disease, gastric ulcers are not commonly associated with cirrhosis and portal hypertension. There is, however, an increased incidence of duodenal ulcers. Esophageal carcinoma does not usually present with massive hematemesis. Dysphagia for solids, weakness, and weight loss are the usual presenting signs and symptoms.

137–140. The answers are: 137-C, 138-C, 139-D, 140-D. *(Pediatrics; cystic fibrosis)*
Cystic fibrosis is a multisystem disease with protean manifestations, and pancreatic exocrine insufficiency is responsible for most of them. Recurrent pulmonary infections, malabsorption, and failure to thrive are hallmarks. It is inherited

as an autosomal recessive trait and is the major cause of lung disease in children.

Recurrent infections result from an inability to clear thick secretions of mucus and bacteria from the respiratory tract. Sputum is positive for *Staphylococcus aureus* and *Pseudomonas aeruginosa*. Malabsorption results from deficiency of the exocrine glands of the pancreas and is present in over 85% of patients with cystic fibrosis. The malabsorption manifests as frequent, fatty stools and failure to thrive in the presence of ingestion of huge amounts of calories, and it can cause iron-deficiency anemia. The abdomen is protuberant, and maturation is delayed. Patients exhibit elevated sweat chloride levels, and a sweat chloride test is indicated to help establish the diagnosis.

Although liver enzymes are elevated and the liver is enlarged, there is no evidence of viral hepatitis. Approximately 30% of patients with cystic fibrosis have fatty infiltration in the liver. Biliary cirrhosis occurs from blockage of intrahepatic bile ducts but is rare early in life. Combined iron and folate deficiency is observed in this particular patient. Hemoglobin is 7.5 g/dl, and mean corpuscular volume is 90 μm³; the smear shows both micro- and macrocytosis. Pneumonia is suspected on physical examination due to the crepitant rales and dullness on percussion, and it is confirmed by x-ray, which shows consolidation of the left lower lobe. Vitamin deficiency results from malabsorption and is suggested by the osteopenia seen on x-ray.

Celiac disease causes malabsorption, fatty stools, a protuberant abdomen, and failure to thrive, but it does not cause recurrent pulmonary infections.

Chronic granulomatous disease (CGD), a disorder of phagocyte function, is characterized by chronic and recurrent pyogenic infections. Patients can have anemia of chronic disease. CGD occurs in X-linked and autosomal forms, and nitroblue tetrazolium aids in diagnosis.

Although Bruton's agammaglobulinemia is characterized by recurrent infections, malabsorption is not a hallmark of this disease. Symptoms appear at 6 to 12 months of age, with loss of maternally acquired antibodies. Panhypogammaglobulinemia is seen.

Nephrotic syndrome produces edema and decreased serum albumin, but protein should be seen in the urine. Malabsorption and failure to thrive do not occur.

141. The answer is B. *(Obstetrics; thromboembolic disorders)*
Appropriate treatment of deep venous thrombosis in pregnancy is critical for both the mother (to prevent pulmonary embolization) and the fetus (to avoid teratogenesis). Heparin is the treatment of choice because it is a large molecule and does not cross the placenta. Coumarin is a small molecule, does cross the placenta, and is implicated in a specific teratogenic syndrome in the fetus. Aspirin, dipyridamole, and streptokinase are not indicated in pregnancy.

142. The answer is C. *(Psychiatry; mania)*
Mania is a syndrome characterized by an irritable, elevated, or euphoric mood, coupled with increased psychomotor activity, decreased need for sleep, grandiosity, and deterioration of judgment. It is seen in the manic phase of bipolar disorder and certain drug-induced mood disorders resulting from psychostimulants or steroids.

143. The answer is D. *(Pediatrics; diphtheria–tetanus–pertussis immunization)*
Most of the reactivity of diphtheria–tetanus–pertussis (DTP) is due to the pertussis component. Serious reactions, such as seizures, contraindicate the further use of the pertussis vaccine. This reaction, however, does not contraindicate the further use of the tetanus and diphtheria toxoids.

144. The answer is D. *(General surgery; complications associated with carotid endarterectomy)*
The most common complication following a carotid endarterectomy is an acute myocardial infarction. Endarterectomy is the standard treatment for atherosclerosis involving the bifurcation of the common carotid artery. Overall, there is approximately a 4% incidence of complications following this procedure. In addition to acute myocardial infarction, complications

include stroke (uncommon), numbness beneath the chin, and weakness of the hypoglossal nerve. A pulmonary embolus is not a common complication of carotid endarterectomy.

Air embolism is a potential problem in surgery or trauma in the head and neck area. Venous injury can result in air being sucked into the right heart from the negative intrathoracic pressure associated with inspiration. Air mixed with blood in the right heart produces a frothy material that blocks the blood entering the pulmonary artery. This can be prevented by keeping the patient supine and applying digital pressure to the injured vessel. Treatment involves placing the patient on the left side and keeping the head lower than the feet, thus trapping the air in the right ventricle. This is followed by administration of 100% oxygen.

145. The answer is C. (Obstetrics; postpartum hemorrhage)

Postpartum hemorrhage is defined as blood loss in excess of 500 ml at the time of vaginal delivery or 1000 ml with cesarean section. Although retained placental tissue, genital tract trauma, uterine inversion, and a coagulation disorder are all explanations for postpartum hemorrhage, uterine atony is the cause of 75% to 80% of cases.

146–148. The answers are: 146-E, 147-D, 148-E. (Endocrinology; Cushing's syndrome)

Cushing's syndrome is a state of hyperadrenocorticism. There are several causes. Iatrogenic Cushing's syndrome, which occurs most commonly in a patient taking corticosteroids, is the major nonpathologic cause. Pituitary adenoma is the most common cause of pathologic Cushing's syndrome; the majority of the adenomas are benign. Adrenal Cushing's can be secondary to a benign adenoma, bilateral hyperplasia, or carcinoma. Ectopic Cushing's is commonly associated with small cell carcinoma of the lung with ectopic adrenocorticotropic hormone (ACTH) secretion.

Clinical findings in Cushing's syndrome are protean and parallel the excessive production of cortisol, weak mineralocorticoids (deoxycorti-

costerone), and weak androgens (dehydroepiandrosterone, androstenedione). Truncal obesity is characteristic. Excess fat is distributed in the face (moon face), cervical area ("buffalo hump"), and abdomen, with sparing of the extremities. This peculiar distribution is due to the lipogenic effect of insulin, which is released in response to hyperglycemia, and the catabolic effect of cortisol on proteins in skeletal muscle in the extremities to provide amino acids for gluconeogenesis. Wide purple striae are secondary to weak subcutaneous tissue and vessel instability, leading to ecchymoses and bleeding into the stretch marks. This tissue instability is the result of the inhibitory effect of cortisol on collagen synthesis. Hypertension is associated with increased release of weak mineralocorticoids (not aldosterone) and subsequent retention of sodium. Hirsutism is due to an increased concentration of 17-ketosteroids, which are weak androgens. Diabetes mellitus is secondary to the gluconeogenic effect of cortisol. The plethoric face is due to vessel engorgement from secondary polycythemia induced by cortisol-enhanced erythropoiesis. Severe osteoporosis can result from cortisol's potentiation of the effects of parathormone (PTH) and vitamin D on bone. Menstrual irregularities (usually amenorrhea) and mental aberrations round out the clinical picture.

Laboratory testing for the hyperadrenocorticism involves the use of screening tests to establish the diagnosis and other tests to determine the type of Cushing's syndrome. After documenting an increased level of serum cortisol, most clinicians screen for Cushing's syndrome with a low-dose (1-mg) dexamethasone (an analog of cortisol) suppression test to see if the high baseline cortisol can be suppressed to less than 5 µg/dl. Patients with pituitary, adrenal, and ectopic Cushing's do not suppress cortisol below 5 µ/dl. False-positives can occur in stressed patients and in obese patients. There is an increased false-positive loss of the normal diurnal rhythm of serum cortisol (high at 8 A.M. and low at 4 P.M.) in stressed or obese individuals. A 24-hour urine test for 17-hydroxycorticosteroids, which are metabolites of 11-deoxycortisol and cortisol, and 17-ketosteroids, representing the metabolites of dehydroepiandrosterone and androstenedione, shows increased levels in patients with Cushing's. However, the urine test for free cortisol (cortisol not bound to protein), is a better all-around urine test for screening purposes. It not only has a higher sensitivity (95% versus 89%) than the other tests but also more clearly differentiates obese patients, who have a normal test, from those with Cushing's syndrome.

To determine the type of Cushing's syndrome, the high-dose dexamethasone test (8 mg/day) has the highest specificity. Hyperadrenocorticism in pituitary Cushing's can be suppressed, whereas that associated with adrenal and ectopic Cushing's cannot be suppressed.

Plasma ACTH is also a useful study. Patients with adrenal Cushing's syndrome have low levels; those with pituitary Cushing's have normal to slightly elevated values; and patients with ectopic Cushing's have extremely high concentrations.

Hyperadrenocorticism has an effect on the leukocyte count. Cortisol decreases neutrophil adhesion to endothelial cells, resulting in a neutrophilic leukocytosis; increases adhesion of lymphocytes in efferent lymphatics, which produces lymphopenia; and is cytotoxic to eosinophils, causing eosinopenia.

Rapid-sequence intravenous pyelography is used to document renovascular hypertension, which is most commonly due to atherosclerosis of the renal artery in elderly men or fibromuscular hyperplasia of the renal artery in young to middle-aged women. It would not be associated with the constellation of findings noted in this patient.

The clonidine suppression test is used to confirm pheochromocytoma caused by a tumor secreting excess catecholamines. Clonidine is a centrally acting adrenergic drug that cannot suppress the excessive catecholamines associated with a pheochromocytoma. Absence of sweating, anxiety, paroxysms of hypertension, and sinus tachycardia in this patient argue against a pheochromocytoma.

A bone marrow examination, ostensibly as a workup of polycythemia in this patient, is not indicated, because the other clinical findings do not suggest a primary problem in the bone marrow (e.g., polycythemia rubra vera).

149. The answer is E. *(Psychiatry; personality disorders)*
This case is most consistent with schizoid personality disorder. Schizotypal personality disorder includes peculiar thinking. Paranoid personality disorder is characterized by unwarranted suspiciousness. Narcissistic personality disorder involves a disdain for most people, but extreme idealization or denigration of a few. Avoidant personality disorder implies that the individual has a need for human contact and feels lonely.

150. The answer is A. *(Gynecology; sexual assault)*
Rape is the fastest growing violent crime in the United States, with one in six women likely to be raped during her lifetime. Although each option may be useful in clearing an accused assailant, the DNA studies check genetic "fingerprints," which are highly specific to the individual and thus provide a high degree of accuracy.

151. The answer is D. *(General surgery; Zollinger-Ellison syndrome)*
The patient has the Zollinger-Ellison syndrome, which is associated with a malignant islet cell tumor that secretes excessive amounts of gastrin, causing the excessive secretion of acid and peptic ulcer disease. Diarrhea is also evident, since acid inactivates the pancreatic enzymes. The best initial screen is a basal acid output, which is usually greater than 20 mEq/hour. The maximal acid output after pentagastrin stimulation is usually greater than 60 mEq/hour. A secretin challenge test is the confirmatory test. It shows a paradoxical increase in gastrin secretion. Total gastrectomy is the treatment of choice. Proton blockers, like omeprazole, are excellent in controlling acid secretion.

Ménétrier's hypertrophic gastritis is characterized by giant rugal hypertrophy secondary to the collection of protein-rich fluid in cysts in the submucosa and glandular epithelium. The mucosa is atrophic, and achlorhydria is the rule. Loss of protein-rich fluid from the mucosa is often associated with hypoalbuminemia (protein-losing enteropathy).

A glucagonoma is a malignant islet cell tumor that presents with diabetes mellitus and migratory necrolytic erythema. It is not associated with increased gastrin release or peptic ulcer disease.

A gastric adenocarcinoma is associated with achlorhydria and would not be expected to be associated with hyperacidity.

152. The answer is C. *(Pediatrics; pertussis)*

Pertussis (whooping cough) is an extremely contagious respiratory disease caused by *Bordetella pertussis*. From 50% to 70% of cases occur in children less than 1 year of age, and most deaths occur in nonimmunized infants. After a 1-week incubation period, children present with three successive stages of the disease. The catarrhal stage consists of symptoms of an upper respiratory infection, thick nasal discharge, and conjunctivitis. The paroxysmal stage is characterized by spasms of forceful coughing ending in an inspiratory whoop. The cough is strong enough to force vomiting, and facial redness and cyanosis are often observed. Often, there is no whoop in infants, but apnea may be manifested. In the convalescent stage, the cough and vomiting gradually subside. Cough can persist for several months. Petechiae and conjunctival hemorrhages can be seen. Otitis media is a common complication. Complete blood count (CBC) usually shows a leukocytosis, predominantly lymphocytes toward the end of the catarrhal stage and during the paroxysmal stage.

153. The answer is B. *(Psychiatry; drug abuse)*

Alprazolam is the benzodiazepine associated with severe withdrawal, perhaps because of its high potency and short half-life. For this reason, it is used less commonly for adjustment disorders or generalized anxiety disorder; it is usually reserved for treatment of panic disorder.

154. The answer is B. *(Gynecology; endometriosis)*

Endometriosis is a benign condition in which endometrial glands and stroma are located outside the endometrial cavity. This condition affects up to 15% of all women in the United States. Although a history and pelvic examination may be suggestive of endometriosis, only a laparoscopy is definitive. A hysterosalpingogram (HSG) is not helpful because the findings are extrauterine. A menstrual culdocentesis lacks specificity and sensitivity.

155. The answer is A. *(Transplantation surgery; hyperacute rejection testing)*

Hyperacute rejections of transplants are due to a mismatch in ABO groups between a recipient and a donor or the presence of anti–human leukocyte antigen (HLA) antibodies in the recipient against HLA antigens in the donor graft. These reactions occur instantaneously once the circulation is established through the graft.

Using an ABO mismatch as an example, if an A person receives a B donor graft, the anti-B IgM antibodies normally present in the A recipient will attack the B antigen in the endothelial cells of the graft. This activates complement, which damages the endothelium, resulting in thrombosis and rejection of the graft. This is an example of a type II hypersensitivity reaction. A proper ABO match between the donor and recipient is the single most important factor for graft survival. A lymphocyte crossmatch between the recipient's serum and donor lymphocytes is used to detect the presence of anti-HLA antibodies in the recipient.

The lymphocyte microcytotoxicity test is a serologic test that identifies HLA-A, B, C, and some D loci on the recipient and donor lymphocytes. Mixed lymphocyte reaction testing further identifies compatibility of the D loci of the donor and recipient. A modification of the test is used to evaluate the potential for a graft-versus-host reaction, which is particularly common in bone marrow transplantation.

Tests that determine the compatibility of the HLA loci are useful in preventing cellular rejection (type IV hypersensitivity) of the graft. However, HLA compatibility is not as critical for graft survival as ABO compatibility and the absence of anti-HLA antibodies in the recipient. This is mainly true because an immunosuppressant, such as cyclosporine, can block the release of interleukin-2 by CD4 T helper cells, which play a pivotal role in graft rejection.

156. The answer is C. (*Behavioral science; stroke*)

The construction apraxia seen in this patient is associated with damage to the nondominant parietal lobe. Damage to the dominant frontal lobe is associated with expressive (Broca's) aphasia. Damage to the dominant temporal lobe is associated with receptive (Wernicke's) aphasia. Damage to the nondominant frontal and temporal lobes is associated with problems of mood, orientation, concentration, and memory.

157. The answer is D. (*Pediatrics; infant botulism*)

Infant botulism usually occurs in infants less than 1 year of age, particularly between 2 and 6 months. It occurs after the ingestion of *Clostridium botulinum* spores, which can be found in honey and corn syrup, as well as in soil and house dust. The course of the disease varies but progresses quickly. Typically the child is afebrile and has been previously healthy. The infant becomes constipated and feeds poorly. A weak cry, hypotonia, and loss of head control are then seen. Descending paralysis progresses over hours to days. Ventilatory support may be necessary.

Gray syndrome is associated with chloramphenicol use. Although hypothyroidism and Werdnig-Hoffmann disease present with hypotonia, it is seen earlier in life, and progression of symptoms occurs more slowly. Hypomagnesemia usually presents in conjunction with hypocalcemia and manifests as tetany.

158. The answer is C. (*Pediatrics; retinopathy of prematurity*)

Retinopathy of prematurity is an angiopathy occurring primarily in preterm infants. Manifestations vary; they range from mild changes to severe vasoproliferation and retinal detachment. Causes include prematurity, hypoxia, hyperoxia, infection, and heart disease. The disease is usually asymmetric, and about 90% of cases show spontaneous arrest. The disease begins peripherally and proceeds centrally, where vasculariza-

tion of the retina can occur. Although the exact role of vitamin E is not known, supplementation to maintain adequate levels is recommended.

159. The answer is D. (*Nephrology; renovascular hypertension*)

This patient has renovascular hypertension secondary to atherosclerotic narrowing of the left renal artery orifice. The diagnosis of renal artery stenosis should always be considered when:

- hypertension develops after 50 years of age
- vascular bruits are heard in the abdomen
- hypertension is resistant to therapy
- advanced retinopathy is present
- the serum creatinine concentration is increased
- abrupt deterioration of renal function occurs after an angiotensin-converting enzyme inhibitor is given
- hypertension is present in patients with peripheral vascular disease

Renovascular hypertension is the most common secondary cause of hypertension. In young to middle-aged women, it is most commonly caused by fibromuscular hyperplasia of one or both renal arteries; whereas in elderly men, it is most commonly caused by atherosclerosis. In fibromuscular hyperplasia, the renal arteriogram shows a characteristic beading effect along the course of the artery.

Stimulation of the renin–angiotensin–aldosterone system is associated with vasoconstriction secondary to angiotensin II and volume overload from aldosterone. The increase in aldosterone is also responsible for hypokalemic metabolic alkalosis due to enhanced exchange of potassium and hydrogen ions for sodium in the distal tubule. Loss of hydrogen ions leaves un-neutralized bicarbonate in the plasma. Captopril in these patients blocks the formation of angiotensin II, which has a negative feedback on renin; therefore, renin levels increase significantly over the baseline high values. However, if the patient has bilateral renal artery stenosis, captopril causes an abrupt deterioration in renal function. This change is caused by the block in angiotensin II, which is important in maintaining renal blood flow.

There are no optimal screening tests for renovascular hypertension. Some clinicians consider the captopril test described previously as a good first step. Angiography is the definitive test and is usually accompanied by a split renal vein sampling of renin from the right and left renal veins. In this patient, the left renal vein renin levels would be increased, whereas those on the right should be suppressed, because the excess angiotensin II and volume overload from aldosterone will shut off renin production from the right kidney. If the ratio of renin from the arteriographically abnormal kidney is 1.5 times higher than that of renin obtained on the normal (uninvolved) side, patients are likely to benefit from surgery or angioplasty. However, if both sides have increased renin levels, the "normal" kidney also has vascular disease, most commonly nephrosclerosis with small vessel disease. These changes occur because the "normal" kidney experiences a significant increase in blood flow and systemic blood pressure because the flow to the stenotic kidney is reduced by the stenotic segment in the artery. In these difficult cases, the "normal" kidney is often removed, and the renal artery is repaired in the involved kidney.

160. The answer is E. (*Pediatrics; Arnold-Chiari syndrome*)
The Arnold-Chiari syndrome consists of hydrocephalus, spina bifida, and meningomyelocele. The hydrocephalus is a communicating one. The fourth ventricle is elongated, there is kinking of the brain stem, and portions of the brain stem and cerebellum are displaced into the cervical spinal canal, causing obstruction of flow of cerebrospinal fluid (CSF). Skull films show a small posterior fossa and widened cervical canal (platybasia). Type I Chiari malformation is not associated with hydrocephalus.

161. The answer is E. (*Obstetrics; hyperemesis gravidarum*)
Hyperemesis gravidarum describes the intractable nausea and vomiting that occur in 1% of pregnancies. Usually a first-trimester phenomenon, the condition also occurs more frequently in first pregnancies. Hypokalemia, weight loss,

ketonemia, and nausea with vomiting are frequent findings of hyperemesis. A change in acid–base status is usually a hypochloremic alkalosis rather than an acidosis.

162. The answer is C. (*Psychiatry; schizophrenia*)
Recent studies have demonstrated that a sizeable number of patients with schizophrenia have an amelioration of symptomatology in later decades of life. This finding contradicts earlier views. A better outcome is correlated with early use of antipsychotic medication and maintenance of social ties.

163. The answer is B. (*Endocrinology; differentiation of central diabetes insipidus, nephrogenic diabetes insipidus, and primary polydipsia*)
Differentiation of the polyuria syndromes is best accomplished with the water deprivation test. The polyuria syndromes include central diabetes insipidus (CDI), which involves an absolute deficiency of antidiuretic hormone (ADH); nephrogenic diabetes insipidus (NDI), in which the kidney tubules are not responsive to ADH; and primary polydipsia, in which a person chronically overingests water.

Patients with CDI and NDI present with polydipsia and polyuria owing to the loss of free water in the urine, which increases their plasma osmolality, which stimulates thirst. However, in primary polydipsia, the patient drinks excessive amounts of water, thus lowering the plasma osmolality. The excess water is removed by the kidneys, which produces a low U_{osm}. Primary polydipsia is usually not difficult to separate from diabetes insipidus because, at the outset, the P_{osm} is decreased, as opposed to CDI and NDI, which have an increased P_{osm}.

The water deprivation test will cause the plasma osmolality in normal controls and in people with primary polydipsia to reach the upper limit of the normal range, which is 275–295 mmol/kg. P_{osm} is increased in both CDI and NDI, because the loss of free water concentrates the plasma. U_{osm} is increased in both normal controls and in primary polydipsia, because ADH is available to reabsorb free water and concentrate the urine. However, in CDI and NDI, the U_{osm} is markedly decreased owing to the loss of free water. Once the maximum U_{osm} is reached (specimens do not differ by more than 30 mmol/kg), intramuscular vasopressin is administered. Normal controls and patients with primary polydipsia have less than a 9% increase in U_{osm}. In CDI, the U_{osm} increases more than 50%, whereas in NDI, it increases less than 45% from the maximum U_{osm}.

Patient A has CDI, because the maximum P_{osm} is increased, the maximum U_{osm} is decreased, and the U_{osm} increase is greater than 50% (160 to 400 mmol/kg) after administration of vasopressin. CDI is associated with hypothalamic lesions where ADH is synthesized; severance of the pituitary stalk, which interrupts the neuron carrying ADH to the posterior pituitary; or destruction of the posterior pituitary, where ADH is stored.

Patient B has NDI, because the maximum P_{osm} is increased, the maximum U_{osm} is decreased, and the U_{osm} does not increase more than 45% (125 to 150 mmol/kg) after administration of vasopressin. NDI can be hereditary or acquired from tubulointerstitial disease (e.g., chronic pyelonephritis) or drugs (e.g., lithium, demeclocycline, alcohol, amphotericin B).

Patient C has primary polydipsia, because the maximum P_{osm} is normal, the maximum U_{osm} is increased, the U_{osm} increases less than 9% (690 to 710 mmol/kg) after vasopressin administration. The normal control has the same findings.

164. The answer is B. (*Psychiatry; psychosis*)
Psychosis can engender anxiety, but anxiety can also accompany a host of other stressors. By contrast, delusions, hallucinations, and loose associations, by definition, indicate the presence of psychosis.

165. The answer is B. (*Obstetrics; multiple gestation*)
Twin gestation occurs in approximately 1% of pregnancies. Although the presence of two placentas indicates the implantation of two different ova (dizygosity), the twins may come from a single ovum that divided prior to implantation (monozygosity).

166. The answer is B. (*Biostatistics; effect of prevalence on the predictive value of positive and negative test results*)
The predictive value (PV) of a negative test is calculated as follows:

$$\frac{\text{true negatives}}{\text{true negatives + false negatives}}$$

The PV of a negative test is more likely to be a false negative than a true negative when there is a high prevalence of disease; therefore, the PV decreases. The PV of a negative test increases with decreasing prevalence of disease because true negatives now outnumber the false negatives. The reverse is true of the PV of a positive test. The PV of a positive test can be calculated as follows:

$$\frac{\text{true positives}}{\text{true positives + false positives}}$$

The PV of a positive test decreases in a low prevalence of disease (i.e., there are more false positives) and increases in a high-prevalence situation (i.e., there are more true positives).

167. The answer is E. (*Psychiatry; depression*)
The depressive mood and lassitude seen in major depression often lessen in intensity over the course of the day, only to return in full force the following morning. The other symptoms are all very characteristic of depressive episodes.

168. The answer is D. (*Genetics; deafness syndromes*)
Alport's syndrome is the most common of the hereditary nephritides. Patients develop nephritis that progresses to renal failure. Some patients develop hearing loss. Approximately 10% have eye abnormalities such as cataracts. Leopard syndrome is autosomal-dominant. It consists of lentigines, electrocardiogram abnormalities, ocular hypertelorism, pulmonary stenosis, abnormal genitalia, growth retardation, and sensorineural deafness. Pendred's syndrome is an autosomal-recessive disorder characterized by deafness and goiter. The goiter appears at puberty; and although most patients are euthyroid, hypothyroidism can occur. Usher's syndrome is characterized by deafness, mental retardation, seizures,

retinitis pigmentosa, and cataracts. Waardenburg's syndrome is autosomal-dominant. Affected persons have a white forelock, patches of hyperpigmentation, defective hearing, and lateral displacement of the inner canthi.

169. The answer is A. *(Pediatrics; orthopedic disorders by age-group)*
Osgood-Schlatter disease is an overuse injury that is more common in physically active boys around puberty. It is characterized by pain and swelling at the tibial tubercle. Radial head subluxation ("nursemaid's elbow") is common in children younger than 4 years of age. It occurs after sudden traction on the hand with the elbow extended and the forearm pronated. Sometimes a click is felt or heard. Gently supining the arm while in 90% flexion causes another click and reduces the subluxation and immediately relieves the pain. Legg-Calvé-Perthes presents with a gradual limp, stiffness, and pain in the groin, hip, thigh, or knee. It is most common in boys 4 to 8 years of age. It is an avascular necrosis of the femoral head. Slipped capital femoral epiphysis typically occurs in overweight adolescent boys. The chronic condition is associated with endocrine abnormalities such as hypothyroidism. Idiopathic scoliosis occurs in 3% to 5% of the general population. It most commonly presents during adolescence. Larger degrees of curvature are more common in girls.

170. The answer is D. *(Laboratory medicine; purpose of tests with high sensitivity)*
Tests with high sensitivity are used to screen for diseases that have a significant morbidity rate, mortality rate, or both if left untreated; diseases that can be detected early in an asymptomatic phase; and diseases that have an effective mode of therapy. Multiple sclerosis does not have an effective therapy; therefore, tests with high specificity (no false positives) are more useful than those with high sensitivity. Rendering a false-positive report of multiple sclerosis to a normal person could be devastating to that patient's psychological well-being. Phenylketonuria, hypothyroidism, pheochromocytoma, and venereal diseases fit the criteria for screening.

171. The answer is E. *(Obstetrics; fetal pulmonary maturity assessment)*
Lung maturity and the ability to maintain successful oxygenation are the major determinants of the degree of morbidity and mortality in the neonate. An immature lecithin/sphingomyelin (L/S) ratio has a high (rather than low) false-negative rate.

172. The answer is B. *(Pediatrics; drug-overdose)*
Adult iron preparations are responsible for most serious poisonings. Symptoms include hemorrhagic gastroenteritis, circulatory collapse, hepatorenal failure, bleeding, metabolic acidosis, and coma. Serum iron levels greater than 400 µg/dl within 4 hours postingestion are indicative of intoxication; greater than 500 µg/dl are considered severe poisoning. Treatment is supportive, and deferoxamine is the recommended drug.

173. The answer is E. *(Pharmacology; anticoagulants)*
Heparin is a large sulfated polysaccharide with poor oral bioavailability. It acts rapidly to activate antithrombin III, both in vivo and in vitro; and its action is antagonized by chemical complexation with protamine. Warfarin, a coumarin anticoagulant, inhibits the vitamin K–dependent hepatic synthesis of clotting factors II, VII, IX, and X. It has good oral bioavailability, but displacement of warfarin from plasma protein binding sites by many drugs can increase its anticoagulant actions.

174. The answer is A. *(Obstetrics; abnormal labor)*
It is important to identify the cause of abnormal labor as accurately as possible so that an effective and safe plan of management can be developed. Assessment of the intensity and frequency of the uterine contractions can help identify causes of arrest of dilation that can be treated nonsurgically. Rupturing the membranes and placing an intrauterine pressure catheter can enhance inadequate uterine contractions, as can administration of intravenous oxytocin. A pelvimetry to determine pelvic adequacy rules out absolute pelvic contraction. Appropriate management would not

include a cesarean delivery for cephalopelvic disproportion.

175. The answer is D. *(Pediatrics; jaundice)*

Physiologic jaundice is the jaundice that appears after the first day of life, peaks at about 3 to 5 days, and does not involve a bilirubin level above 12.9 mg/dl. Prematurity predisposes an infant to jaundice. Sepsis, ABO and Rh incompatibility, and cytomegalovirus (CMV) are all examples of pathological jaundice and most commonly present in the first 24 hours of life.

176. The answer is A. *(Pharmacology; chemotherapy)*

Methotrexate (MTX) is an inhibitor of dihydrofolate reductase (DHFR), and tumor cell resistance can develop either by changes in enzyme sensitivity to the drug or by gene amplification that results in marked increases in the messenger RNA (mRNA) for dihydrofolate (DHF) reductase. In other instances, a multidrug-resistant (MDR) phenotype occurs in association with increased expression of the normal MDR 1 gene for the P glycoprotein involved in drug efflux. Decreased activity of hypoxanthine–guanine phosphoribosyl transferase (HGPRT) is associated with resistance to 6-mercaptopurine and 6-thioguanine, which require this enzyme for their bioactivation.

177. The answer is E. *(Genetics; lysosomal storage disease)*

Von Gierke's disease is a glycogen storage disease. It is due to a deficiency of glucose-6-phosphatase and results in enlarged kidneys and liver; hypoglycemia is common. Tay-Sachs disease involves the central nervous system (CNS). There is a defect in the lysosomal enzyme β-hexosaminidase. Gaucher's disease is one of the lipidoses, or lysosomal lipid storage diseases, as is Niemann-Pick disease. The enzyme defect in Gaucher's disease is β-glucosidase; the enzyme defect in Niemann-Pick disease is sphingomyelinase. Tay-Sachs, Gaucher's, and Niemann-Pick diseases are all more common in Ashkenazic Jews than in other ethnic groups. Hurler syndrome is the most severe of the mucopolysaccharidoses. A deficiency of α-L-iduronidase leads to mucopolysaccharide-engorged lysosomes.

178. The answer is A. *(Dermatology; pruritus)*

Pruritus, or itching, is the most common symptom in dermatology. In polycythemia rubra vera, there is an increase in basophils in the peripheral blood. These basophils degranulate and release histamine, which produces generalized pruritus. Lukewarm baths often precipitate this reaction in the skin because heat degranulates basophils.

Pruritus is one of the first manifestations of primary biliary cirrhosis, an autoimmune disease in middle-aged women. The autoimmune destruction of bile ducts in the portal triads hampers the excretion of bile salts. The excess bile salts deposited in the skin produce intense itching. Cholestyramine therapy is used to bind bile salts in the intestine, thereby enhancing their excretion.

Atopic dermatitis is a chronic, inherited form of irritation of the skin (eczema), usually associated with a strong history of allergies and type I hypersensitivity. It occurs in infants, children, and adults. In infants, it presents as an acute, oozing, erythematous dermatitis on the face, neck, and scalp. Children typically have a more chronic presentation, with thickening of the skin from scratching (lichenification). Atopic dermatitis classically involves the flexor creases. In adults, it tends to be either generalized or localized to areas such as the hands.

One of the most common systemic diseases associated with pruritus is uremia in conjunction with hemodialysis. This type of pruritus is usually resistant to all therapies. It may relate to metastatic calcification of the skin because of the driving force of the elevated phosphate, which pushes calcium into tissue.

Carcinoid syndrome is usually secondary to metastatic carcinoid tumor to the liver from a primary site in the small intestine. In the liver, the metastatic nodules secrete serotonin and other chemicals directly into the blood. Flushing is the most common symptom and is due to the vasodilatation effects of serotonin. Pruritus is not a feature of the syndrome.

179. The answer is E. *(Pediatrics; galactosemia)*
Classic galactosemia results from a deficiency of galactose-1-phosphate uridyltransferase. Galactose, derived from lactose, is not metabolized past galactose-1-phosphate, which then accumulates and damages the liver, kidney, and brain. Galactitol, a polyol by-product of galactose, can accumulate, causing cataracts. Among other manifestations are jaundice, hepatomegaly, hypoglycemia, vomiting, aminoaciduria, and failure to thrive. Early diagnosis is important, and dietary management contributes to a good prognosis.

180. The answer is E. *(Genetics; Klinefelter's syndrome)*
Klinefelter's syndrome with a 47, XXY chromosome complement occurs in 1/1000 males. The incidence is 1/100 among the mentally retarded. The two X chromosomes indicate one Barr body. The diagnosis is seldom made before puberty. Patients are mentally retarded, tall, slim, underweight, and long-legged. In addition, 80% of adults have gynecomastia. Testicular biopsy after puberty shows adematous Leydig cells. Azoospermia is present, and patients are infertile.

181. The answer is C. *(Pediatrics; phenylketonuria)*
Phenylketonuria (PKU) is caused by a deficiency in phenylalanine hydroxylase. The normal pathway is disrupted, so phenylalanine and other metabolites accumulate and cause brain damage. Clinically, affected infants are blond, with fair skin and blue eyes. A mild eczematous rash disappears with age. Vomiting can be confused with pyloric stenosis. Mental retardation is usually severe. The infants have a musty, mousey odor of phenylacetic acid. Screening is recommended after 72 hours of age and after feeding of proteins. Early institution of a diet low in phenylalanine is essential in preventing brain damage. Women who have PKU and want to have children should go on a low-phenylalanine diet prior to conception and throughout pregnancy to reduce the risk of spontaneous abortion and birth defects.

182. The answer is A. *(General medicine; gold standard tests)*
The gold standard test for primary syphilis is dark-field examination of serous fluid expressed from a chancre in the genital area, with identification of the tight coils of *Treponema pallidum*. Dark-field examination is not recommended for lesions in the mouth, because of the potential for false-positives from other spirochetes that are normally present in this location. The rapid plasma reagin (RPR) and Venereal Disease Research Laboratories (VDRL) are nontreponemal serologic tests, which, when positive, must be confirmed as a true-positive with a treponemal test like the fluorescent treponemal antibody absorption (FTA-ABS) test.

Measurement of creatine kinase isoenzymes (CK-MB) is the gold standard test for an acute myocardial infarction. CK-MB first becomes elevated in 4 to 8 hours, peaks in 24 hours, and is gone in 1.5 to 3 days. It has a sensitivity of 100%, particularly if performed on admission and at intervals of 12 and 24 hours. It has a specificity of 98%. Because the electrocardiogram (ECG) is negative for acute myocardial injury in up to 50% of cases, it is not the primary test.

Venography is the gold standard for diagnosing deep venous thrombosis in the legs. Noninvasive methods include impedance plethysmography (overall, the most sensitive and specific noninvasive test), Doppler ultrasonography, and nuclear fibrinogen scanning.

Ultrasound is the gold standard for diagnosing gallstones and duct dilatation. Computed tomography (CT) scan is not as sensitive in detecting stones and is more expensive than ultrasound. Oral cholecystography requires a patent cystic duct for visualization of the gallbladder. A radionuclide (HIDA) scan is the gold standard for cystic duct obstruction.

Pulmonary angiography is the gold standard for diagnosing a pulmonary embolism if perfusion scans are inconclusive.

183. The answer is D. *(Pediatrics; alpha-fetoprotein level)*
Alpha-fetoprotein (AFP) is found in the amniotic fluid. It is synthesized in the fetal liver, gastroin-

testinal tract, and yolk sac. Its level is elevated in open neural tube defects, anencephaly, meningomyelocele, encephalocele, omphalocele, and twin gestation. The AFP level is useful in evaluating subsequent pregnancies if a prior child had the same defects. However, this is not true in cases of omphalocele, which is not hereditary. Decreased AFP levels can be seen in 20% of fetuses with trisomy 21 and trisomy 18.

184. The answer is C. *(Gastroenterology; malabsorption secondary to chronic pancreatitis)*
Malabsorption refers to increased fecal excretion of fat and concurrent deficiencies of vitamins, minerals, carbohydrates, and proteins. Pathophysiologically, it can be the result of small bowel disease, ending in reduced absorption of fat; pancreatic insufficiency, leading to the improper breakdown of fat by lipases; and bile salt deficiency, which interferes with the micellarization of fat and its absorption by the villi in the small intestine.

The screening test of choice for documenting malabsorption is analyzing the quantitative stool for fat, which is greater than 6 g per day in these patients. Localization studies to isolate the cause(s) of malabsorption include the D-xylose test and more sophisticated tests that are not commonly available in hospitals (e.g., radioactive bile breath test).

The D-xylose test differentiates small bowel disease from pancreatic disease or bile salt deficiency that is not related to bacterial overgrowth. Orally administered xylose does not require pancreatic enzymes for reabsorption by the small bowel. Decreased levels of xylose in the blood or urine after an orally administered dose indicates small bowel disease (e.g., celiac disease, which is most common), whereas normal levels indicate pancreatic disease or bile salt deficiency.

The radioactive bile breath test is useful in documenting bacterial overgrowth as a cause of bile salt deficiency. Bacteria break down the radioactive bile salt into radioactive carbon dioxide, which is detected in the breath.

Pancreatic insufficiency, as is exhibited in this patient, is difficult to document. However, the presence of calcifications in the pancreas visual-

ized by routine x-ray (less sensitive), or by ultrasound or computed tomography (CT) scan (higher sensitivity), plus a clinical history suggestive of malabsorption is highly predictive of significant pancreatic disease.

Clinical findings parallel the disease responsible for the malabsorption and the deficiency states that are produced. Malabsorption of fat results in the loss of fat-soluble vitamins A, D, E, and K. Hypovitaminosis A is associated with night blindness and squamous metaplasia of the respiratory tract, leading to infections. Vitamin D deficiency produces rickets in children and osteomalacia in adults; both conditions result from excess buildup of unmineralized osteoid secondary to hypocalcemia and hypophosphatemia. Vitamin K deficiency results in a hemorrhagic diathesis secondary to inactivation of the vitamin-K–dependent factors, which are factors II (prothrombin), VII, IX, and X. The prothrombin time (PT) would be prolonged in this patient because it is a measure of the extrinsic system (factor VII) down to the formation of a clot (X, V, II, and fibrinogen → fibrin clot).

Loss of proteins reduces the total protein and albumin concentrations. Hypoalbuminemia results in a decreased plasma oncotic pressure and loss of a transudate into the interstitial tissue, producing clinical evidence of pitting edema. In addition, the hypoproteinemia leads to reduced synthesis of apolipoproteins that are necessary to surround lipid (e.g., very low-density lipoprotein [VLDL]) before it is excreted into the blood; therefore, hepatomegaly due to fatty change is commonly present in patients.

Other problems include water-soluble vitamin deficiencies (e.g., thiamine deficiency), trace metal deficiencies (e.g., hypomagnesemia), hematologic problems (combined iron, folate, and B_{12} deficiencies), and electrolyte disturbances (e.g., isotonic loss of sodium, hypokalemia, normal anion gap metabolic acidosis).

In summary, this patient with chronic pancreatic disease and malabsorption would be expected to have a prolonged PT from vitamin K deficiency, because there is clinical evidence of a bleeding diathesis (ecchymoses in areas of trauma); increased fat in stool; a normal D-xylose test, because the small bowel biopsies are normal; hypoalbuminemia from protein loss, because pitting edema is present; and hypocalcemia, due to either vitamin D deficiency or the effect of hypoalbuminemia in lowering the total calcium concentration, because 40% of calcium is normally bound to albumin.

185. The answer is E. *(Pediatrics; characteristics of postterm infants)*
Term babies are defined as those who are born at 38 to 42 weeks' gestation. Postterm babies are born after 42 weeks' gestation. They tend to be large for gestational age and hyperalert. Lanugo is absent, and the skin is cracked and peeling. Fingernails are long. They are at increased risk for meconium aspiration.

 186–188. The answers are: 186-B, 187-E, 188-D. *(Laboratory medicine; serum protein electrophoresis patterns in sarcoidosis, alcoholic cirrhosis, and alpha$_1$-antitrypsin deficiency)*
A serum protein electrophoresis (SPE) separates proteins on the basis of charge in the presence of an alkaline pH. Albumin moves the fastest to the anode (positive pole) because it has the most negative charges, whereas gamma globulins, with the least number of negative charges, remain at the cathode (negative pole). The five components of an SPE—in order of decreasing negative charge—are albumin, alpha$_1$, alpha$_2$, beta, and gamma globulins. The most common indication for ordering an SPE is to rule out a monoclonal gammopathy, like multiple myeloma. However, there are many other uses.

Sarcoidosis is a chronic granulomatous inflammatory disease (CGD) of unknown cause that has a predilection for the black population. The diagnosis requires the demonstration of noncaseating granulomas plus the appropriate clinical picture. The lungs are involved in 90% of patients who produce a restrictive type of lung disease with prominent perihilar adenopathy, the latter known as "potato nodes." Since it is a chronic inflammatory disease, there is polyclonal stimulation of B cells by unknown antigens, with subsequent formation of predominantly immunoglobulin G (IgG) antibodies. These antibodies produce a diffuse enlargement of the gamma globulin curve, called a polyclonal peak. Furthermore, albumin concentration is decreased in any acute or chronic inflammatory state because interleukins produced by macrophages decrease the synthesis of albumin in the liver in favor of synthesizing other proteins, called acute-phase reactants. Other causes of polyclonal gammopathy are tuberculosis, autoimmune disease, and cirrhosis of the liver.

Alcoholic cirrhosis is the most common cause of cirrhosis in the United States. It produces a very characteristic SPE pattern, called the beta–gamma bridge. This pattern is due to an increased production of IgG, which migrates in the middle of the gamma globulin curve, and IgA, which migrates at the junction of the beta and gamma curves. Therefore, the increase in IgG produces a polyclonal peak, whereas the increase in IgA fills in the valley between the beta and gamma curves to produce a beta–gamma bridge. In addition, the cirrhotic liver is unable to synthesize albumin, resulting in hypoalbuminemia.

The presence of panacinar emphysema involving the lower lobes in a nonsmoking young adult is classic for alpha$_1$-antitrypsin deficiency, which has an autosomal-recessive inheritance pattern. Alpha$_1$-antitrypsin is the main globulin beneath the alpha$_1$-globulin curve. It is an antiprotease that is synthesized by the liver, the main function of which is to neutralize the elastases and collagenases emitted by neutrophils and other inflammatory cells in order to prevent destruction of structural tissue.

Starch electrophoresis techniques have determined many different phenotypes. The MM phenotype has 100% alpha$_1$-antitrypsin activity, whereas the ZZ phenotype produces only 15% of the normal quantity of alpha$_1$-antitrypsin. Only Z and S alleles are associated with disease when they are present in the homozygous state. Approximately 10% of children with the ZZ phenotype develop serious liver disease, including neonatal hepatitis and cirrhosis. Adults with the same phenotype most commonly present with an asymptomatic cirrhosis, which can develop into hepatocellular carcinoma, or lower-lobe panacinar emphysema at an early age. The diagnosis is suggested by the absence of the alpha₁ peak on an SPE, which should be followed up by direct measurement of alpha₁-antitrypsin. Once a deficiency has been established, the patient and family members should be phenotyped. Aerosol therapy with alpha₁-antitrypsin is available for those patients with lung disease.

The SPE pattern depicted in choice A exhibits a reduction in albumin and a normal gamma globulin peak—the characteristic pattern of acute inflammation. As previously mentioned, inflammation causes reduced synthesis of albumin in favor of other proteins, called acute-phase reactants. These reactants include fibrinogen (nonspecific opsonin), C-reactive protein (CRP) [opsonin, complement cascade activator], ferritin (storage form of iron), and the complement component, C3 (opsonin). The primary immunoglobulin on first exposure to an antigen is IgM, which is not generated in sufficient amounts to alter the shape of the gamma globulin curve. This pattern is in contrast to the SPE patterns in choices B and E, which show chronic inflammation and increased production of IgG.

The SPE pattern depicted in choice C is a monoclonal spike. Monoclonal spikes are the result of clonal proliferation of a neoplastic plasma cell, with production of its immunoglobulin and corresponding light chain (e.g., IgG kappa). Suppressor T cells prevent synthesis of immunoglobulins by the other plasma cells, so the uninvolved immunoglobulins are decreased. Multiple myeloma is an example of a malignant plasma cell disorder that produces monoclonal spikes due to IgG (most common), IgA, or light chains alone. Waldenström's macroglobulinemia is characterized by a monoclonal proliferation of lymphoplasmacytoid cells that produce IgM, which predisposes to the hyperviscosity syndrome. Monoclonal spikes that are unassociated with the preceding diseases are called monoclonal spikes of undetermined significance. Some of these patients later develop multiple myeloma or malignant lymphomas, so they should be carefully followed.

189–190. The answers are: 189-B, 190-C. *(Psychiatry; sleep disorders)*

Diazepam decreases stage 4 sleep, which makes the drug useful in treating sleep disorders characterized by pathology during this stage. Sleep terror and sleepwalking are examples.

Benzodiazepine rebound causes increased sleep latency, which is one mechanism that leads to addiction. Graph A represents normal sleep architecture. Graph D represents early morning awakenings, which are often associated with major depression. Graph E represents suppression of rapid eye movement (REM) sleep, which is caused by barbiturates and some antidepressants.

191–193. The answers are: 191-D, 192-E, 193-B. *(Pharmacology; antibiotics)*

It must be assumed that the patient had an allergic reaction to a penicillin, although a maculopapular skin rash associated with ampicillin may not be a hypersensitivity reaction. Thus, ampicillin–sulbactam would not be an appropriate drug for this patient, even though the sulbactam inhibits penicillinases produced by *Escherichia coli*. It is important to recall that some cross-allergenicity exists between penicillins and cephalosporins.

Hemolysis following the use of antimalarial drugs suggests that this patient has glucose-6-phosphate dehydrogenase (G6PD) deficiency. If so, there is enhanced sensitivity of erythrocyte membranes to drugs that can act as oxidizing agents (e.g., chloroquine, primaquine, isoniazid, nitrofurantoin, and the sulfonamides). Although trimethoprim–sulfamethoxazole (TMP-SMZ) is often effective in urinary tract infections of the type described in this patient, the sulfa drug may cause hemolysis.

The penicillin and the TMP–SMZ combination should be ruled out based on the potential for adverse effects. Cefaclor, ciprofloxacin, and gentamicin are theoretically appropriate based on the results of susceptibility testing. However, gentamicin can only be administered parenterally, and this mode of administration would not be appropriate in an ambulatory patient. Cefaclor, which is given orally, is a second-generation cephalosporin with activity against strains of *Haemophilus influenzae* and *E. coli,* but it is susceptible to β-lactamases produced by some Enterobacteriaceae, and (as mentioned previously) there is the problem of potential cross-allergenicity. The fluoroquinolones are effective orally and penetrate the prostate well. Cure rates in prostatitis with ciprofloxacin are high and similar to those achieved with TMP–SMZ. However, resistance has emerged during the course of therapy for urinary tract infections with fluoroquinolones.

194–195. The answers are: 194-J, 195-K.
(Psychiatry; anxiety disorders)
Separation anxiety disorder is a childhood illness characterized by fear of separation from caregivers. It can manifest itself as worry about separation, severe protest over separation, or severe anxiety after separation. Often, the presenting complaint involves marital problems caused by these behaviors.

Social phobia is characterized by fear and avoidance of social situations. Individuals with this disorder tend to be solitary and reclusive. Their presenting complaint is often depression and loneliness.

196–198. The answers are: 196-B, 197-A, 198-E. *(Pharmacology; chemotherapy)*
Hemorrhagic cystitis during cyclophosphamide therapy is due to the formation of the metabolite acrolein. This compound may accumulate in the bladder to toxic levels, especially following high doses of cyclophosphamide. Vigorous hydration is useful in decreasing the occurrence of this problem.

In addition to causing myelosuppression, the anthracyclines (doxorubicin and daunorubicin) are toxic to myocardial cells through a free radical mechanism. Clinical effects include conduction abnormalities, arrhythmias, and a pericarditis-like syndrome. Congestive heart failure may occur within 1 month of therapy; and once it occurs, the mortality rate is high.

Asparaginase, a protein of bacterial origin, is used to treat childhood acute leukemias. Allergic reactions range from urticaria to anaphylaxis

with hypotension, laryngospasm, and cardiac arrest. Patients should be observed carefully for several hours after dosing, and epinephrine should be available.

199–200. The answers are: 199-J, 200-G.
(Psychiatry; defense mechanisms)
Regression is characterized by a return to less mature levels of functioning. This defense mechanism appears when levels of anxiety become high and are not alleviated by more mature defenses, such as intellectualization and humor. In medically ill patients presented with a very poor prognosis, regression is often manifested by the use of denial or fantasy.

Projection involves attributing to others one's uncomfortable internal feelings, especially anger and guilt. As a result, the person transforms anger at self into anger toward others. Such people often seem bitter or suspicious.

Test III

QUESTIONS

DIRECTIONS: Each of the numbered items or incomplete statements in this section is followed by answers or by completions of the statement. Select the ONE lettered answer or completion that is BEST in each case.

1. Which gynecologic malignancy has no official staging criteria?

(A) Oviductal
(B) Ovarian
(C) Uterine
(D) Vaginal
(E) Vulvar

2. A 45-year-old man complains to his family physician of pain in his left calf. Physical examination reveals some swelling of the left ankle, a reddish-brown discoloration of the skin around the ankle, and a small area of ulceration over the medial malleolus. Nontender superficial varicosities are also noted. The femoral, popliteal, and dorsalis pedis pulses are equal and strong. This patient most likely has

(A) superficial thrombophlebitis
(B) deep venous insufficiency
(C) arterial insufficiency
(D) an immune vasculitis

3. A 40-year-old, happily married man sometimes fantasizes that his wife is wearing high-heeled shoes when they have sex. The best description of this man's response is

(A) exhibitionism
(B) fetishism
(C) frotteurism
(D) voyeurism
(E) normal

4. A 13-year-old boy has a history of recurrent upper and lower respiratory infections that began at 3 years of age. Physical examination reveals a transverse nasal crease; pale, boggy, grayish-pink nasal mucosa; and infraorbital edema with dark pigmentation beneath the eyes. The boy's respiratory rate is increased, and he is barrel-chested. Expiratory wheezes are noted in all lung fields. A posteroanterior chest x-ray reveals radiolucency of the lungs, widening of the intercostal spaces, and flattening of the diaphragm. Which test result would be expected in this patient?

(A) Abnormal sweat chloride test
(B) Low C3 complement level
(C) Abnormal nitroblue tetrazolium (NBT) dye test
(D) Increased serum immunoglobulin E (IgE) levels
(E) Sputum with gram-positive diplococci

5. The potential loss of blood from a closed fracture is greatest in fractures of the

(A) humerus
(B) tibia and fibula
(C) pelvis
(D) spine
(E) femur

6. A 19-year-old female law student becomes very concerned that a small lump in her left breast is malignant cancer. Workup and biopsy show it to be entirely benign, but she remains excessively worried in spite of reassurance by her physician. The best treatment would be

(A) a careful explanation of the benign nature of the physical complaint
(B) use of a benzodiazepine
(C) skillful physician reassurance
(D) use of placebo medication
(E) psychotherapy to explore her current life circumstances

7. An 80-year-old man with a history of coronary artery disease and prostate cancer presents with weakness of both legs for 1 week. He has sensory loss from T10 downward and is barely able to move his legs. He has new onset of bladder dysfunction. What is the proper treatment strategy?

(A) Order emergency myelogram after bolusing with intravenous steroids
(B) Admit the patient and schedule magnetic resonance imaging (MRI) the next day
(C) Schedule plasmapheresis for Guillain-Barré syndrome
(D) Order electromyograph (EMG)
(E) Send for radiation therapy over lumbar and sacral levels

8. A newborn female infant at 1 minute after birth is noted to have acral cyanosis and a weak respiratory effort at a rate of 30 breaths/min. Her heart rate is 105 beats/min and a systolic murmur is heard. She flexes all four extremities weakly, but only after external stimulation. When her nose and mouth are suctioned, she shows no response. She keeps her eyes closed. What is her assigned Apgar score at 1 minute?

(A) 4
(B) 5
(C) 6
(D) 7
(E) 8

9. Which injury is the most common in large-for-gestational-age newborns?

(A) Cephalhematoma
(B) Brachial plexus injury
(C) Intraventricular hemorrhage
(D) Brain contusion
(E) Fractured clavicle

10. A radiograph of the pelvis from a 25-year-old patient of West Indian origin shows bilateral hip deformities with increased density of the bone. Her hemoglobin (Hgb) electrophoresis reveals predominantly Hgb S, slightly increased Hgb F, and no Hgb A. This patient most likely has

(A) osteomyelitis
(B) aseptic necrosis of the femoral heads
(C) pathological bone fractures
(D) osteoarthritis
(E) Legg-Calvé-Perthes disease

11. Somatoform pain disorder is distinguished from chronic pain syndromes by

(A) pain that is disproportionate to the physical lesions
(B) the presence of obvious worker's compensation issues
(C) the absence of physical lesions
(D) good response to biofeedback therapy
(E) the presence of personality pathology

12. A 65-year-old man with a 40 pack-year history of smoking presents with right costovertebral angle pain, hematuria, fever, and a palpable mass on deep palpation of the right lower quadrant. A chest x-ray reveals multiple nodular masses in the lungs. These findings most strongly suggest

(A) renal tuberculosis
(B) renal adenocarcinoma
(C) primary lung cancer with metastasis to the kidney
(D) transitional cell carcinoma of the bladder with metastasis to the lung
(E) acute pyelonephritis with metastatic abscesses in the lung

13. Which drug used in neonatal resuscitation reverses narcotic-induced respiratory depression?

(A) Naloxone
(B) Sodium bicarbonate
(C) Epinephrine
(D) Plasma protein fraction
(E) Beractant

14. Which statement about type I error and the null hypothesis is true?

(A) A true null hypothesis is rejected
(B) A true null hypothesis is accepted
(C) A false null hypothesis is rejected
(D) A false null hypothesis is accepted
(E) A null hypothesis is neither accepted nor rejected

15. A 2-year-old child who plays in a sandbox presents with wheezing, hepatosplenomegaly, and prominent peripheral blood eosinophilia. Which diagnosis is most likely in this child?

(A) Pinworm infestation
(B) Löffler's syndrome
(C) Ascariasis
(D) Visceral larva migrans
(E) Strongyloidiasis

16. A 60-year-old woman presents with bone pain over the sternum and pelvic area. A skeletal survey reveals radiolucent areas in the sternum, ribs, and pelvic bones. Her complete blood count (CBC) shows a hemoglobin (Hgb) of 8.0 g/dl (normal: 12–16 g/dl), normal red blood cell (RBC) indices, a leukocyte count of 3000 cells/μl (normal: 4500–11,000 cells/μl), and a platelet count of 50,000 cells/μl (normal: 150,000–400,000 cells/μl). The peripheral smear shows prominent rouleaux. A bone marrow aspirate exhibits sheets of cells with eccentric nuclei, perinuclear clearing, and basophilic-staining cytoplasm. The physician would expect

(A) the cells in the marrow to be estrogen and progesterone receptor–positive
(B) a normal erythrocyte sedimentation rate (ESR)
(C) hypocalcemia
(D) a monoclonal spike on a serum protein electrophoresis
(E) an excellent response to tamoxifen therapy

17. Which statement about maternal respiratory physiology during pregnancy is true?

(A) Respiratory rate increases
(B) Vital capacity decreases
(C) Minute ventilation increases
(D) Functional residual capacity remains unchanged
(E) Tidal volume decreases

18. A pathology report on a colon biopsy states that "sheets of malignant cells without gland or mucin formation infiltrate the muscle wall and serosal fat. Three out of ten lymph nodes contain metastatic tumor." Which of the following choices concerning grade and stage of cancer is correct?

(A) Well-differentiated; not in report
(B) High-grade; modified Dukes' C2
(C) Low-grade; modified Dukes' B2
(D) Poorly differentiated; not in report

19. In the pediatric population, which extraocular palsy is most commonly associated with a brain tumor?

(A) Superior oblique palsy
(B) Lateral rectus palsy
(C) Inferior oblique palsy
(D) Medial rectus palsy
(E) Superior rectus palsy

20. Which location in the fetal–placental circulation has the highest Po_2 level?

(A) Right atrium
(B) Inferior vena cava
(C) Left ventricle
(D) Ductus arteriosus
(E) Umbilical vein

21. A 6-month-old infant presents to the emergency room with fever, intermittent inspiratory stridor, retraction of the intercostal muscles, and flaring of the nostrils. The mother states that the child has had an upper respiratory infection for the last 1 or 2 days. Which diagnosis is the most likely in this patient?

(A) Laryngotracheobronchitis (croup)
(B) Whooping cough
(C) Acute epiglottitis
(D) Bronchiolitis
(E) Acute bronchial asthma

22. A 15-year-old female patient has frequent occurrences of supraventricular tachycardia, but no evidence of an abnormal conducting pathway of the Wolff-Parkinson-White type. Which regimen is most appropriate for conversion of the arrhythmia and for maintenance?

(A) Flecainide for conversion; adenosine for maintenance
(B) Adenosine for conversion; lidocaine for maintenance
(C) Digoxin for conversion; adenosine for maintenance
(D) Adenosine for conversion; quinidine for maintenance
(E) Digoxin for conversion; quinidine for maintenance

23. A 30-year-old man presents to the emergency room with an acute onset of severe, colicky left flank pain, with radiation of the pain down the abdomen into the groin. He has increased frequency of urination and dysuria. Physical examination shows tenderness in the left costovertebral angle. Urinalysis shows a positive dipstick for blood. Sediment examination confirms the presence of hematuria. The most common metabolic abnormality associated with this patient's disease is

(A) hypercalciuria

(B) increased urine citrate

(C) hyperuricemia

(D) alkaline urine pH

(E) distal renal tubular acidosis

24. A 55-year-old woman goes into shock 24 hours after abdominal surgery for chronic cholecystitis. The most likely cause of the shock is

(A) endotoxic

(B) hemoperitoneum

(C) an acute myocardial infarction

(D) a pulmonary embolus

25. A 43-year-old patient with end-stage renal disease has the following electrocardiogram (ECG).

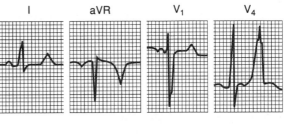

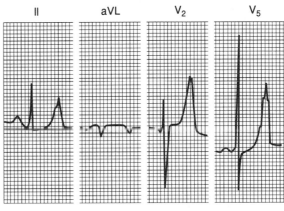

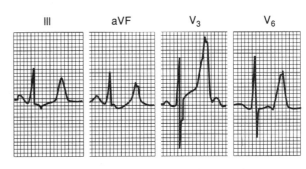

For specifically reversing the effect on the cardiac muscle in this patient, the physician should administer

(A) sodium bicarbonate

(B) furosemide

(C) calcium gluconate

(D) glucose plus insulin

(E) a cation-exchange resin

26. A 42-year-old woman complains of aching in the shoulder muscles and pelvis, with difficulty in climbing stairs. She has a "butterfly rash" over her nose and cheeks, with erythema and edema over the eyelids and knuckles. An electromyograph (EMG) reveals low-amplitude polyphasic potentials, and laboratory testing reveals an elevated creatine phosphokinase (CPK). The most likely diagnosis is

(A) polymyalgia rheumatica
(B) rheumatoid arthritis
(C) polymyositis
(D) dermatomyositis
(E) systemic lupus erythematosus (SLE)

27. Which maternal condition is associated with development of polyhydramnios?

(A) Asthma
(B) Diabetes mellitus
(C) Hyperthyroidism
(D) Seizure disorder
(E) Sickle cell anemia

28. A 48-year-old man complains of memory impairment. Mental status examination reveals an alert and attentive patient with average vocabulary. He remembers one out of three objects after 5 minutes and has marked difficulties with reasoning and abstraction. This combination suggests

(A) delirium
(B) organic amnesic syndrome
(C) dementia
(D) major depression
(E) mental retardation

29. Which statement about hirsutism in women is true?

(A) Race or ethnicity is not a factor
(B) Hirsutism can lead to serious health problems
(C) Treatment is frequently disappointing
(D) Female body contours may disappear
(E) The voice may become deeper

30. A 65-year-old man with a long history of constipation presents with cramping left lower quadrant pain. Physical examination reveals a low-grade fever, midabdominal distention, and left lower quadrant rebound tenderness. An absolute neutrophilic leukocytosis and a shift to the left is noted on a complete blood count (CBC). The patient most likely has

(A) colon cancer
(B) irritable bowel syndrome
(C) acute diverticulitis
(D) ulcerative colitis

31. A 5-year-old child with severe asthma is being treated with an intravenous drip of aminophylline in the emergency room. The child is slowly becoming sleepy and less responsive. Examination of the chest reveals less wheezing than on admission. Which action is the most appropriate in the care of this patient?

(A) Send the child home with the mother
(B) Order a chest x-ray
(C) Measure the theophylline level
(D) Order arterial blood gas studies immediately

32. A 35-year-old man presents to the office with a history of abrupt onset of fever, chills, a productive cough, and chest pain on inspiration. Physical examination shows dullness to percussion, increased tactile fremitus, bronchophony, egophony, and fine, crepitant rales anteriorly over the right lung. A neutrophilic leukocytosis with greater than 20% bands is present. A chest x-ray reveals a lobar consolidation obliterating the outline of the right-heart silhouette. The patient most likely has

(A) pneumococcal pneumonia involving the right upper lobe
(B) *Klebsiella pneumoniae* of the right lower lobe
(C) viral pneumonia of the right middle lobe
(D) *Streptococcus pneumoniae* infection involving the right middle lobe
(E) primary tuberculosis involving the right upper lobe

33. A 65-year-old woman presents to the emergency room with a distended, diffusely painful abdomen. She has not had any bowel movements or passed gas for the past 3 days. An abdominal x-ray reveals distended loops of small bowel with a stepladder pattern of differential air–fluid levels. The mechanism that most likely produced these findings is

(A) ischemia secondary to thrombosis of the superior mesenteric artery
(B) adhesions from previous surgery
(C) torsion of the bowel around the mesenteric root
(D) intussusception of the terminal ileum into the cecum

34. A 5-year-old child presents with occipital headache, an ataxic gait, nystagmus, and papilledema. Which diagnosis is most likely?

(A) Pontine astrocytoma
(B) Pilocytic astrocytoma of the cerebellum
(C) Craniopharyngioma
(D) Colloid cyst of the third ventricle
(E) Medulloblastoma

35. Which statistical test would be most appropriate for assessing the differences in age among three groups of patients?

(A) Student's *t*-test
(B) Analysis of variance
(C) Correlation coefficient
(D) Chi-squared test
(E) Logistic regression

36. A 55-year-old black man with a 5-year history of essential hypertension has a retinal examination revealing an irregular caliber of the arterioles, "copper wiring," and a focal area of arteriovenous nipping. No flame hemorrhages or exudates are present. This patient most likely has

(A) a normal retina
(B) grade I hypertensive retinopathy
(C) grade II hypertensive retinopathy
(D) grade III hypertensive retinopathy
(E) grade IV hypertensive retinopathy

37. A 28-year-old mother of two children undergoes a Pap smear as part of an annual examination. She is taking oral contraceptives. The report shows cytologic atypia. Colposcopically directed biopsy is consistent with condylomata acuminata. Which statement about her condition is true?

(A) The etiologic agent is a herpes virus
(B) Transmission is by infected fomites
(C) Oral contraception increases extent of lesions
(D) Her condition shows no relationship to vaginal infections
(E) Treatment of choice is topical metronidazole

38. A 12-month-old child presents with iron deficiency anemia and a history of rectal bleeding unassociated with pain. Which diagnosis is the most likely in this patient?

(A) Intussusception
(B) Duodenal ulcer
(C) Angiodysplasia
(D) Meckel's diverticulum
(E) Ulcerative colitis

39. The most common fistula in the gastrointestinal tract usually results from

(A) Crohn's disease
(B) ulcerative colitis
(C) diverticular disease
(D) childbirth
(E) peptic ulcer surgery

40. A highly anxious woman complains of seeing gruesome murders committed in alleyways all over the city and believes that her landlord is pumping poisonous gas into her apartment. Which condition is causing her symptoms?

(A) Dementia
(B) Obsessive-compulsive disorder
(C) Panic disorder
(D) Posttraumatic stress disorder
(E) Generalized anxiety disorder

41. A 32-year-old Mexican-American woman who lives in Phoenix, Arizona, presents with fever, a nonproductive cough, flu-like symptoms, chest pain, and painful red nodules on both lower extremities. A chest x-ray shows a left lower lobe cavitation and a small pleural effusion. A mild eosinophilia is noted in the peripheral blood. This patient most likely has

(A) histoplasmosis
(B) *Klebsiella pneumoniae*
(C) tuberculosis
(D) *Mycoplasma pneumoniae*
(E) coccidioidomycosis

42. A 58-year-old man with a 20 pack-year history of smoking is being evaluated for a coronary artery bypass graft. The best preoperative screen of pulmonary function for this patient would be

(A) arterial pH
(B) arterial carbon dioxide tension (P_{CO_2})
(C) arterial oxygen tension (P_{O_2})
(D) forced expiratory volume in 1 second/forced vital capacity (FEV_1/FVC) ratio

43. Which combination suggests "cause and effect"?

(A) Aluminum toxicity—parkinsonism
(B) Carbon monoxide—Huntington's disease
(C) Head trauma—multiple sclerosis
(D) Genetic trait—infantile spasms
(E) Preceding viral illness—Guillain-Barré syndrome

44. A 51-year-old mother of four children underwent a radical hysterectomy for cervical carcinoma 3 weeks ago. She now complains of painless, continuous urine leakage through her vagina. Which test would best assess the cause of this complaint?

(A) Cystometric studies
(B) Urine culture
(C) Intravenous indigo–carmine
(D) Pelvic ultrasonography
(E) Urethral pressure measurements

45. A patient with diabetic ketoacidosis (DKA) is being treated with insulin. During therapy, the patient develops respiratory paralysis requiring intubation and assisted ventilation. What is the mechanism for the patient's respiratory failure?

(A) An anaphylactic reaction against insulin
(B) Glucose toxicity
(C) Ketoacidosis
(D) Hypophosphatemia
(E) Hyperkalemia

46. A 21-year-old woman presents with complaints of painful intercourse on vaginal entry since she got married, as a virgin, 1 month ago. Which condition is the most likely cause of her pain?

(A) Narrow hymen
(B) Psychogenic problem
(C) Endometriosis
(D) Pelvic inflammatory disease (PID)
(E) Atrophic vaginitis

47. Which inborn error of metabolism is associated with thromboembolism, which could predispose to infantile hemiplegia?

(A) Phenylketonuria
(B) Galactosemia
(C) Homocystinuria
(D) Tyrosinemia
(E) Histidinemia

48. A 60-year-old man with intermittent, cramping abdominal pain and obstipation has a barium enema that reveals a massively dilated sigmoid colon with a column of barium resembling a "bird's beak" or an "ace of spades." This patient most likely has

(A) an intussusception
(B) volvulus of the sigmoid colon
(C) toxic megacolon
(D) Ogilvie's syndrome

49. Disturbed recall is an essential feature of

(A) organic psychosis
(B) conversion disorder
(C) dissociative fugue
(D) major depression
(E) delirium

50. Which fetal condition is associated with development of oligohydramnios?

(A) Duodenal atresia
(B) Open spina bifida
(C) Tracheoesophageal fistula
(D) Renal agenesis
(E) Atrial flutter

51. An obese 45-year-old woman develops fever 24 hours after an elective cholecystectomy. The fever is most likely due to

(A) a urinary tract infection secondary to catheterization
(B) a wound infection
(C) atelectasis
(D) intravenous catheter-related sepsis
(E) a normal postoperative finding

52. A child with hemiparesis following a focal or jacksonian seizure plus weakness and neurologic deficits that disappear within 24 hours most likely has which disorder?

(A) Hemiplegia complicating a migraine headache
(B) Acute infantile hemiplegia
(C) Postviral encephalitis
(D) Todd's paralysis
(E) Infratentorial tumor

53. Bipolar disorder is distinguished from schizophrenia by the

(A) course of the illness
(B) presence of depression
(C) presence of anxiety
(D) presence of psychosis
(E) presence of mania

54. A 23-year-old black man has an intermittent history of respiratory difficulties, swelling of the extremities and face, along with abdominal cramps since childhood. There is a strong family history for similar problems in both men and women. Which test would be the best screen for this disease?

(A) C3 complement
(B) C4 complement
(C) Quantitative immunoglobulins
(D) Serum antinuclear antibody test
(E) Sweat test

55. A 58-year-old woman presents with vaginal bleeding of 1 week. She went through menopause 7 years ago. She is 5′ 3″ tall and weighs 190 pounds. The diagnostic method of choice is

(A) Pap smear
(B) endometrial biopsy
(C) pelvic examination under anesthesia
(D) laparoscopy
(E) colposcopy

56. A 56-year-old man develops symptoms of acute pancreatitis postoperatively, including epigastric pain and elevation of serum amylase. This is most likely due to

(A) a reaction to anesthetic drugs
(B) hypovolemia
(C) total parenteral nutrition
(D) a common bile duct exploration for gallstones

57. A 3-year-old child presents with convulsions followed by coma. Cerebrospinal fluid (CSF) findings include a total white blood cell (WBC) count of 250 cells/µl with predominantly lymphocytes and monocytes, glucose of 20 mg/dl, and a protein concentration of 80 mg/dl. A Gram's stain of a spun-down sediment is negative. A computed tomography (CT) scan with contrast shows enhancement at the base of the brain. Which diagnosis is the most likely?

(A) Eastern equine encephalitis
(B) Subacute sclerosing panencephalitis
(C) Tuberculous meningitis
(D) Cryptococcal meningitis
(E) Meningococcal meningitis

58. A 40-year-old man who is a real estate broker complains of excessive worry, jumpiness, feelings of impending doom, feelings of being unable to get enough air, and restlessness. Which condition does this combination suggest?

(A) Depersonalization
(B) Anxiety
(C) Delirium
(D) Depression
(E) Psychosis

59. A 35-year-old man with duodenal ulcer disease had a 10-U blood transfusion for upper gastrointestinal bleeding 3 months ago. He presents with flu-like symptoms, malaise, and tender hepatomegaly. Laboratory studies show an atypical lymphocytosis, a serum alanine aminotransferase (ALT) of 1200 U/L (normal: 8–20 U/L), a serum aspartate aminotransferase (AST) of 800 U/L (normal: 8–20 U/L), a serum alkaline phosphatase of 110 U/L (normal: 20–70 U/L), and a normal total bilirubin. This patient most likely has

(A) infectious mononucleosis
(B) hepatitis A
(C) hepatitis B
(D) hepatitis C
(E) a cytomegalovirus infection

60. A 44-year-old man with scoliosis has wasting of both hands, with loss of pinprick sensation in the hands, arms, and shoulders, but normal proprioception. He has diminished reflexes in the arms, increased reflexes in the legs. There is a right Horner's syndrome. A magnetic resonance imaging (MRI) scan of the cervical and thoracic spine should show

(A) a syrinx
(B) cervical spine stenosis
(C) herniated cervical disc at C7
(D) myelitis from multiple sclerosis
(E) normal result

61. Cytogenetic studies on "complete" hydatidiform moles show that the karyotype for most is

(A) 46 XX
(B) 69 XXX
(C) 46 XY
(D) 45 X
(E) 69 XXY

62. A 46-year-old man underwent an emergency operation to repair a left lung laceration from a knife wound to the chest received during a brawl in a bar. A few days later, he develops anxiety, tremor, hallucinations, overactivity, and seizure activity. The most likely diagnosis is

(A) a reaction to anesthetic drugs
(B) delirium tremens (DTs)
(C) postoperative psychosis
(D) intensive care unit syndrome

63. A child with short stature, polyuria, bitemporal hemianopia, and calcifications above the sella turcica on a computed tomography (CT) scan most likely has

(A) an astrocytoma of the third ventricle
(B) a pinealoma
(C) a craniopharyngioma
(D) a chromophobe adenoma
(E) Hand-Schüller-Christian disease

64. A 62-year-old man with Parkinson's disease, but with no previous psychiatric history, is admitted to the hospital because of the onset, 1 week ago, of emotional lability, disinterest in personal appearance, intermittent inattention and confusion, peculiar beliefs about his wife poisoning his food, and intermittent visual hallucinations concerning insects in the house. He is currently taking carbidopa (Sinemet) and trihexyphenidyl (Artane). He reportedly has a history of alcohol abuse and has been drinking more lately. Mental status examination reveals that the patient is oriented to year but not month. The most likely psychiatric diagnosis in this patient is

(A) alcoholic hallucinosis
(B) organic mood syndrome
(C) delirium of unknown etiology
(D) dementia owing to Parkinson's disease
(E) alcoholic dementia

65. A 33-year-old woman complains of severe agoraphobia. She also has a history of childhood anxiety. The disorder most likely associated with these symptoms is

(A) panic disorder
(B) somatization disorder
(C) obsessive-compulsive disorder
(D) schizophrenia
(E) major depression

66. An appropriate indication for cesarean delivery of a fetus through a transverse low segment uterine incision is

(A) coexistent invasive cervical cancer
(B) transverse lie, back down
(C) arrest of active phase of labor
(D) dead mother with live child
(E) shoulder presentation with arm in vagina

67. A 65-year-old man with multiple myeloma presents with confusion, severe depression, vomiting, constipation, and polyuria. His electrocardiogram (ECG) follows.

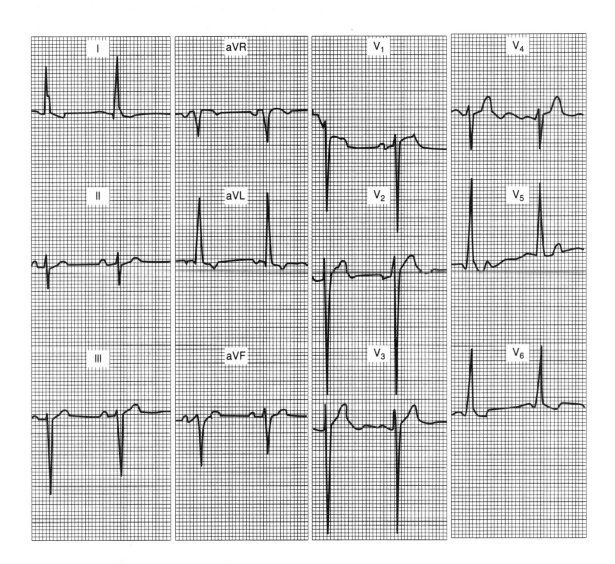

The first step in the management of this patient is to

(A) give calcium gluconate
(B) infuse saline
(C) administer sodium bicarbonate
(D) infuse furosemide
(E) initiate mithramycin therapy

68. Which statistical test would be most appropriate for assessing the differences in height between two groups of patients?

(A) Student's *t*-test
(B) Analysis of variance
(C) Correlation coefficient
(D) Chi-squared test
(E) Logistic regression

69. A 26-year-old man with multiple fractures and soft-tissue injuries from a motorcycle accident has diffuse bleeding from all needle puncture sites and open wounds on the second day of hospitalization. His prothrombin time is 20 seconds (normal: 11–15 seconds), his partial thromboplastin time is 100 seconds (normal: 60–85 seconds), and his platelet count is 45,000 cells/μl (normal: 150,000–400,000 cells/μl). This patient most likely has

(A) thrombotic thrombocytopenic purpura (TTP)
(B) disseminated intravascular coagulation (DIC)
(C) fat embolism syndrome
(D) primary fibrinolysis

70. An advantage of a classic uterine incision for cesarean delivery is

(A) decreased chance of scar rupture
(B) less operative blood loss
(C) fewer subsequent bowel adhesions
(D) reduced risk of paralytic ileus
(E) least delivery trauma risk to fetus

71. A 23-year-old woman presents with suprapubic pain, dysuria, and increased frequency of urination. A urinary sediment examination reveals clumps of neutrophils, occasional red blood cells (RBCs), and rod-shaped bacteria. No casts or crystals are present. Assuming that this sediment is representative of the entire specimen, the patient would be expected to have

(A) excessive proteinuria
(B) a positive dipstick for nitrite and leukocyte esterase
(C) a nephritic type of glomerulonephritis
(D) acute pyelonephritis
(E) a renal stone

72. A child with mental retardation, eczema, hypopigmentation, and blue eyes most likely has which disorder?

(A) Down syndrome
(B) Tuberous sclerosis
(C) Phenylketonuria
(D) Cretinism
(E) Galactosemia

73. A 49-year-old man complains of a 6-month history of worrying about his health, increased desire to sleep, demoralization, and difficulty focusing attention on tasks. These symptoms are most commonly associated with

(A) mania
(B) somatization disorder
(C) anxiety
(D) depression
(E) delirium

74. A previously healthy patient weighing 170 pounds is lying quietly in bed, receiving controlled mechanical ventilation via an endotracheal tube at a rate of 16 breaths/min with a tidal volume (V_T) of 700 ml. Which maneuver would most likely cause an arterial $Paco_2$ of 25 mm Hg to increase to 50 mm Hg?

(A) Add 150 ml of dead space
(B) Decrease the ventilatory rate to 12 breaths/min
(C) Decrease the V_T to 500 ml
(D) Decrease the ventilatory rate to 14 breaths/min and the V_T to 600 ml

75. Which feature is associated with a serum prolactin level that is lower than normal?

(A) Craniopharyngioma
(B) Sheehan's syndrome
(C) Tricyclic antidepressants
(D) Acromegaly
(E) Chest surgery

76. What is the most common brain tumor in children?

(A) Medulloblastoma
(B) Pilocytic astrocytoma of the cerebellum
(C) Ependymoma
(D) Neuroblastoma
(E) Oligodendroglioma

77. Mania is distinguished from depression by

(A) an altered level of activity
(B) the presence of psychosis
(C) the quality of mood
(D) the presence of insomnia
(E) the presence of known pathophysiology

78. A 38-year-old man presents with bouts of severe, right retro-orbital pain lasting one-half hour or more, up to several times a day. The pain often occurs at night and is associated with nasal congestion on the right and right conjunctival injection. A possibly effective acute treatment would be

(A) sublingual nitroglycerin
(B) an alcoholic beverage
(C) vigorous exercise
(D) nasal oxygen
(E) a warm pack over the eye

79. A 2-year-old boy presents with recurrent and severe paroxysmal colicky pain accompanied by straining efforts, loud cries, and vomiting. A stool with red blood mixed with mucus is passed. An oblong mass is palpated in the mid-epigastrium. The most likely diagnosis is

(A) a Meckel's diverticulum
(B) congenital pyloric stenosis
(C) an intussusception
(D) meconium ileus
(E) necrotizing enterocolitis

80. Which gynecologic malignancy is surgically staged?

(A) Cervical
(B) Ovarian
(C) Uterine
(D) Vaginal
(E) Vulvar

81. A 23-year-old medical student expresses concern that the lump he has discovered in his neck is an indication of Hodgkin's disease. A routine workup is completely negative, but the patient says that he cannot stop worrying about it. The most likely diagnosis is

(A) conversion disorder
(B) hypochondriasis
(C) delusional disorder, somatic type
(D) somatization disorder
(E) factitious disorder

82. A 65-year-old patient develops aspiration pneumonitis following general anesthesia. Twenty-four hours later, there is a rapid onset of dyspnea, tachypnea, cyanosis, and intercostal retractions. A chest x-ray shows diffuse, bilateral infiltrates with both an interstitial and alveolar pattern. There is sparing of the costophrenic angles. Air bronchograms are noted. The arterial blood gases on room air show a pH of 7.50 (normal: 7.35–7.45), a Pa_{CO_2} of 29 mm Hg (normal: 33–44 mm Hg), a Pa_{O_2} of 40 mm Hg (normal: 75–105 mm Hg), and a bicarbonate of 21 mEq/L (normal: 22–28 mEq/L). The mechanism most responsible for this patient's clinical and laboratory findings is

(A) depression of the respiratory center
(B) intrapulmonary shunting
(C) increased compliance of the lungs
(D) increased elasticity of the lungs
(E) atelectasis with respiratory acidosis

83. A 75-year-old man with a 35 pack-year history of smoking presents with puffiness of the face, arms, and shoulders associated with a bluish to purple discoloration of the skin. In addition, he complains of dizziness, dyspnea, and cough. Neck vein distention is noted on physical examination. The pathogenesis for this patient's findings most likely results from

(A) primary lung cancer
(B) a pericardial effusion
(C) sclerosing mediastinitis
(D) polycythemia rubra vera

84. Which gynecologic malignancy has the best 5-year survival rate for stage I disease?

(A) Cervical
(B) Vaginal
(C) Endometrial
(D) Ovarian
(E) Oviductal

85. Which pathogen is the most common cause of neonatal meningitis?

(A) *Escherichia coli*
(B) *Listeria monocytogenes*
(C) *Streptococcus agalactiae*
(D) *Streptococcus pneumoniae*
(E) *Neisseria meningitidis*

86. Which statistical test would be most appropriate for assessing the differences in 1-minute Apgar scores between infants born by emergency cesarean section and those born by spontaneous vaginal delivery?

(A) Student's *t*-test
(B) Analysis of variance
(C) Correlation coefficient
(D) Chi-squared test
(E) Logistic regression

87. Malingering is distinguished from factitious disorder by

(A) volitional nature of symptoms
(B) the duration of the complaints
(C) the presence of secondary gain
(D) the resemblance of the complaints to believable pathology
(E) the type of physical complaints

88. A 60-year-old man who had been treated for leukemia is admitted to the hospital with malaise, chills, and high fever. His chest is clear to percussion and auscultation, with no heart murmurs. His abdomen is free of masses or tenderness. Extensive erythematous lesions are present on his trunk and extremities, some of which have progressed to the hemorrhagic stage with necrosis. Skin scrapings and blood samples are obtained for Gram's stain and microbiologic culture. Which action is most appropriate?

(A) Withhold antibiotics until all microbiologic results are available
(B) Prescribe erythromycin orally
(C) Start treatment with intravenous (IV) ampicillin
(D) Administer tetracycline IV to cover for both gram-positive and gram-negative organisms
(E) Initiate treatment with parenteral cefazolin and tobramycin

89. A 31-year-old woman complains of an overwhelming number of physical problems involving practically every organ system. She has seen numerous physicians over the last 10 years and describes them all as "quacks." The most appropriate treatment for her is

(A) regularly scheduled medical visits
(B) trials of various medications
(C) a refusal to see her again
(D) referral to another clinician
(E) a warning to use medical resources more sparingly

90. A 56-year-old, asymptomatic man from Ohio has a concentrically calcified solitary coin lesion in the right upper lung lobe. This lesion most likely represents

(A) a primary lung cancer
(B) a bronchial hamartoma
(C) metastatic cancer
(D) a granuloma

91. Three men ranging from 35 to 55 years of age are brought to the emergency room in an ambulance after their friends found them in a hunting lodge that morning. Because of the cold weather that evening, they started a fire in a wood-burning stove vented to the outside of the building. Two of the three men are dead on arrival. The third man is unresponsive to verbal commands. Physical examination shows an obese male with alcohol on his breath and a ruddy complexion. Arterial blood gases on room air are reported as normal. The first step in the management of this patient is to

(A) administer methylene blue intravenously
(B) give amyl nitrite, sodium nitrite, and sodium thiosulfate
(C) intubate the patient and administer 100% oxygen
(D) administer activated charcoal

92. Which cause of infertility has the highest incidence?

(A) Ovulatory factor
(B) Cervical factor
(C) Uterine factor
(D) Tubal factor
(E) Male factor

93. A 3-year-old child develops fever, listlessness, and nuchal rigidity. A spinal tap would most likely reveal

(A) *Haemophilus influenzae* type B
(B) *Escherichia coli*
(C) *Neisseria meningitidis*
(D) *Streptococcus pneumoniae*
(E) group B streptococcus

94. A 17-year-old boy with a low-grade fever and pain in the right lower quadrant on palpation of the left lower quadrant of the abdomen most likely has

(A) ulcerative colitis
(B) Crohn's disease
(C) acute appendicitis
(D) irritable bowel syndrome
(E) psychogenic pain

95. An 18-year-old woman is sluggish during the day and has had two motor vehicle accidents related to falling asleep at the wheel. She also has abrupt sleep attacks during which she collapses to the ground briefly without loss of consciousness, and on several occasions has had episodes of terrifying hallucinations just as she is falling asleep. What should her polysomnogram show?

(A) Normal sleep
(B) Sleep-onset rapid eye movement (REM)
(C) Episodic obstructive sleep apnea
(D) Periodic leg movements during sleep
(E) Delta wave sleep onset (stages III and IV)

96. Which gynecologic malignancy has a staging category of IA_2?

(A) Vulvar
(B) Vaginal
(C) Cervical
(D) Endometrial
(E) Trophoblastic

97. Delirium and schizophrenia both commonly present with a history of

(A) social withdrawal
(B) memory impairment
(C) hallucinations
(D) a family history of psychopathology
(E) waxing and waning of symptoms over hours

98. A 3-year-old child has gait abnormalities, absent deep tendon reflexes bilaterally, increased cerebrospinal fluid (CSF) protein with a normal glucose and cell count, and urinary sediment that stains positively with toluidene blue. Which disease is the most likely diagnosis in this child?

(A) Phenylketonuria
(B) Metachromatic leukodystrophy
(C) Krabbe's disease
(D) Fabry's disease
(E) Adrenoleukodystrophy (Schilder's disease)

99. Which pathogen is most commonly associated with sterile effusions complicating meningitis?

(A) *Neisseria meningitidis*
(B) *Streptococcus pneumoniae*
(C) *Escherichia coli*
(D) *Haemophilus influenzae*
(E) *Staphylococcus aureus*

100. Conversion disorder is distinguished from factitious disorder by

(A) the presence of emotional distress
(B) the presence of unconscious psychological conflict
(C) physical symptoms involving loss of function
(D) a lengthy clinical course
(E) involuntary production of symptoms

101. Which gynecologic malignancy is considered an epidemiologic venereal disease?

(A) Vulvar
(B) Vaginal
(C) Cervical
(D) Endometrial
(E) Ovarian

102. Several months after a Billroth II procedure for intractable peptic ulcer disease, a 48-year-old woman has palpitations, sweating, diarrhea, and flushing of the face 30 minutes after eating. This is most likely secondary to

(A) gastroparesis
(B) dumping syndrome
(C) afferent loop syndrome
(D) efferent loop syndrome

103. A young male patient comes to the clinic with complaints of dysuria and urethral discharge of yellow pus. A Gram's stain of exudate shows gram-negative cocci, subsequently confirmed as *Neisseria gonorrhoeae* by the laboratory. The patient is out of work and appears to be malnourished. He has no drug allergies. The most appropriate treatment for this patient would be

(A) a single injection of ceftriaxone plus a single oral dose of azithromycin
(B) procaine penicillin G by injection plus oral probenecid
(C) oral amoxicillin for 7 days
(D) spectinomycin as a single intramuscular injection
(E) oral tetracycline for 7 days

104. Which statement about validity is correct? It

(A) expresses the degree to which two things are related

(B) implies that the results of a test can be reproduced

(C) concerns how well a study measures what it purports to measure

(D) measures the strength of relationship between cause and effect

(E) indicates the probability of obtaining a given result by chance alone

105. A woman's family sues a physician for malpractice after she dies while in his care. For this claim, the family must prove that the doctor

(A) was improperly educated

(B) intended to cause the patient harm

(C) committed a crime

(D) overcharged the patient for the care given

(E) deviated from the established standard of care

106. What is the primary purpose for performing a Pap smear during the annual pelvic examination?

(A) Screening asymptomatic patients for preinvasive cervical malignancy

(B) Evaluating the probable cause for vaginal infections

(C) Evaluating the probable cause for postmenopausal bleeding

(D) Screening asymptomatic patients for ovarian malignancy

(E) Confirming the diagnosis of suspicious cervical lesions

107. A child with known neurofibromatosis presents with unilateral decrease in visual acuity, pallor of the disc, and exophthalmos. Which diagnosis is the most likely in this child?

(A) Craniopharyngioma

(B) Optic nerve glioma

(C) Medulloblastoma

(D) Cavernous sinus thrombosis

(E) Cerebellar astrocytoma

108. Schizotypal personality disorder is distinguished from schizophrenia by the absence of

(A) a family history of schizophrenia

(B) a good response to antipsychotic medications

(C) any history of psychosis

(D) bizarre preoccupations

(E) severe social impairment

Questions 109–110

A 9-year-old girl had been treated with erythromycin for a respiratory tract infection, but she continued to have headaches and stuffy nose. A facial x-ray suggested maxillary sinusitis, but this diagnosis could not be confirmed following sinus puncture. Amoxicillin was prescribed for 10 days; but on day 9 the child developed abdominal pain, with diarrhea that was initially watery but then became mucoid with blood. She had these symptoms for several days before her physician was informed. A toxin titer for *Clostridium difficile* was requested; and on hospitalization, sigmoidoscopy revealed colitis, with pseudomembranes confirmed histologically. The patient was treated with oral vancomycin for 7 days and discharged following rectoscopic examination that proved normal and a negative stool culture.

109. Which of the following antibiotics are reported to be involved in gastrointestinal super-infections of this type?

(A) Ampicillin
(B) Clindamycin
(C) Tetracycline
(D) Cefazolin
(E) All of the above

110. Vancomycin is a glycopeptide that in some patients may be antigenic. If the child in this case is known to be allergic to vancomycin, management of her pseudomembranous colitis should involve

(A) treatment with vancomycin because allergic reactions do not occur following oral administration
(B) treatment with amoxicillin plus clavulanic acid
(C) administration of oral metronidazole
(D) management of the patient symptomatically, withholding all antibiotics because they have the potential to exacerbate the colitis
(E) administration of trimethoprim—sulfamethoxazole (TMP–SMZ)

111. A 35-year-old man with a long history of epigastric distress experiences sudden onset of severe epigastric distress with associated pain in the left shoulder. Physical examination reveals a rigid abdomen with rebound tenderness. The first step in the management of this patient is to

(A) order a barium study of the upper gastrointestinal system
(B) order an upright and supine abdominal film
(C) perform a peritoneal lavage
(D) administer antacids

112. Which gynecologic malignancy has lactate dehydrogenase (LDH) as a tumor marker?

(A) Endodermal sinus tumor
(B) Dysgerminoma
(C) Embryonal cell carcinoma
(D) Choriocarcinoma
(E) Immature teratoma

113. A 9-year-old boy constantly tests the limits of discipline with parents and teachers. He gets along well with his peers, however, and he seems to be able to complete projects that he likes. The most likely diagnosis is

(A) oppositional defiant disorder
(B) mental retardation
(C) conduct disorder
(D) childhood disintegrative disorder
(E) attention-deficit hyperactivity disorder

114. A child with sinusitis presents with fever, confusion, extraocular palsies, and proptosis of the eye. Which condition is the most likely diagnosis?

(A) Hand-Schüller-Christian disease
(B) Graves' disease
(C) Cavernous sinus thrombosis
(D) Acute bacterial conjunctivitis
(E) Temporal lobe abscess

115. Which cancer is responsible for the most deaths in women each year?

(A) Endometrial
(B) Breast
(C) Lung
(D) Colon
(E) Cervical

Questions 116–117

A 64-year-old man with carcinoma of the tongue was hospitalized and received chemotherapy. He was brought to the operating room for radical neck dissection and received 2 g of cefoxitin intravenously. Within 10 minutes the patient was wheezing and had developed an urticarial rash. His systolic blood pressure had dropped to 40–50 mm Hg. The operation was postponed; and the patient was given intravenous epinephrine, dexamethasone, diphenhydramine, and fluids. Blood pressure was restored and maintained by intravenous dopamine. In the intensive care unit (ICU), the electrocardiogram (ECG) revealed cardiac injury; and a subsequent x-ray showed bilateral pulmonary edema, which responded to supportive care over the next 5 days.

116. Which statement regarding the use of cefoxitin in this patient is most accurate?

(A) Cefoxitin is not appropriate in a patient who is likely to be immunosuppressed

(B) The prophylactic use of an antibiotic during surgery is valid in this patient

(C) The reaction could have been avoided with a lower dose of cefoxitin

(D) In this patient, erythromycin would have provided more effective coverage against postoperative infection

(E) It would have been better to have used penicillin G in this patient

117. Regarding the drug reaction in this patient, all of the following statements are accurate EXCEPT

(A) it was a type I (immediate) allergic reaction

(B) the cardiovascular changes were probably secondary to hypoxia

(C) skin testing with a dilute solution of cefoxitin would have revealed hypersensitivity

(D) the reaction was IgE-mediated

(E) reactions of this type occur more frequently after administration of penicillins than after cephalosporins

118. A 16-year-old boy who is married and self-supporting requires surgery. Who must give consent for the surgery?

(A) One parent

(B) The spouse

(C) Both parents

(D) A court-appointed legal guardian

(E) The 16-year-old boy himself

119. Which one of the following is the most physiologic shunt used in the treatment of portal hypertension?

(A) Mesocaval shunt

(B) Side-to-side portacaval shunt

(C) End-to-side portacaval shunt

(D) Distal splenorenal shunt

120. Which mechanism gives estrogen its protective effect against osteoporosis?

(A) Enhanced bone formation

(B) Decreased bone formation

(C) Enhanced bone resorption

(D) Decreased bone resorption

(E) Enhanced formation and decreased resorption

121. Which bias is most effectively reduced by double-blinding investigators in a randomized prospective study design?

(A) Measurement bias
(B) Selection bias
(C) Analysis bias
(D) Recall bias
(E) Ascertainment bias

122. A 38-year-old man seeks treatment for a depressive episode. His initial complaints involve feelings of hopelessness and despair, with marked lack of energy. The greatest risk for suicide during the course of treatment occurs

(A) when the patient admits his feelings of guilt
(B) when the patient completes a course of electroconvulsive therapy
(C) at the start of treatment
(D) when the patient develops untoward effects to antidepressants
(E) when the patient begins to respond to antidepressant medication

123. Which risk factor is associated with development of osteoporosis in women?

(A) Low dietary animal protein
(B) Increase in body mass index
(C) Multiparity
(D) Cigarette smoking
(E) Exercise

124. A 63-year-old woman who was given high doses of analgesics and a benzodiazepine postoperatively develops mild confusion, disorientation, and anxiety. Her behavioral symptoms are best managed by

(A) attempts at guided imagery
(B) soft restraints to a stationary bed
(C) a well-lighted room with frequent interaction
(D) adequate doses of benzodiazepines for sedation
(E) a darkened room with decreased interaction

125. A 45-year-old obese woman enters the emergency room complaining of steady, severe, aching pain in the right upper quadrant that radiates to the right scapula. The onset was acute and occurred 15 minutes after eating. She has nausea and vomiting, but the pain is not relieved by vomiting. Palpation after inspiration reveals right upper quadrant tenderness. Laboratory studies reveal an absolute leukocytosis and a shift to the left. The mechanism most likely responsible for her condition is

(A) an impacted stone in the cystic duct
(B) chemically induced inflammation of the gallbladder
(C) an impacted stone in the common bile duct
(D) biliary dyskinesia

126. Designating legal representatives to make decisions concerning one's health care in the event that one can no longer do so is most correctly known as

(A) a living will
(B) a durable power of attorney
(C) managed care
(D) involuntary treatment
(E) informed consent

127. Which endocrinologic profile including follicle-stimulating hormone (FSH), gonadotropin-releasing hormone (GnRH), and sex hormone–binding globulin (SHBG) is characteristic of postmenopausal women?

	FSH	GnRH	Estrogen	SHBG
(A)	Increased	Decreased	Increased	Increased
(B)	Increased	Increased	Decreased	Decreased
(C)	Increased	Decreased	Decreased	Decreased
(D)	Decreased	Decreased	Decreased	Decreased
(E)	Increased	Increased	Increased	Increased

128. A 32-year-old man with eunuchoid proportions and arachnodactyly comes to the emergency room complaining of sudden onset of severe substernal chest pain with searing pain radiating down his back. An immediate chest x-ray reveals widening of the aortic diameter. The pathogenesis of this man's disease is most closely related to

(A) atherosclerosis
(B) cystic medial necrosis
(C) vasculitis secondary to syphilis
(D) granulomatous inflammation

129. Autism is distinguished from mental retardation by

(A) a more severe prognosis
(B) a progressive deterioration of function over the developmental period
(C) a qualitative disturbance of normal development
(D) the presence of areas of brilliant accomplishment
(E) the presence of normal intelligence

130. Which factor in the woman's history is the most likely cause for the postpartum hemorrhage?

(A) Size of the baby
(B) Multiparity
(C) Length of labor
(D) Duration of oxytocin administration
(E) Maternal age

131. The psychotherapeutic exploration of unconscious conflict might be most useful for a patient suffering from

(A) social phobia
(B) enuresis
(C) schizophrenia
(D) obsessive-compulsive disorder
(E) dysthymia

132. The most significant health hazard of menopause is

(A) osteoporosis
(B) genital atrophy
(C) urinary tract atrophy
(D) depression
(E) cardiovascular disease

133. A 50-year-old woman presents with fever, jaundice, and colicky, right upper quadrant pain. The most likely diagnosis is

(A) amebic liver abscess
(B) acute hepatitis
(C) acute pancreatitis
(D) ascending cholangitis

134. Which statement about rape is true?

(A) Approximately 25% of rapists are white

(B) Rape is frequently associated with the use of weapons

(C) Rapists usually rape women of a different race

(D) The "rape trauma syndrome" typically lasts less than 3 months

(E) Most rapists are older than 25 years

Questions 135–136

A 5-year-old child awakens at night with a high fever, sore throat, drooling, inspiratory stridor, and respiratory distress.

135. The first step in the management of this child is to

(A) order a lateral soft-tissue x-ray of the neck structures

(B) prepare to establish an airway

(C) treat the patient immediately with aerosolized racemic epinephrine

(D) procure a throat swab and do a Gram's stain

(E) obtain arterial blood gas values to evaluate the degree of hypoxemia

136. Which pathogen is the most likely cause of the child's disease?

(A) Respiratory syncytial virus

(B) Parainfluenza virus

(C) *Haemophilus influenzae* type B

(D) *Staphylococcus aureus*

(E) Group A streptococcus

Questions 137–138

137. Test X for systemic lupus erythematosus (SLE) is positive in 60 out of 100 patients with known SLE and is normal in 80 out of 100 controls. If test X returns positive in a person who is randomly selected in this population under study, what is the percent chance that the person has SLE?

(A) 60%

(B) 65%

(C) 70%

(D) 75%

(E) 80%

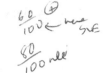

138. Assume that test X for SLE is being used in a patient population where SLE has a prevalence of 10%. If the test returns positive in a person who is randomly selected in this population under study, what is the percent chance that the person has SLE?

(A) 25%

(B) 50%

(C) 60%

(D) 75%

(E) 80%

Questions 139–140

A 35-year-old man complains of stomach pain. When the clinician tries to ask him questions, he answers, "You're the doctor; you figure it out." He also states that he does not like the clinician's attitude and will sue if he is not treated appropriately. "If you make me leave the hospital," he adds, "I'll cut my wrists in the parking lot and it will be your fault."

139. The personality trait that best describes this patient's style of interaction is

(A) antisocial
(B) passive–aggressive
(C) passive–dependent
(D) avoidant
(E) narcissistic

140. The best first response to this patient would be to say

(A) "Without better cooperation, I'll be forced to order a stat barium enema and then probably have to do exploratory surgery"
(B) "You make me feel unable to help you, and that hurts me personally"
(C) "You seem angry with me, and I'd like to know why"
(D) "You're an irritating person, and that makes me angry"
(E) "I'm sure that you'd like my colleague better—I'll page her right away"

141. Which gynecologic malignancy is staged surgically?

(A) Vulvar
(B) Vaginal
(C) Cervical
(D) Endometrial
(E) Trophoblastic

142. A 35-year-old man complains of rapid onset of midepigastric pain with radiation into the back after eating a large meal. He has nausea and vomiting. Physical examination reveals low-grade fever, epigastric tenderness, and decreased bowel sounds. An abdominal film shows a localized dilatation of the upper duodenum and a small collection of fluid in the left pleural cavity. Which of the following tests would be most useful and cost-effective in confirming the diagnosis?

(A) Upper gastrointestinal barium study
(B) Endoscopy
(C) Serum amylase or lipase
(D) Oral cholecystogram
(E) HIDA radionuclide scan

143. A random sample of 100 female students is selected from the freshman class of a large university. The women are followed prospectively over 4 years to see if use of oral contraceptive pills is associated with a decrease in ovarian cysts. What is the study design?

(A) Cohort study
(B) Case-control study
(C) Randomized controlled trial
(D) Cross-sectional study
(E) Crossover prospective study

144. An 8-year-old girl worries every day that she will be abducted after classes and never see her family again. This worrying interferes with her ability to work or play in school. She voices no other worries. This symptom is most consistent with

(A) overanxious disorder of childhood
(B) simple phobia
(C) pervasive developmental disorder
(D) social phobia
(E) separation anxiety disorder

145. Which histologic type of endometrial carcinoma is associated with the best prognosis?

(A) Secretory carcinoma
(B) Grade III adenocarcinoma
(C) Adenosquamous carcinoma
(D) Clear cell carcinoma
(E) Papillary serous carcinoma

146. A 65-year-old man with a 40 pack-year history of smoking associated with productive cough presents with a 15-pound weight loss over the last 3 months and recent onset of streaks of blood in the sputum. Physical examination reveals a thin, afebrile man with clubbing of the fingers, an increased anteroposterior diameter, scattered coarse rhonchi and wheezes over both lung fields, and distant heart sounds. A chest x-ray exhibits left hilar adenopathy, dilated tubular markings, and flattened diaphragms. A sputum cytology using a Papanicolaou stain is reported to show eosinophilic staining cells, with irregular, hyperchromatic nuclei intermixed with inflammatory cells. The most likely diagnosis in this patient is

(A) tuberculosis
(B) small cell carcinoma of the lung
(C) a pulmonary embolism with infarction
(D) bronchiectasis
(E) a squamous cell carcinoma of the lung

147. Which gynecologic malignancy has staging categories Ic, IIc, and IIIc?

(A) Vulvar
(B) Vaginal
(C) Cervical
(D) Endometrial
(E) Ovarian

148. Antisocial personality disorder is best distinguished from other conditions by

(A) membership in cults with destructive ideologies and plans for future warfare
(B) a belief that other people are unimportant, coupled with an idealization of past tyrants such as Hitler and Genghis Khan
(C) a childhood history of enuresis, fire-setting, and cruelty to animals
(D) a history of abuse during childhood, impulsivity and anger, and incarceration for substance-abuse–related crimes
(E) a long and pervasive pattern of disregard for and violation of the basic rights of others

149. A 45-year-old afebrile man with chronic pancreatitis has a palpable abdominal mass and a persistently elevated serum amylase. This is most consistent with a pancreatic

(A) cystadenoma
(B) pseudocyst
(C) carcinoma
(D) abscess

DIRECTIONS: Each of the numbered items or incomplete statements in this section is negatively phrased, as indicated by a capitalized word such as NOT, LEAST, or EXCEPT. Select the ONE lettered answer or completion that is BEST in each case.

150. All of the following laboratory findings would be expected in an 88-year-old man EXCEPT

(A) plasma hemoglobin in the adult female range
(B) slightly increased alkaline phosphatase
(C) slightly decreased arterial oxygen partial pressure (Pa_{O_2})
(D) slightly increased serum albumin
(E) slightly decreased gonadotropins

151. Characteristics of vitamin-D–resistant rickets include all of the following EXCEPT

(A) inability to reabsorb phosphate in the renal tubules
(B) hypocalcemia
(C) hypophosphatemia
(D) excess osteoid
(E) sex-linked dominant inheritance

152. A 52-year-old man who is a cattle rancher complains that he has become terrified of flying in private planes since an acquaintance of his was killed in one. However, flying is a necessary part of running his enterprise. All of the following statements indicate a phobia EXCEPT that the

(A) patient always avoids flying
(B) patient believes that his fears are realistic
(C) patient's fears are grounded in reality
(D) patient has no unconscious symbolism behind his fear

153. Prenatal diethylstilbestrol (DES) exposure can predispose to all of the following conditions in female offspring EXCEPT

(A) vaginal adenosis
(B) koilocytic cervical dysplasia
(C) spontaneous abortion
(D) clear cell vaginal adenocarcinoma
(E) anomalous uterus

154. Specific evidence of child abuse in a 7-year-old child includes all of the following conditions EXCEPT

(A) old healed fractures
(B) bruised buttocks
(C) rupture of the liver
(D) bruised knees
(E) subdural hematoma

155. Presumptive evidence for menopause includes all of the following EXCEPT

(A) elevated gonadotropins
(B) hot flashes
(C) night sweats
(D) metromenorrhagia
(E) decreased vaginal secretions

156. All of the following conditions may present with psychosis EXCEPT

(A) schizoid personality disorder
(B) major depression
(C) cocaine delirium
(D) bipolar disorder (manic)
(E) Alzheimer's dementia

157. Adult females differ from adult males in all of the following laboratory parameters EXCEPT

(A) they have lower hemoglobin concentration than men
(B) they have more estradiol than men
(C) they have slightly higher serum creatinine levels than men
(D) they have fewer iron stores than men

158. All of the following genetic disease relationships are correct EXCEPT

(A) Tay-Sachs—cherry red macula
(B) homocystinuria—dislocated lens
(C) phenylketonuria—vomiting resembling pyloric stenosis
(D) maple syrup urine disease—abnormal crystals in the urine
(E) trisomy 18—rocker-bottom feet

159. All of the following adverse effects are common complications of lithium therapy EXCEPT

(A) abnormal liver function tests
(B) tremor
(C) hypothyroidism
(D) polyuria
(E) leukocytosis

160. All of the following conditions are predisposing causes of endometrial adenocarcinoma EXCEPT

(A) obesity
(B) diabetes mellitus
(C) early menopause
(D) history of breast cancer
(E) unopposed estrogen

161. Which sign or symptom is LEAST likely to be present in neonatal meningitis?

(A) Temperature instability
(B) Lethargy
(C) Jaundice
(D) Nuchal rigidity
(E) Respiratory distress

162. A 39-year-old woman states that she has been living with another woman for the past 5 years in a stable, sexual relationship. All of the following statements about this patient are likely to be true EXCEPT

(A) she has had sex with a man in the past
(B) she would like to have a sex-change operation
(C) she has had children
(D) she has normal estrogen levels
(E) she has a homosexual relative

163. All of the following diseases in the bowel commonly present with obstruction EXCEPT

(A) carcinoid tumor of the small bowel
(B) intussusception
(C) volvulus
(D) Hirschsprung's disease
(E) angiodysplasia

164. The LEAST likely risk factor for primary breast cancer in a woman is

(A) history of endometrial carcinoma
(B) low-fiber diet
(C) first-degree relative with breast cancer
(D) previous history of contralateral breast cancer
(E) history of taking combination-type oral contraceptives

165. A 7-year-old boy is referred from a school because of poor reading ability and disruptiveness in class. All of the following indicators are productive components of testing EXCEPT

(A) lead levels
(B) food allergies
(C) hearing acuity
(D) family stress markers
(E) IQ

166. Signs and symptoms of heroin addiction in the newborn include all of the following EXCEPT

(A) low birth weight and prematurity
(B) withdrawal, usually within the first 48 hours of birth
(C) acceleration of surfactant synthesis
(D) generalized hypotonia
(E) high-pitched cry

167. A 53-year-old patient who was diagnosed with diabetes at 45 years of age complains that he is having sexual problems. All of the following are likely to be true EXCEPT

(A) he is not maintaining optimal blood sugar levels
(B) erection is normal but ejaculatory problems are present
(C) microscopic nerve damage is present
(D) psychological problems are present
(E) vascular changes in the penis are present

168. Which condition is LEAST likely to present with polyarthritis?

(A) Rheumatic fever
(B) Wilson's disease
(C) Whipple's disease
(D) Gout
(E) Juvenile rheumatoid arthritis

169. Each condition listed is an indication for postmenopausal estrogen replacement therapy EXCEPT

(A) cystocele
(B) urethritis
(C) osteoporosis
(D) hepatitis

170. A 51-year-old woman stopped menstruating at 49 years of age. Which symptom is LEAST likely to occur?

(A) Reduced vaginal lubrication
(B) Hot flashes
(C) Reduced libido
(D) Thinning of the vaginal mucosa
(E) Pain on intercourse

171. A 40-year-old man complains of increased hat size and headaches when he wakes up in the morning. Physical examination reveals a mild diastolic hypertension, a prominent jaw with spaces between the teeth, large hands and feet, and generalized muscle weakness. Which finding would be LEAST expected in this patient?

(A) Cardiomegaly
(B) Enlargement of the sella turcica
(C) Suppression of glucose with an oral glucose challenge
(D) Elevation of somatomedins
(E) Increased serum phosphate

172. Which sexual dysfunction is LEAST common?

(A) Premature ejaculation
(B) Primary erectile dysfunction
(C) Secondary erectile dysfunction
(D) Delayed ejaculation

Questions 173–174

173. An 8-year-old child with pes cavus and kyphoscoliosis develops an explosive dysarthric speech. This disease may be associated with all of the following EXCEPT

(A) nystagmus
(B) severe mental retardation
(C) absent deep tendon reflexes
(D) hypertrophic cardiomyopathy
(E) positive Romberg test

174. The most likely diagnosis is

(A) Friedreich's ataxia
(B) juvenile pilocytic astrocytoma of the cerebellum
(C) overdose of chlorpromazine
(D) abetalipoproteinemia
(E) chickenpox encephalitis

175. An 80-year-old male patient complains that his sex life is "not as good as it used to be." This statement is LEAST likely to refer to

(A) decreased interest in sex
(B) reduced intensity of ejaculation
(C) slower erection
(D) longer refractory period
(E) illness

176. A 32-year-old woman complains of weight loss in association with a good appetite and a sensation of her heart beating at night. Physical examination reveals exophthalmos and lid retraction. In addition, all of the following conditions would be expected in this patient EXCEPT

(A) a nodular toxic goiter
(B) sinus tachycardia
(C) systolic hypertension
(D) a low serum thyroid-stimulating hormone (TSH) level
(E) an increased iodine-131 (^{131}I) uptake

177. All of the following statements regarding twin-to-twin intrauterine transfusions are correct EXCEPT

(A) the donor twin is more likely to develop hyperbilirubinemia than the recipient twin
(B) twin-to-twin exchange is more likely to occur with monochorionic placentas
(C) the hematocrit should differ by 15% and the body weight by 20% between the twins
(D) maternal polyhydramnios suggests the syndrome
(E) the recipient twin often develops signs of volume overload (e.g., heart failure, convulsions)

178. Characteristics of obstructive sleep apnea include all of the following EXCEPT

(A) pectus excavatum
(B) dental malocclusion
(C) mouth-breathing
(D) pulmonary hypertension with right ventricular hypertrophy
(E) respiratory alkalosis

179. Complications of cyanotic congenital heart disease include all of the following EXCEPT

(A) cerebral thrombosis
(B) secondary polycythemia
(C) cerebral abscess
(D) persistence of hemoglobin F
(E) patent ductus arteriosus

180. All of the following newborn physical examination relationships are correct EXCEPT

(A) umbilical hernias are common in black infants
(B) absence of meconium in the rectal vault suggests Hirschsprung's disease
(C) caput succedaneum is commonly associated with an underlying skull fracture
(D) a palpable abdominal mass is commonly associated with infantile polycystic kidney disease
(E) a dermal sinus with a tuft of hair in the middle of the lower back may be associated with spina bifida occulta

181. A patient with pulmonary involvement from sarcoidosis is differentiated from a patient with obstructive lung disease by all of the following parameters EXCEPT

(A) total lung capacity (TLC)
(B) forced expiratory volume in 1 second (FEV$_1$)
(C) residual volume (RV)
(D) FEV$_1$/forced vital capacity (FVC) ratio
(E) partial pressure of arterial CO$_2$ (Paco$_2$)

182. Complications associated with respiratory distress syndrome in the newborn include all of the following EXCEPT

(A) patent ductus arteriosus
(B) intraventricular hemorrhage
(C) necrotizing enterocolitis
(D) pulmonary infarction
(E) bronchopulmonary dysplasia

183. All of the following tumors are more commonly noted in the pediatric than adult population EXCEPT

(A) osteogenic sarcoma
(B) Ewing's sarcoma
(C) pilocytic astrocytoma of the cerebellum
(D) embryonal rhabdomyosarcoma
(E) chondrosarcoma

DIRECTIONS: Each set of matching questions in this section consists of a list of four to twenty-six lettered options (some of which may be in figures) followed by several numbered items. For each numbered item, select the ONE lettered option that is most closely associated with it. To avoid spending too much time on matching sets with large numbers of options, it is generally advisable to begin each set by reading the list of options. Then, for each item in the set, try to generate the correct answer and locate it in the option list, rather than evaluating each option individually. Each lettered option may be selected once, more than once, or not at all.

Questions 184–186

Match each description with the drug it best describes.

(A) Isoflurane	(H) Fentanyl
(B) Meperidine	(I) Amphetamine
(C) Propoxyphene	(J) Pancuronium
(D) Naloxone	(K) Glycopyrrolate
(E) Ketamine	(L) Flumazenil
(F) Ibuprofen	(M) Nalbuphine
(G) Haloperidol	(N) Midazolam

184. In many patients with moderate to severe pain, this drug has analgesic efficacy similar to that of morphine. It activates κ opioid receptors and is a weak antagonist at μ receptors. Its abuse liability is considered to be substantially less than that of morphine.

185. This drug antagonizes the receptor actions of benzodiazepines. Its main applications are in emergency medicine and anesthesia.

186. Used in anesthesia, this drug has analgesic actions. Its clinical use is limited by a high incidence of disorientation, sensory and perceptual illusions, and vivid dreams in the postanesthetic recovery period.

Questions 187–189

The following are examples of glucose abnormalities encountered in type I diabetics on a split-dose mixed-insulin regimen of NPH and regular insulin given 30 minutes before breakfast and dinner. For each set of treatment options, select the glucose abnormality that would benefit most by the change.

(A) 10 P.M. glucose 90 mg/dl, 3 A.M. glucose 40 mg/dl, and 7 A.M. glucose 200 mg/dl

(B) 10 P.M. glucose 110 mg/dl, 3 A.M. glucose 110 mg/dl, and 7 A.M. glucose 150 mg/dl

(C) 10 P.M. glucose 110 mg/dl, 3 A.M. glucose 160 mg/dl, and 7 A.M. glucose 220 mg/dl

(D) 12 P.M. glucose 200 mg/dl

(E) 5 P.M. glucose 220 mg/dl

(F) 9 P.M. glucose 200 mg/dl

187. Increase the morning dose of regular insulin

188. Decrease the NPH dose at dinner, give a portion of it at bedtime, or give more food at bedtime

189. Increase the NPH dose at dinner or give the dose at bedtime

Questions 190–192

Match each description with the drug it best describes.

(A) Epinephrine   (H) Captopril
(B) Furosemide   (I) Dobutamine
(C) Digoxin   (J) Spironolactone
(D) Phenoxybenzamine (K) Propranolol
(E) Desmopressin   (L) Mannitol
(F) Acetazolamide   (M) Nifedipine
(G) Clonidine   (N) Hydrochlorothiazide

190. This drug has been used extensively in the management of hypertension, in patients with ischemic heart disease including postmyocardial infarction, and in hyperthyroidism. It should be avoided in the asthmatic or diabetic patient.

191. This synthetic catecholamine is a relatively selective β_1-adrenoceptor activator. Tachyphylaxis to its cardiac effects occurs with chronic use, but intermittent infusion may benefit some patients with chronic heart failure.

192. This drug inhibits the $Na^+/K^+/2\ Cl^-$ cotransport system located in the luminal membrane of the renal tubule. It also causes a large increase in the fractional excretion of sodium. The chemical structure of the drug is related to that of sulfonamides.

Questions 193–194

Match each author with the development stages he described.

(A) Sensory–motor, preoperational–operational, formal operational
(B) Paranoid–schizoid position, depressive position
(C) Trust/mistrust, autonomy/shame, initiative/guilt, industry/inferiority
(D) Autism, symbiosis, differentiation
(E) Oral, anal, phallic, genital

193. Erikson

194. Piaget

Questions 195–197

The diagram, a simplified representation of the pathophysiology of asthma, provides a framework for illustrating the primary sites of action of drugs used in the management of the disease. Match each site of action with the proper drug name.

IgE + Antigen

↓ **1**

Release of mediators

2 ↙   ↘ **3**

Early responses   Late responses
↓   ↓

Inflammation,   Bronchoconstriction,
bronchial reactivity   bronchospasm

(A) Terbutaline
(B) Ipratropium
(C) Triamcinolone
(D) Cromolyn
(E) Aminophylline

195. This drug acts at site 3. To avoid oropharyngeal candidiasis when using the aerosol form of the drug, patients should gargle and spit after each inhalation.

196. This drug acts at site 2. It is an inhibitor of phosphodiesterase and may increase tissue levels of cyclic adenosine monophosphate (cAMP). However, recent evidence suggests that it may exert bronchodilating effects via inhibition of cell surface receptors for adenosine.

197. This drug acts at site 1. It inhibits the synthesis and release of mediators of inflammatory responses, including the leukotrienes, thus blocking early responses in asthmatic attacks.

Questions 198–200

(A) Health maintenance organization (HMO)
(B) Independent practice association (IPA)
(C) Preferred provider organization (PPO)
(D) Hospice
(E) Intermediate-care facility

198. A union trust fund contracts with physicians in private practice to provide medical care to the fund's subscribers

199. This type of nursing home is designed to provide restorative nursing care and assistance with self-care

200. Physicians are paid a yearly salary to provide medical services to a group of people who have paid a yearly premium in advance

ANSWER KEY

1-A	31-D	61-A	91-C	121-A
2-B	32-D	62-B	92-E	122-E
3-E	33-B	63-C	93-A	123-D
4-D	34-B	64-C	94-C	124-C
5-C	35-B	65-A	95-B	125-A
6-E	36-C	66-C	96-C	126-B
7-A	37-C	67-B	97-C	127-B
8-B	38-D	68-A	98-B	128-B
9-E	39-C	69-B	99-D	129-C
10-B	40-A	70-E	100-E	130-A
11-A	41-E	71-B	101-C	131-E
12-B	42-D	72-C	102-B	132-A
13-A	43-E	73-D	103-A	133-D
14-A	44-C	74-C	104-C	134-B
15-D	45-D	75-B	105-E	135-B
16-D	46-A	76-B	106-A	136-C
17-C	47-C	77-C	107-B	137-D
18-B	48-B	78-D	108-C	138-A
19-B	49-C	79-C	109-E	139-B
20-E	50-D	80-B	110-C	140-C
21-A	51-C	81-B	111-B	141-D
22-D	52-D	82-B	112-B	142-C
23-A	53-A	83-A	113-A	143-A
24-B	54-B	84-A	114-C	144-E
25-C	55-B	85-C	115-C	145-A
26-D	56-D	86-D	116-B	146-E
27-B	57-C	87-C	117-C	147-E
28-C	58-B	88-E	118-E	148-E
29-C	59-D	89-A	119-D	149-B
30-C	60-A	90-D	120-D	150-E

151-B	161-D	171-C	181-B	191-I
152-B	162-B	172-B	182-D	192-B
153-B	163-E	173-B	183-E	193-C
154-D	164-E	174-A	184-M	194-A
155-D	165-B	175-A	185-L	195-C
156-A	166-D	176-A	186-E	196-E
157-C	167-B	177-A	187-D	197-C
158-D	168-D	178-E	188-A	198-C
159-A	169-D	179-D	189-C	199-E
160-C	170-C	180-C	190-K	200-A

ANSWERS AND EXPLANATIONS

1. The answer is A. *(Gynecology; oviductal cancer)*
Fallopian tube malignancies are extremely rare and have no official International Federation of Gynecology and Obstetrics staging criteria. However, because they are intraperitoneal organs, intimately related to the ovaries, with a similar mode of metastasis, they are staged with criteria similar to those for ovarian carcinoma.

2. The answer is B. *(General surgery; stasis dermatitis)*
The patient has deep venous insufficiency, as indicated by the stasis dermatitis and superficial varicosities. Stasis dermatitis is a rusty discoloration of the skin, with or without ulceration, that is located around the ankles. The rupture of vessels around the ankles leads to hemosiderin deposition in the skin, which causes the rusty discoloration. Ischemia predisposes to ulceration of the skin as well. Deep venous insufficiency is also associated with secondary development of superficial varicosities. The increased hydrostatic pressure, which is transmitted through incompetent valves in the penetrating branches back into the superficial saphenous system, causes the varicosities.

Superficial thrombophlebitis presents with pain and erythema along the course of the superficial saphenous vein. It is not associated with stasis dermatitis. Arterial insufficiency is not associated with stasis dermatitis or superficial varicosities. The normal pulses in this patient also exclude that diagnosis. Rheumatoid arthritis can present with immune vasculitis in the lower extremities, but the patient history argues against that diagnosis.

3. The answer is E. *(Psychiatry; sexual issues)*
This man is showing normal behavior. In order to qualify as a paraphilia, a person must not only have an unusual object of sexual desire but must also have acted on the fantasy or have problems forming relationships because of it. Paraphilias include exhibitionism, in which an individual exposes his genitals to others; fetishism, in which sexual pleasure is gained from inanimate objects; frotteurism, in which sexual pleasure is gained by rubbing the penis against a clothed woman; and voyeurism, in which a person secretly observes people dressing or engaging in sexual activity.

4. The answer is D. *(Clinical immunology; patient with perennial allergic rhinitis and bronchial asthma)*
The patient has classic findings of an allergic diathesis (type I hypersensitivity) including infraorbital edema with discoloration ("allergic shiners"); allergic rhinitis (pale, boggy, grayish-pink nasal mucosa); an allergic crease on the nose (constant rubbing of the nose—"allergic salute"); and a chest x-ray with radiolucency of the lungs, widening of the intercostal spaces, and flattening of the diaphragm secondary to trapping of air from bronchial asthma. Type I hypersensitivity conditions are characterized by an increase in immunoglobulin E (IgE) antibodies.

Allergic shiners in the infraorbital area result from a combination of venous stasis from submucosal edema and spasm of the unstriated muscle of Müller, which impedes venous drainage from the infraorbital area. Other physical findings encountered in the facial area include a gaping mouth with associated mouth breathing and dental malocclusion, pharyngeal congestion and erythema with hyperplastic lymphoid follicles, allergic conjunctivitis with itchiness and cobblestoning of the conjunctiva, and atopic dermatitis of the upper eyelids.

Bronchial asthma is an exaggerated bronchoconstrictor response to many stimuli. This response induces dyspnea and expiratory wheezing as a result of small-airway resistance to airflow, which is related to inflammation and submucosal edema. It is a reversible airway disease with an obstructive pattern on pulmonary function studies. Lung compliance (inflation of the lung on inspiration) is decreased secondary to increased fluid in the interstitial tissue.

Pathogenesis is complex and involves neutrophils, mast cells, and platelets, which elaborate a variety of chemical mediators that increase vessel permeability and produce bronchoconstriction. Some of these mediators include histamine, bradykinin, leukotrienes, platelet activating factor (PAF), prostaglandins, and thromboxane A_2 (TXA_2). Complex neural factors and neuropeptides such as substance P have also been implicated. Regardless of the cause, inflammation is the most important pathophysiologic event.

Asthma is frequently subdivided into extrinsic and intrinsic types, the latter not associated with type I hypersensitivity. Agents that induce asthmatic attacks include antigens (e.g., pollens, occupational exposure to chemicals, *Aspergillus* spores), aspirin (nonimmunologic; also associated with nasal polyps), exercise (nonimmunologic), viral infections (nonimmunologic), and drugs (β-blockers, nonsteroidals, nebulized medications).

Laboratory tests for type I hypersensitivity–related disease include:

- Measurement of the serum IgE concentration using the PRIST test (the best initial management step in proving an allergic diathesis)
- Evaluating the peripheral blood for eosinophilia
- Scratch-testing the skin with various antigens and noting the presence or absence of a wheal and flare reaction
- Radioallergosorbent tests (RAST), which are serologic tests that react the patient's serum with IgE antibodies against known antigens for a positive match
- Nasal smears for eosinophils
- Provocative tests, where patients are challenged with a specific allergen, for example, food, to see if it provokes symptoms. Bronchial provocation with methacholine or histamine identifies subtle cases of bronchial asthma

Patients presenting with an asthma attack have expiratory wheezes, high-pitched sibilant rhonchi, dyspnea, persistent cough, and hyperinflation of the lungs. Arterial blood gases initially show a respiratory alkalosis with mild to moderate hypoxemia. In more severe cases, there is retention of CO_2 with development of respiratory acidosis.

Modalities of treatment vary depending on the severity of the disease. One of the mainstays for treatment is the use of sympathomimetic bronchodilators, such as albuterol and metaproterenol, administered through metered-dose inhalers, via aerosols, or parenterally. Inhaled corticosteroids, like beclomethasone, are also considered a mainstay for therapy in patients with moderate to severe asthma. In patients resistant to sympathomimetic agents in the emergency room, methylprednisolone is frequently given intravenously. Cromolyn sodium is the preferred treatment for exercise-induced asthma. Theophylline is no longer a mainline drug in the treatment of asthma, particularly in an emergency room setting. Ipratropium bromide is an anticholinergic that inhibits smooth-muscle contraction in the airways. It is used in the treatment of elderly patients with an asthmatic component to their chronic obstructive pulmonary disease (COPD). Ancillary measures include adequate hydration and the administration of oxygen to keep the oxygen saturation above 90%.

An abnormal sweat chloride test is expected in cystic fibrosis. Lung disease is complicated by bacterial infections with *Staphylococcus aureus, Haemophilus influenzae,* and *Pseudomonas aeruginosa.*

A low C3 complement level is an uncommon cause of severe infections. Because C3 is an important opsonizing agent, these patients are prone to bacterial infections.

The nitroblue tetrazolium (NBT) dye test is an in vitro test for a respiratory burst in neutrophils. The respiratory burst occurs when molecular oxygen is converted by nicotinamide–adenine dinucleotide phosphate (NADPH) oxidase in the neutrophil membrane into the superoxide free radical. When NBT is added to a test tube of the patient's blood and is phagocytized by neutrophils, the normally colorless dye is converted into a colored dye if the respiratory burst mechanism is intact. After the respiratory burst, superoxide is converted by superoxide dismutase into peroxide, which combines with chloride ions via myeloperoxidase to form bleach (hypochlorite → HOCl). Hypochlorite destroys the cell walls of bacteria. This entire process is called the oxygen-dependent myeloperoxidase system, which is the most important bactericidal mechanism available to neutrophils and circulating monocytes. Patients with chronic granulomatous disease (CGD) of childhood, a sex-linked recessive disease, lack the NADPH oxidase and cannot form the peroxide that is necessary for the reaction to form hypochlorite.

The clinical findings of chronicity and the lack of consolidation in the chest x-ray argue against this case representing a *Streptococcus pneumoniae* infection, which would be expected to have gram-positive diplococci in the sputum.

5. The answer is C. *(Orthopedics; pelvic fractures and blood loss)*
Pelvic fractures have the greatest potential for blood loss (> 1 L) of all fractures because of a large venous and arterial blood supply. This underscores why most trauma centers are prepared to place external fixators to tamponade pelvic bleeding in the emergency room. Bladder injury and transection of the urethra are also common injuries associated with pelvic fractures. The femur is the second most common fracture site associated with massive blood loss. Closed fractures in the spine, humerus, tibia and fibula, and other sites are usually associated with a blood loss of less than 450 ml.

6. The answer is E. *(Psychiatry; somatoform disorder)*
This patient's worrying suggests hypochondriasis, which is characterized by excessive worry about the meaning of a physical symptom. Moreover, this patient does not respond to physician reassurance after an adequate workup. Hypochondriacal symptoms usually become evident during periods of psychological stress. By definition, reassurance and explanations are ineffective. Resolution of the stressor through brief psychotherapy usually results in symptom resolution. Placebo response is usually temporary, at best.

7. The answer is A. *(Neurology; emergent myelography)*
With a history of prostate cancer, the presumptive diagnosis is subacute cord compression from metastatic prostate cancer at T10. Plain films will likely show bony destruction, but emergent myelography is indicated. Steroids may reduce the tumor edema during the workup, and arrangements should be made for radiation therapy after the diagnosis is confirmed, but not before. Because of the high risk of permanent paraplegia if acute action is not taken, waiting for magnetic resonance imaging (MRI) is unacceptable. Guillain-Barré syndrome would not present with a sensory level, and an electromyograph (EMG) would not be diagnostic and would not be expected to show abnormalities for approximately 3 weeks after the onset of weakness.

8. The answer is B. *(Obstetrics; neonatal evaluation)*
The Apgar score is assigned on the basis of five parameters: skin color, respiratory effort, heart rate, muscle tone, and reflex irritability. This infant will be assigned 1 point for pink body but blue extremities, 1 point for weak respiratory effort, 2 points for heart rate (because it is over 100), 1 point for muscle tone, and 0 for reflex irritability.

9. The answer is E. *(Pediatrics; macrosomic newborns)*
The clavicle is the most commonly fractured bone in infants during delivery. This fracture is more common in macrosomic newborns (e.g., infants of diabetic mothers). The infant generally does not move the arm, giving an absent Moro reflex on the affected side. Crepitus is felt on palpation. Treatment is usually unnecessary, and the prognosis is good.

10. The answer is B. *(Hematology; aseptic necrosis of the femoral head)*
This patient has bilateral aseptic necrosis of the femoral heads secondary to sickle cell disease. Aseptic necrosis occurs in 10% to 25% of patients with sickle cell disease, with the hip joint being the most common joint involved. It has an even higher incidence in patients with Hgb sickle cell disease.

The Hgb electrophoresis in sickle cell disease shows predominantly Hgb S (valine for glutamic acid substitution in the sixth position of the β chain), variable increase in Hgb F (fetal Hgb), and no Hgb A (adult Hgb).

Salmonella osteomyelitis has an increased propensity at all stages of the disease. Autosplenectomy due to repeated splenic infarcts reduces the phagocytic capabilities of the patient as well as the opsonizing potential. Ischemia in the bowel predisposes to *Salmonella* septicemia and the potential for seeding to necrotic bone. An acute onset of bone pain must be differentiated from ischemic necrosis of bone, but the latter condition is 50 times more common than osteomyelitis. A combined technetium and gallium scan usually shows an increased uptake in osteomyelitis, whereas infarction of bone shows avascularity near painful joints.

A pathological bone fracture would show a defect in the bone and a discontinuity in the periosteum. They are commonly due to osteoporosis or metastatic disease to bone.

Osteoarthritis commonly occurs in weight-bearing joints. Characteristic radiologic findings in the hip joint are segmental narrowing of the interosseous space, subchondral sclerosis due to wearing down of the articular cartilage, subchondral cysts with sclerotic margins, and the formation of osteophytes along the lateral borders of the joint from reactive bone formation.

Legg-Calvé-Perthes disease, an avascular necrosis of the femoral head, shows a predilection for boys between 4 and 10 years old. Insidious development of a limp, with pain in the groin, anterior thigh, or knee is what initially brings the patient to a physician. The process is self-limited and its cause is unknown. Approximately 55% of patients have a full recovery with revascularization of bone, whereas 45% of patients have a permanent hip deformity.

11. The answer is A. *(Psychiatry; somatoform disorder)*
In somatoform pain disorder, a painful lesion is often present, but the resultant pain is disproportional. Both somatoform pain disorder and chronic pain syndromes can respond to biofeedback therapy, and personality pathology can also be seen in both. Worker's compensation issues

can exist in both conditions, but both can also raise additional concerns about malingering.

12. The answer is B. *(Urology; renal adenocarcinoma)*
The patient has metastatic renal adenocarcinoma. This cancer, which affects men more often than women, most commonly arises in the sixth to seventh decade of life. Smoking is a predisposing factor. Hematuria is the most consistent sign (seen in 90% of cases), followed by pain (45% of cases), a palpable mass (30% of cases), and fever (20% of cases). "Cannon ball" metastases to the lung occur in 60% of cases. Fever is not related to infection but results from chemicals released by the tumor.

The tumors can ectopically secrete erythropoietin (leading to secondary polycythemia), parathormone-like peptide (leading to hypercalcemia), renin (leading to hypertension), gonadotropins (leading to feminization or masculinization), or cortisol (leading to Cushing's syndrome). Needle aspiration of the mass using computerized tomography for needle guidance is usually performed to obtain a histologic diagnosis. Angiograms reveal a vascular pattern. Radical nephrectomy is the treatment of choice. The presence or absence of renal vein or capsular invasion affects overall survival—45% of patients without renal vein or capsular invasion achieve a 5-year survival rate, as opposed to 15% to 30% of those with invasion.

The kidney is the most common extrapulmonary site for tuberculosis; however, nodular masses in the lung argue against this diagnosis. Acute pyelonephritis producing metastatic abscesses in the lung would be very unlikely. In addition, pyuria is the predominant urinary finding. Transitional cell carcinomas of the bladder usually involve the renal pelvis and produce obstruction. They are not as common as renal cell adenocarcinoma.

13. The answer is A. *(Obstetrics; neonatal resuscitation)*
Respiratory depression due to maternal narcotics is unusual with the increased use of conduction anesthesia. However, treatment using naloxone is highly effective. Sodium bicarbonate, epineph-

rine, plasma protein fraction, and beractant are all useful in neonatal resuscitation, but only naloxone is specific for reversal of narcotic depression.

14. The answer is A. (*Biostatistics; type I error and null hypothesis*)

Type I and type II errors describe faulty outcomes when a statistical test is performed on a null hypothesis. Type I error is the chance that a true null hypothesis is rejected. Type II error is the chance that a false null hypothesis is accepted.

15. The answer is D. (*Pediatrics; visceral larva migrans*)

Visceral larva migrans is caused by infection with *Toxocara* larvae. It is most common in children 1 to 4 years of age, especially if they have pica and have close contacts with dogs and cats, because *Toxocara* are common parasites of both. Sandboxes are common areas for both pets and children. Symptoms include fever, hepatomegaly, wheezing, pulmonary disease, and eosinophilia.

16. The answer is D. (*Hematology; multiple myeloma*)

This patient has multiple myeloma, which is the most common malignant plasma-cell disorder. It is also the most common primary hematologic malignancy of bone. It is more common in men than in women and in blacks than in whites. The onset is between 50 and 70 years of age. Chromosomal abnormalities, radiation, and chronic antigenic stimulation have been implicated in its pathogenesis. Any middle-aged to elderly patient with an unexplained anemia, bone pain, pathological fracture, recurrent infection, unexplained hypercalcemia, renal failure without hypertension, or a monoclonal protein in the serum or urine is suspect for having multiple myeloma.

Bone pain is the initial manifestation in 70% of patients. Osteolytic lesions occur in 70% of patients because osteoclast activating factor is released by the neoplastic plasma cells. Scans are less sensitive than x-rays in identifying lytic areas in bone.

Hematologic findings include a normocytic anemia (60%), pancytopenia in advanced cases, and rouleaux (stack-of-coins effect) of the red blood cells (RBCs). The erythrocyte sedimentation rate (ESR) is increased because of the increase in gamma globulins. It is frequently over 100 mm/hour. Coagulation studies commonly document qualitative platelet defects associated with a prolonged bleeding time. A bone marrow examination reveals sheets of neoplastic plasma cells with eccentrically located nuclei and perinuclear clearing.

A serum protein electrophoresis frequently exhibits a monoclonal spike owing to a malignant clone of plasma cells synthesizing a single immunoglobulin (most commonly IgG) and its light chain. There is T-cell suppression for synthesis of other immunoglobulins by B cells. Excess light chains are filtered into the urine, where they are identified as Bence Jones protein by urine electrophoresis.

Infection is very common. Nearly 70% of patients die from infections in the lung, urinary tract, or both. *Staphylococcus aureus* and *Streptococcus pneumoniae* are the most common pathogens.

Renal dysfunction is present in 30% to 50% of patients at the time of diagnosis. Extreme caution should be exercised in performing an intravenous pyelogram, because it can precipitate renal failure. Problems include:

- Metastatic calcification with subsequent nephrocalcinosis and renal failure
- Renal tubular acidosis from nephrotoxicity secondary to light chains
- Urate nephropathy from excessive uric acid formation due to breakdown of neoplastic cells
- Primary amyloidosis with proteinuria in the nephrotic range
- A giant-cell reaction against Bence Jones protein producing tubulointerstitial disease

Neurologic problems consist of carpal tunnel syndrome and polyneuropathies from compression fractures of the vertebrae.

Hypercalcemia from the release of excess calcium in the lytic areas occurs in approximately 20% of cases.

Treatment of multiple myeloma is with alkylating agents. The median survival is 2 to 3 years.

Breast cancer also produces lytic lesions in the bone, but the neoplastic cells have a glandular appearance. Stains for carcinoembryonic antigen (CEA) and estrogen and progesterone receptors (ERA and PRA, respectively) are frequently positive. Tamoxifen, an antiestrogen agent, is effective alone or in combination with chemotherapeutic agents, particularly in postmenopausal women, who are ERA- or PRA-positive, or both.

Hypocalcemia is rarely caused by bone metastases, which are invariably osteoblastic.

17. The answer is C. *(Obstetrics; maternal physiology)*
Because respiratory rate is unchanged, but tidal volume is increased, the vital capacity increases. Therefore, minute ventilation increases. The enlarging uterus elevates the resting position of the diaphragm, resulting in a less negative intrathoracic pressure and a decreased resting lung volume (functional residual capacity). Because the enlarging uterus does not impair diaphragmatic or thoracic muscle motion, the vital capacity is unchanged.

18. The answer is B. *(General surgery; colon cancer staging)*
The pathology report indicates a high-grade colon cancer that is a modified Dukes' stage C2, because it infiltrates the muscle wall and involves lymph nodes. Grading and staging of cancer are extremely important in determining the prognosis and treatment options for a patient.

Grade of cancer refers to what the tumor looks like. If the tumor is easily identified as a squamous carcinoma (presence of keratin) or adenocarcinoma (glandular epithelium), it is low-grade or well-differentiated. If it is not possible to tell its tissue of origin, the tumor is high-grade, poorly differentiated, or anaplastic.

Staging is the most important factor for patient prognosis, because it describes the size of the tumor, whether it has metastasized to lymph nodes, and whether it has metastasized to other locations. The report in this case establishes the pathologic stage of the cancer, because the actual extent of bowel involvement can be ascertained. Regardless of stage, the overall 5-year survival rate for colorectal cancer is 35%. The modified Dukes' staging system is commonly used for the staging of colorectal cancers.

Dukes' Staging System for Colorectal Cancer

Stage	Description	5-Year Survival Rate
A	Tumor limited to mucosa and submucosa	80%
B1	Tumor into, but not through, muscle wall; no lymph node or distant involvement	60%
B2	Tumor penetrates entire wall; no lymph nodes involved	55%
C1	Tumor into, but not through, muscle wall; lymph node involvement	30%
C2	Tumor penetrates entire wall; lymph node involvement	20%
D	Distant metastasis; any level of invasion; may or may not be lymph node involvement	< 5%

Note that the key difference between stages B and C is lymph node status and the key criterion for stage D is distant metastasis.

19. The answer is B. *(Pediatrics; extraocular palsy)*
Children rarely complain of diplopia (double vision) because they suppress the image of the affected eye. With brain tumors, diplopia is a sign of increased intracranial pressure. Eye examination may reveal strabismus from palsy of the lateral rectus secondary to involvement of the abducens. Many children tilt their heads in an effort to compensate for the diplopia. Other affected nerves are the oculomotor and, rarely, the trochlear.

20. The answer is E. *(Obstetrics; fetal physiology)*
Because the umbilical vein carries blood directly from the placenta to the fetal body, it has the highest level of Po_2. The other locations carry blood that is downstream from the umbilical vein and, as such, is mixed with unoxygenated fetal blood.

21. The answer is A. *(Pediatrics; croup)*
Croup, or laryngotracheobronchitis, is most common between 6 months and 6 years of age. Caused primarily by parainfluenza virus, it typically presents with prodromal symptoms of an upper respiratory infection. The child then develops fever and a brassy, barking, seal-like cough, with intermittent inspiratory stridor. Acute respiratory distress can develop. Pertussis usually occurs in unimmunized infants and is usually preceded by a prodromal catarrhal stage with conjunctivitis. Spasms of coughing end with an inspiratory whoop. In younger infants the whoop is not present and the signs are more subtle, for example, apnea and cyanosis. Acute epiglottitis is more common in the 3- to 7-year age-group, and usually drooling is present, but the barking cough is absent. Bronchiolitis and asthma can present with retractions and nasal flaring, but wheezing is usually present.

22. The answer is D. *(Pharmacology; cardiac drugs)*
Adenosine given as an intravenous (IV) bolus is currently the drug of choice for immediate management of paroxysmal supraventricular tachycardia because it is highly effective (90%–95%) and has a very short duration of action (< 30 seconds). Because the oral bioavailability of lidocaine is only 3%, it must be given parenterally, a mode of administration inappropriate for maintenance therapy. Quinidine is effective orally, and its half-life is appropriate for dosing at intervals of 4 to 6 hours.

23. The answer is A. *(Nephrology; renal stones)*
This patient has renal colic secondary to a renal stone. Renal colic characteristically has an abrupt onset in the flank, with radiation of the pain toward the abdomen and into the groin. It is associated with urinary frequency, dysuria, and hematuria. Men are more frequently affected than women.

The most common metabolic abnormality in stone-formers is idiopathic hypercalciuria. Calcium oxalate stones account for the majority of stones (60%). There is an increased incidence of these stones in patients on megadoses of vitamin C and in Crohn's disease, the latter due to increased reabsorption of oxalate in the damaged mucosa of the terminal ileum. Other factors that predispose to stones are low urine citrate levels, because citrate is necessary to bind stone constituents; reduced urine volume; and incomplete distal renal tubular acidosis (phosphate stones in children). The recurrence rate for stone-formers is 75%.

Only stones that contain calcium, such as calcium oxalate or calcium phosphate, are radiopaque. However, uric acid, xanthine, and ammonium nitrate stones are radiolucent on x-ray and show up as a filling defect.

The laboratory workup for stones involves

- urinalysis, which checks urine pH
- urine culture, if pyuria is present; urease splitters increase stone formation
- serum calcium and serum phosphate to rule out primary hyperparathyroidism
- serum uric acid to rule out hyperuricemia
- electrolytes to identify metabolic acidosis due to distal renal tubular acidosis
- serum creatinine to evaluate renal function status

- a flat plate of the abdomen, which identifies radiopaque stones or locates filling defects
- an intravenous pyelogram to rule out stones (staghorn calculi) in the renal pelvis and medullary sponge kidney, which is commonly associated with stones
- a 24-hour urine for calcium to detect hypercalciuria
- a 24-hour urine for uric acid to detect uricosuria
- a 24-hour urine for citrate, because low levels predispose to stones
- a 24-hour urine for sodium, because increased levels contribute to increased calcium excretion
- a 24-hour urine for phosphates, which are an indirect measure of dairy product ingestion

Urine should always be strained to identify the stones, which must be submitted for analysis, so that appropriate treatment modalities can be employed. X-ray diffraction is the gold standard for stone analysis.

The mainstay of therapy is increased water intake (2.5–3 L/day). Hydrochlorothiazide is the treatment of choice for hypercalciuria, because volume contraction increases calcium reabsorption. Alkalinizing the urine pH is useful in the treatment of uric acid, oxalate, and cystine stones.

The best overall management of stones is waiting for spontaneous passage. Extracorporeal shock wave lithotripsy is most useful for stones that are less than 2 cm. A combination of percutaneous lithotripsy and shock wave therapy is used for larger stones. Staghorn calculi (struvite stones) in the renal pelvis are best removed by surgery.

24. The answer is B. *(General surgery; shock after abdominal surgery)*
Hemoperitoneum (i.e., an intraabdominal bleed) is the most common cause of shock in the first 24 hours after abdominal surgery. This problem is most commonly a technical one, as opposed to one related to a platelet disorder or a coagulopathy. The manifestations of hemoperitoneum are those of hypovolemic shock, mainly hypotension, sinus tachycardia, oliguria, and peripheral vasoconstriction resulting in cold, clammy skin. The bleeding is not usually reflected by a drop in the hematocrit in the first few hours. If other causes of shock are eliminated, reoperation is mandatory. Immediate postoperative circulatory collapse can also be due to a massive pulmonary embolus, a cardiac arrhythmia, pneumothorax, an acute myocardial infarction, a transfusion reaction, or an allergic reaction to some medication.

25. The answer is C. *(Cardiology; treatment of hyperkalemia)*
The electrocardiogram (ECG) reveals tall, slender, tented T waves in leads I, II, aVF, and V_{2-6}. In general, the serum potassium levels correlate well with the ECG findings, but the ECG more accurately reflects the gradient between the myocardial intracellular and extracellular potassium. Peaking of the T waves is a more important criterion of hyperkalemia than is the wave amplitude.

Hyperkalemia is common in end-stage renal disease, because potassium is normally excreted in the kidney. Hyperkalemia is associated with dangerous cardiac arrhythmias and, if high enough, stops the heart in diastole. Calcium antagonizes cardiac conduction abnormalities and specifically reverses the effect of hyperkalemia on cardiac muscle. Sodium bicarbonate and insulin plus glucose increase the uptake of potassium into cells. Sodium bicarbonate also produces metabolic alkalosis, which shifts potassium into cells in exchange for hydrogen ions coming out of the cells. Furosemide is a loop diuretic that increases the distal exchange of sodium ions for potassium ions, therefore losing significant amounts of potassium in the urine. Cation-exchange resins given as enemas also remove potassium from the body.

26. The answer is D. *(Neurology; dermatomyositis)*
Dermatomyositis peaks in two age-groups, prepuberty and at approximately 40 years of age (the latter usually women). The elevated creatine phosphokinase (CPK) and proximal myopathic features are common, with the rash readily differentiating from polymyositis. Polymyalgia rheu-

matica may be associated with proximal aching, but would not fit well with the elevated muscle enzymes and the myopathic features on electromyograph (EMG). Likewise, rheumatoid arthritis would explain only the discomfort, and is generally distal rather than proximal. Finally, systemic lupus erythematosus (SLE) could easily explain the butterfly rash, but would not explain the myopathic features expressed in the EMG and the elevated muscle enzymes. A muscle biopsy may be necessary to solidify the diagnosis.

27. The answer is B. *(Obstetrics; polyhydramnios)*
Excessive amniotic fluid is a result of an imbalance of secretion and absorption. The only option listed that is associated with increased polyhydramnios is diabetes mellitus. It appears to be related to the degree of glucose control.

28. The answer is C. *(Psychiatry; cognitive disorder)*
Dementia is characterized by memory disturbance coupled with other cognitive disturbances, including problems with abstraction, aphasia, apraxia, or agnosia. In delirium, awareness and attention are also disturbed. In organic amnestic syndrome, both awareness and cognition are generally intact.

29. The answer is C. *(Gynecology; hirsutism)*
The only option that is true is that unsatisfactory treatment is a frequent possibility with hirsutism. Ethnicity is very much a factor, with Mediterranean heritage showing a prominence. Hirsutism is largely a cosmetic problem, with few serious health problems. Loss of female body contours and voice deepening are characteristics of virilization, not hirsutism.

30. The answer is C. *(General surgery; acute diverticulitis)*
The patient has acute diverticulitis, the most common complication of diverticulosis in the sigmoid colon. Clinically, it replicates the findings in acute appendicitis, except that they are located in the left lower quadrant. The patient has

a low-grade fever, left lower quadrant rebound tenderness, and absolute neutrophilic leukocytosis with a shift to the left. Occasionally, a tender mass can be palpated. Computerized tomography is particularly useful in making the diagnosis of diverticulitis. Low pressure barium studies using water-soluble contrast can also be used, but perforation is a risk. The type of management varies with the severity of the attack and depends on whether peritonitis is present. Ampicillin, tetracycline, or amoxicillin clavulanate can be administered orally. Pentazocine is useful in treating pain. If symptoms do not subside, then surgical options include primary resection with anastomosis or primary resection and colostomy with anastomosis at a later date, once inflammation has subsided.

Ulcerative colitis most often occurs in young adults and involves bloody diarrhea and rectal bleeding. Irritable bowel syndrome is an abnormality of electrical rhythm in the bowel that is commonly related to stress. Patients have alternating diarrhea and constipation with cramping abdominal pain, tenesmus, and mucus in the stool. Administering anticholinergics and increasing insoluble fiber are methods of treatment. Colon cancer in a patient with known diverticulosis should be suspected if there is a change in bowel habits or an onset of pain. Colonoscopy is indicated in these situations. A neoplasm is discovered in up to 30% of cases.

31. The answer is D. *(Pediatrics; severe asthma)*
A child with severe asthma who is becoming sleepy and less responsive is most likely tiring and retaining carbon dioxide. In addition, if less wheezing is heard, it should not be assumed that the patient is improving. On the contrary—air exchange is diminished because of severe bronchospasm and decreased respiratory effort. Arterial blood gas measurement should be ordered to evaluate acid–base status and carbon dioxide content.

32. The answer is D. *(Pulmonary medicine; right middle lobe pneumonia due to pneumococcus)*
This 35-year-old patient has the classic findings of a bacterial pneumonia. They include a history

of abrupt onset of fever, chills, a productive cough, and chest pain on inspiration, which correlates with pleuritic inflammation. Physical examination findings of lung consolidation in bacterial pneumonia are dullness to percussion, increased tactile fremitus (increased tactile vibration when a person speaks), bronchophony ("99" becomes clear through the stethoscope), egophony ("eeeee" sounds like "aaaaa" through the stethoscope), and fine, crepitant rales.

Streptococcus pneumoniae (pneumococcus) is the most common cause of community-acquired bacterial pneumonia. Obliteration of the right-heart silhouette (the silhouette sign) indicates involvement of the right middle lobe. A neutrophilic leukocytosis with left shift (greater than 10% band neutrophils) provides additional evidence of a bacterial pneumonia. A Gram's stain of sputum would likely show gram-positive diplococci. Penicillin G is the drug of choice.

Klebsiella is more commonly associated with alcoholics and presents with a mucoid-appearing sputum, often tinged with blood. Fat gram-negative rods with a capsule are noted in the Gram's stain of sputum.

Viral pneumonias are usually associated with a nonproductive cough and have an interstitial pattern on chest x-ray rather than a consolidation.

Primary tuberculosis is rare in a 35-year-old man and occurs more frequently in children or immunocompromised patients. It involves the periphery of the lower part of the upper lobe or upper part of the lower lobe in the lungs.

33. The answer is B. (General surgery; small bowel obstruction)

The patient has a small bowel obstruction, which is most commonly caused by adhesions from a previous surgery. Characteristic physical findings in small bowel obstruction are vomiting, colicky midabdominal pain, abdominal distention, hyperperistalsis, obstipation (i.e., absence of stool and flatus), and a lack of rebound tenderness. Abdominal x-rays show distended loops of bowel with a stepladder pattern of differential air–fluid levels. In some cases, intestinal intubation relieves the entrapped gas and fluids, causing the obstruction to subside. Other cases require surgical intervention.

Torsion of the bowel around the mesenteric root is referred to as a volvulus. It produces obstruction and strangulation of bowel. Intussusception is uncommon in adults and produces a combination of obstruction and infarction. Small bowel infarction resulting from thrombosis of the superior mesenteric artery causes a bloody diarrhea. "Thumbprinting" from submucosal edema is noted on abdominal films.

34. The answer is B. (Pediatrics; posterior fossa tumors)

Astrocytoma is the most common posterior fossa tumor of childhood. Posterior fossa tumors are more common in children than in any other age group, whereas posterior fossa and supratentorial tumors are equal in frequency in infants less than 2 years of age and adolescents. Ataxia and nystagmus are often associated with posterior fossa tumors. Headache and papilledema are common signs of increased intracranial pressure.

35. The answer is B. (Biostatistics; analysis of variance)

The question relates to assessing group differences of a continuous variable, which in this question is age. If the comparison were between two groups with a continuous variable, a Student's *t*-test would be correct. With more than two groups, it is necessary to use analysis of variance. A correlation coefficient assesses the strength of association, not the differences among groups. The chi-squared test assesses differences among groups of categorical variables. Logistic regression is used to assess a categorical outcome for a continuous predictor.

36. The answer is C. *(Nephrology; hypertensive retinopathy)*
According to the Keith-Wagener-Barker classification of the retinal changes in hypertension, the irregular arterial caliber, "copper wiring," and arteriovenous nipping of this patient's retina would indicate grade II hypertensive retinopathy.

The sequence of events in hypertensive retinopathy is focal spasm of the arterioles, followed by progressive sclerosis and narrowing of the arterioles, leading eventually to flame hemorrhages from rupture of the vessels, formation of exudates, and papilledema. Grayish white exudates that are soft, like cotton wool, are due to microinfarctions, whereas exudates that have clear margins (hard exudates) are due to leakage of protein from increased vessel permeability. Sclerotic changes in the vessels are first described as "copper wiring," because blood is still visible through the vessel wall. When the vessel wall is thickened enough to prevent visualization of the blood, the light reflects back from the vessel wall to produce a "silver wiring" effect. Because the arterioles cross over the venules, the wall of the venule is depressed as arterioles thicken, and arteriovenous nipping defects are produced. Papilledema refers to swelling of the optic disc.

Keith-Wagener-Barker Classification

	Normal	**Grade I**	**Grade II**	**Grade III**	**Grade IV**
A/V ratio*	3/4	1/2	1/3	1/4	Fine cords
Flame hemorrhages	None	None	None	Present	Present
Exudates	None	None	None	Present	Present
Papilledema	None	None	None	None	Present
Copper wiring	None	None	Present	None	None
Silver wiring	None	None	None	Present	None
AV nipping	None	Slight depression	Depression with humping at ends	Right-angle deviation; vein disappears underneath	Same as grade III

*A/V ratio refers to the ratio of the diameter of the arteriole to the venule.

37. The answer is C. *(Gynecology; benign cervical lesions)*
Genital condylomata acuminata are caused by the human papillomavirus subtypes 6 and 11. Transmission is usually by direct sexual contact. Often these condylomata acuminata are associated with vaginitis. Treatment is by surgical excision or ablative therapy. Oral contraception increases the extent of lesions.

38. The answer is D. *(Pediatrics; Meckel's diverticulum)*
Meckel's diverticulum usually presents as painless rectal bleeding. The condition is best remembered as the disease of twos; it affects 2% of the population, occurs in the first 2 years of life, and is a sacculation 2 feet proximal to the ileocecal junction. Iron deficiency anemia can result from chronic blood loss. The diverticulum usually consists of ectopic gastric tissue. Diagnosis is made by technetium scan. Excision is the treatment of choice.

39. The answer is C. *(General surgery; colovesical fistula secondary to diverticular disease)*
Fistulas are abnormal communications between two hollow organs or between a hollow organ and the exterior. The most common fistulas in the gastrointestinal tract are colovesical fistulas and the most common cause is diverticular disease complicated by diverticulitis. Colovesical fistulas are more common in men. Air and fecal material in the urine suggest the diagnosis. Methylene blue instilled into the rectum or bladder can identify these fistulas. Surgery is required if they persist.

Rectovaginal fistulas are most commonly caused by trauma secondary to childbirth. Anorectal fistulas can be associated with inflammatory bowel disease. Small intestine fistulas are common in Crohn's disease. Gastrocolic fistulas can occur after peptic ulcer surgery.

40. The answer is A. *(Psychiatry; psychosis)*
This patient's symptoms consist of delusions. Delusions always indicate the presence of psychosis. Of the choices, only dementia can present with psychosis, often consisting of persecutory delusions. Other disorders with similar psychotic symptoms include schizophrenia and delusional disorder.

41. The answer is E. *(Pulmonary medicine; coccidioidomycosis)*
Coccidioides immitis is a soil saprophyte predominantly found in the Southwestern United States. It is contracted by breathing in arthrospores from the soil, particularly a few days after a rain. Only 40% of patients develop a symptomatic infection. Blacks, Mexicans, and Filipinos are particularly prone to disseminated disease.

Clinical presentation consists of fever, cough, chest pain, malaise, and hypersensitivity reactions such as erythema nodosum and eosinophilia. Erythema nodosum presents as raised, erythematous, painful nodules, usually involving the lower extremities. It is not diagnostic of *Coccidioides* infection but is also associated with tuberculosis, sarcoidosis, various drug reactions (sulfonamides, iodides, birth control pills), inflammatory bowel disease, and malignancy (Hodgkin's disease). Biopsies of these lesions show an inflammatory panniculitis.

Coccidioides is the most common systemic fungal infection to produce cavitary lesions in the lower lobes. Pleural effusions are commonly present as well. Serologic tests are very useful in screening for coccidioidomycosis. Skin testing is less useful as a screen. Sputum cultures frequently isolate the organism.

Primary pulmonary disease usually resolves spontaneously without treatment. More severe cases require amphotericin B. Ketoconazole can also be used.

Histoplasmosis is the most common systemic fungal disease, but it is more common in the central states. There is an association with bird and bat droppings in moist soil. It can be associated with erythema nodosum. Serologic tests and culture confirm the diagnosis.

Mycoplasma pneumoniae is the most common cause of atypical pneumonia. It does not produce cavitary lesions in the lungs.

Klebsiella pneumoniae lung infections are usually seen in alcoholics. These infections frequently produce lung abscesses.

Tuberculosis is also a cavitary disease, but reactivation tuberculosis is most commonly located in the upper lobes.

42. The answer is D. *(General surgery; preoperative pulmonary function testing)*
Patients with lung disease prior to operation are at increased risk for atelectasis, pneumonia, and hypoxemia [i.e., a low arterial O_2 tension (P_{O_2})]. Chest x-rays, electrocardiograms, and arterial blood gases are all useful preoperative screens, but pulmonary function studies provide the best preoperative screen, because they reflect dynamic measurements of pulmonary function in the patient. The forced expiratory volume in 1 second (FEV_1) indicates how much air can be expelled from the lungs in 1 second after a maximal inspiration (normally 4 liters). The forced vital capacity (FVC) represents the entire amount of air that can be expelled (normally 5 liters). The ratio of the FEV_1 to the FVC (normally 80%) is considered the best overall screen. Values less than 50% of predicted outcome correlate with a high risk for postoperative pulmonary complications.

Arterial blood gas measurements reflect primary acid-base disorders (e.g., acidosis or alkalosis), but they do not predict pulmonary complications in the postoperative state. Respiratory acidosis secondary to retention of CO_2 is the main reason for evaluating arterial blood gases, because acidosis is always associated with hypoxemia. In addition, treatment with high-flow oxygen could potentially cause respiratory arrest and further retention of CO_2, because the low arterial O_2 tension (P_{O_2}), which serves as a stimulus for breathing, is lost.

43. The answer is E. *(Neurology; Guillain-Barré syndrome)*
Many cases of Guillain-Barré syndrome are preceded by a virus or vaccination. Multiple sclerosis is believed to be an autoimmune disorder, not posttraumatic. Parkinson's disease might easily arise from neurotoxins affecting the cells of the substantia nigra, but aluminum is not currently suspected (although it has been suspected in the past as contributing to Alzheimer's disease).

Infantile spasms are generally associated with acquired central nervous system injury; they are not genetic. Finally, Huntington's disease is clearly a genetic trait, the autosomal dominant gene localized to chromosome 4.

44. The answer is C. *(Gynecology; urinary incontinence)*
The history of painless, continuous vaginal leakage of urine with a recent pelvic surgery suggests the diagnosis of a fistula between the vagina and the urinary tract. Intravenous (IV) indigo–carmine, which is excreted in the urine and discolors a vaginal pack, is the diagnostic modality of choice. Cystometry, urine culture, pelvic sonogram, and urethral pressure measurements contribute nothing toward ruling out a fistula.

45. The answer is D. *(Endocrinology; hypophosphatemia and respiratory failure)*
In diabetic ketoacidosis (DKA), glucosuria results in the loss of significant amounts of sodium, potassium, and phosphate in the urine. When insulin is used in the treatment of DKA, phosphorus is normally transported along with glucose into muscle and adipose cells so that glucose can be phosphorylated and used for glycolysis. However, the presence of insulin also enhances glycolysis in the liver. The liver begins to remove massive amounts of glucose and phosphorus from the blood, thereby depleting the already-low blood concentration of phosphate. This depletion of phosphate decreases the amount of phosphorus available to accompany glucose into the muscle, which causes a depletion of adenosine triphosphate (ATP) within the muscle, leading to paralysis of the respiratory muscles and death of the patient. This sequence is the rationale for providing phosphate supplementation in the treatment of DKA.

Glucose toxicity refers to the effect of hyperglycemia in reducing the sensitivity of tissues to insulin therapy in both type I and type II diabetes mellitus.

Although hyperkalemia is commonly seen in the setting of DKA, it is not due to an excess of potassium stores but is the result of a transcellular shift of potassium out of cells as excess hydrogen ions in ketoacidosis are buffered intracellularly. This transcellular shift often disguises the marked deficits in total body potassium that these patients have because of loss of potassium in the urine, resulting from the osmotic effect of glucosuria. Therefore, potassium supplementation is extremely important in the treatment of DKA and can be given as potassium phosphate rather than as potassium chloride.

46. The answer is A. *(Gynecology; dyspareunia)*
Although most sexual problems are psychological, organic causes must still be ruled out. Of the options listed, the most likely cause of painful vaginal entry with intercourse in a virginal woman is a narrowed hymen. This situation can be easily treated by surgical incision in the office. Endometriosis and pelvic inflammatory disease (PID) can be causes of deep, not superficial, dyspareunia. Atrophic vaginitis is unlikely in a premenopausal woman.

47. The answer is C. *(Pediatrics; homocystinuria)*
Homocystinuria results from abnormalities in the metabolism of methionine. Classic homocystinuria (cystathione synthase deficiency) is the most common form. It is transmitted as an autosomal recessive trait, and its incidence is 1/200,000. Heterozygote carriers are asymptomatic. Thromboembolic disease is more common in homocystinuria than in the general population. Infants are normal at birth, but they show failure to thrive and developmental delay during infancy. Lens dislocation, astigmatism, glaucoma, and cataracts are seen. Mental retardation is common. Seizures occur in approximately 20%. Patients appear marfanoid. They have fair skin, blue eyes, and a malar flush. Some patients respond to treatment with high doses of vitamin B_6.

48. The answer is B. *(General surgery; volvulus)*
The patient has volvulus, or twisting of the bowel around the mesenteric root. It is most common in the sigmoid colon (65% of patients) and is most often seen in the elderly population. Obstruction and strangulation with infarction are potential sequelae. Clinical signs include colicky abdominal pain with persistence of pain between spasms, abdominal distention, and vomiting. In a sigmoid volvulus, there is a single dilated loop of bowel resembling a "coffee bean" rising up out of the pelvis. The concavity of the coffee bean points toward the left lower quadrant. Barium studies reveal a "bird's beak" or "ace of spades" appearance, with the lumen of the bowel tapering toward the volvulus. A volvulus can frequently be decompressed with a flexible colonoscope, but it often recurs. If it cannot be decompressed, then surgery should be performed with removal of the redundant bowel.

Intussusception is uncommon in adults. It refers to the telescoping of one segment of proximal bowel into the distal bowel. In adults, it commonly results from an underlying mucosal lesion that serves as the nidus for the intussusception, producing obstruction and strangulation of the bowel. Bloody diarrhea and a palpable mass are usually present. Toxic megacolon is primarily associated with ulcerative colitis. The bowel diameter exceeds 6 cm. Perforation is a common complication. Ogilvie's syndrome is a pseudo-obstruction of the right colon in elderly people. There is an acute, massive distention of the colon without pain or tenderness. The right colon is distended with a cutoff at the splenic flexure. Barium studies are negative for obstruction.

49. The answer is C. *(Psychiatry; cognitive disorder)*
Dissociative fugue is characterized by sudden travel away from home, inability to recall one's past, and a disturbance of identity. It often occurs during the course of severe stress. Memory impairment may or may not be present with organic psychoses, conversion disorder, or delirium. Subjective memory problems sometimes occur during major depression.

50. The answer is D. *(Obstetrics; oligohydramnios)*
Marked deficiency in amniotic fluid volume may occur with decreased production or excessive removal of fluid. Fetal hypoxia can occur from umbilical cord compression. Meconium passed by the fetus is not diluted, therefore increasing

the risk of fetal respiratory compromise. With the exception of renal agenesis, all the conditions listed are associated with polyhydramnios.

51. The answer is C. *(General surgery; postoperative atelectasis)*
Atelectasis is the most common cause of fever in the first 24 hours of the postoperative state. Atelectasis refers to collapse of the lung distal to an area of obstruction in the airway. In the postoperative state, the dry secretions imposed by anesthesia and pain-restricted clearance of pulmonary secretions predispose the patient to segmental atelectasis and a nidus of inflammation, resulting in fever. Deep inspiration on standing is the most effective way of minimizing this complication. Intermittent positive-pressure breathing treatments are too expensive and impose the risk of *Pseudomonas* infection in the lungs. Wound infections are more common in the 5- to 10-day postoperative period. Urinary tract infections from indwelling catheters are common but do not usually cause fever unless pyelonephritis is a complication. *Candida albicans* is a common cause of intravenous catheter-related sepsis. Fever is not a normal postoperative finding.

52. The answer is D. *(Pediatrics; Todd's paralysis)*
Todd's paralysis commonly occurs after a seizure. The hemiparesis lasts minutes to hours but resolves within 24 hours. It can easily be confused with a stroke except for its duration. Hemiplegia complicating migraine headaches also shows recovery within a few hours, but residual neurologic effects contribute to permanent hemiparesis. The disorder usually involves a strong maternal history of classic migraine.

53. The answer is A. *(Psychiatry; schizophrenia)*
Schizophrenia is distinguished from bipolar disorder by its different clinical course. In schizophrenia, psychotic symptoms are present during times when mood disturbances are minimal. Although mania is more common in bipolar disorder, both illnesses can present with depression, anxiety, psychosis, and mania.

54. The answer is B. *(Clinical immunology; hereditary angioedema due to C1 esterase deficiency)*
A family history with an autosomal dominant pattern of inheritance of recurrent swelling of the face, upper airways, and extremities along with abdominal cramps from submucosal edema would indicate hereditary angioedema due to C1 esterase inhibitor deficiency. Absence of this inhibitor results in excessive stimulation of C4 and C2, resulting in the release of breakdown products that cause the release of histamine and other vasodilators. The vasodilators increase vessel permeability, resulting in swelling of soft tissue. Edema of the upper airway is the most common cause of death in these patients.

The best screen is a C4 assay, which is low in these patients even when they are in a quiescent period. A normal C4 essentially excludes the disease. C2 is also decreased, whereas C3 is normal. The diagnosis is confirmed with a C1 esterase inhibitor assay.

In acute attacks, maintenance of the upper airways is the most important factor. Fresh frozen plasma (which supplies the inhibitor), ε-aminocaproic acid, and androgens (e.g., stanozolol) are also used. Androgens are also useful as maintenance therapy because they stimulate the synthesis of C1 esterase inhibitor.

Quantitative immunoglobulins, C3 assay, serum antinuclear antibody test, and the sweat test for cystic fibrosis are not indicated with this clinical history.

55. The answer is B. *(Gynecology; postmenopausal bleeding)*
The diagnosis to rule out is endometrial carcinoma; therefore, endometrial biopsy is the diagnostic method of choice. Cytologic screening by Pap smear misses 60% of endometrial carcinoma cases. The diagnosis is a histologic one; therefore, pelvic examination under anesthesia, laparoscopy, and colposcopy are of limited value in this case.

56. The answer is D. *(General surgery; postoperative pancreatitis)*

Postoperative pancreatitis is most commonly seen in the setting of common bile duct exploration for a stone during a cholecystectomy. Both the pancreatic duct and the common bile duct empty into the ampulla of Vater. Emptying is determined by the sphincter tone in the ampulla. Low obstruction in the common bile duct by a stone causes reflux from the bile duct into the pancreatic duct, which can lead to pancreatitis. Endoscopic retrograde cholangiopancreatography is also a cause of pancreatitis. Hypovolemia, anesthetic agents, and total parenteral nutrition do not predispose to acute pancreatitis.

57. The answer is C. *(Pediatrics; tuberculous meningitis)*

Tuberculous meningitis usually presents in recently infected individuals and is usually considered a disease of infants and children. The symptoms develop slowly during three stages. Seizures are common in stage 2; coma occurs in stage 3. A high index of suspicion is necessary for rapid diagnosis. A computed tomography (CT) scan of the head may show periventricular lucencies, edema, infarctions, and hydrocephalus. Cerebrospinal fluid (CSF) findings show a slight elevation in white blood cells (WBCs), usually 250 to 500, predominantly lymphocytes. The CSF glucose is less than 40 mg/dl or less than half the serum glucose performed simultaneously. Protein concentration is normal or slightly high. Gram's stain is negative since the bacilli are acid-fast. CSF chloride is low.

58. The answer is B. *(Psychiatry; anxiety)*

Anxiety is characterized by excessive worry, hypervigilance, motor tension, and autonomic symptoms such as dyspnea, tachycardia, and diaphoresis. Although anxiety can occur during the course of the other conditions listed, the presence of depersonalization, delirium, depression, or psychosis is unlikely.

59. The answer is D. *(Gastroenteritis; hepatitis C post-transfusion)*

Hepatitis C virus (HCV) is the most common cause of posttransfusional hepatitis (90% of cases). There is a 0.3%/U chance of contracting HCV. HCV has an incubation period ranging from 2 weeks to 6 months. The majority of cases are anicteric. Approximately 60% of cases progress into chronic hepatitis. There is also a risk for developing cirrhosis and hepatocellular carcinoma.

Transaminasemia is the best marker for hepatitis, with serum alanine aminotransferase (ALT) usually higher than serum aspartate aminotransferase (AST). Alkaline phosphatase and γ-glutamyltransferase are better indicators of cholestasis. These enzymes are only mildly elevated in hepatitis unless they are in a transient cholestatic phase. The antibody test for HCV is useful in detecting early disease, but is highly specific when it is positive. Atypical lymphocytosis is seen in any viral hepatitis and should not always be construed as representing infectious mononucleosis.

Alpha interferon (IFN-α) is useful in the treatment of chronic HCV infections.

Hepatitis A is rarely contracted by blood transfusion. Hepatitis B can be transmitted from blood transfusion, but the screening of blood for hepatitis B surface antigen has markedly decreased the incidence of the disease. Cytomegalovirus can be transmitted by blood transfusion because it is present in lymphocytes, but it is more commonly seen in immunocompromised hosts.

60. The answer is A. *(Neurology; syrinx)*

The dissociated sensory loss (preserved posterior column, absent spinothalamic tract) is classic for syringomyelia. A Horner's syndrome would suggest intrinsic disease of the upper thoracic spine as well. Spinal stenosis and a herniated cervical disc, although causing weakness and sensory loss, do not fit with dissociated loss or a Horner's syndrome, because they are extrinsic processes. Myelitis is possible, although less likely and difficult to demonstrate by magnetic resonance imaging (MRI). In addition, multiple sclerosis would not likely cause the signs of lower motor neuron dysfunction suggested by loss of reflexes in the upper extremities and hand wasting. With such profound neurologic deficits localized to the cervical spine, a normal MRI is unlikely.

61. The answer is A. *(Obstetrics; gestational trophoblastic disease)*
The majority of hydatidiform moles are "complete," have a 46 XX karyotype, and derive both X chromosomes paternally. "Incomplete," or partial, moles often present with a coexistent fetus and have triploid karyotypes, most commonly 69 XXY.

62. The answer is B. *(General surgery; postoperative delirium tremens)*
The patient is an alcoholic who has delirium tremens (DTs) as a result of the abrupt withdrawal of alcohol. Hyperventilation during surgery and the resultant respiratory alkalosis along with nutritional deficits frequently precipitate a full-blown attack. The attack is characterized by anxiety, tremor, hallucinations, overactivity, and seizure activity and may result in dehiscence of the wound.

Management of DTs is geared toward reducing agitation and anxiety. This is accomplished with the administration of chlordiazepoxide. In addition, attention must be given to correcting underlying nutritional deficiencies. Hypomagnesemia is particularly common in alcoholics and is associated with tetany secondary to hypocalcemia (magnesium normally enhances parathormone activity). Thiamine deficiency is also common in alcoholics. Infusion of an intravenous solution containing glucose can precipitate acute Wernicke's encephalopathy (characterized by confusion, agitation, and nystagmus). The glucose is converted into pyruvate, which uses thiamine to enter into the citric acid cycle. The conversion of pyruvate into acetylcoenzyme A (acetyl-CoA) can consume the already low thiamine stores, creating the potential for acute Wernicke's encephalopathy. Intensive care unit syndrome is associated with the typical intensive care unit environment of bright lights, noise, and sleep deprivation, which can produce confusion and subsequent development of delirium in

patients. Postoperative psychosis is an uncommon stress-induced psychosis that is seen particularly in elderly patients with chronic disease. Many of these patients have preexisting mood disturbances. Stress, drugs, and high β-endorphin levels are also contributing factors. Delirium occurs in approximately 20% of cases. Although uncommon, it is most commonly associated with thoracic or abdominal surgery.

63. The answer is C. *(Pediatrics; craniopharyngioma)*
Craniopharyngioma is the most common supratentorial tumor of children. About 90% of these tumors show calcifications on plain skull films or on computed tomography (CT) scan. Many cases are originally discovered during an endocrine workup for short stature secondary to pituitary–hypothalamic involvement. Bitemporal field defects occur because of pressure or injury to the optic chiasm. The tumor can also compress the third ventricle, causing hydrocephalus. With prominent hydrocephalus, papilledema is evident. Polyuria from diabetes insipidus results from interruption of the supraoptic–hypophyseal tract. Treatment consists of surgical removal of the tumor and hormone replacement.

64. The answer is C. *(Psychiatry; cognitive disorder)*
Delirium is characterized by disturbances of awareness or attention, cognitive problems, rapid onset, and fluctuations in severity. Associated findings such as hallucinations and persecutory ideation are common. The possible physiologic causes include L-dopa or anticholinergic toxicity and alcohol withdrawal. Patients who are elderly or who have preexisting dementia are much more likely to develop delirium.

65. The answer is A. *(Psychiatry; anxiety)*
Agoraphobia is often associated with panic disorder. Patients with panic disorder often have a history of separation anxiety disorder in childhood. The presence of the other disorders listed is unlikely, although patients with anxiety often develop depression.

66. The answer is C. *(Obstetrics; cesarean delivery)*
Classification of cesarean types refers to the uterine incision rather than the skin incision. Most cesareans are performed through a transverse low segment uterine incision. Active phase arrest is a frequent indication for a transverse incision. A classic uterine incision, made vertically in the upper segment and fundus, has specific indications. The other four options are examples of indications for a classic incision.

67. The answer is B. *(Hematology; treatment of hypercalcemia)*
This patient has clinical and electrocardiographic (ECG) evidence of hypercalcemia. The hypercalcemia is due to the production of osteoclast activating factor by myeloma cells in the bone marrow.

The ECG shows shortening of the QT interval (0.28–0.3), which is the characteristic finding in hypercalcemia. Neuropsychiatric findings in hypercalcemia involve personality changes, confusion, depression, acute psychosis, or coma. Cardiovascular changes include hypertension, potentiation of cardiac glycosides, and shortening of the QT interval. Gastrointestinal signs and symptoms consist of nausea, constipation, peptic ulcer disease (calcium stimulates gastrin release), and acute pancreatitis. Pseudogout can occur in the joints. Metastatic calcification in the kidney produces nephrocalcinosis (calcification in the basement membranes of the tubules), which produces polyuria, natriuresis (leading to volume contraction), and problems with urine concentration.

Saline infusion is the first step in management of hypercalcemia, because it corrects volume contraction, which is a stimulus for further calcium reabsorption, and enhances calciuresis. Once hydration is achieved, a loop diuretic, for example, furosemide, is added to potentiate the calciuresis.

If saline administration and furosemide are ineffective or if chronic hypercalcemia is anticipated, a number of other options are available. Bisphosphonates are particularly useful in malignancy-induced hypercalcemia because they inhibit bone resorption. Corticosteroids are recommended in hypercalcemia associated with hypervitaminosis D, sarcoidosis, hematologic malignancies, and breast cancer. Mithramycin, an antineoplastic antibiotic, is generally effective, but requires close monitoring because of its toxicity. Calcitonin is only effective for 1 or 2 weeks; then, hypercalcemia reappears.

Sodium bicarbonate and calcium gluconate are useful in the treatment of hyperkalemia.

68. The answer is A. *(Biostatistics; Student's t-test)*
The question relates to assessing group differences of a continuous variable which in this question is height. If the comparison were among three groups with a continuous variable, analysis of variance would be correct. With two groups, it is necessary to use Student's t-test. A correlation coefficient assesses the strength of association, not the differences between groups. The chi-squared test assesses differences between groups of categorical variables. Logistic regression is used to assess a categorical outcome for a continuous predictor.

69. The answer is B. *(General surgery; disseminated intravascular coagulation)*
The patient has disseminated intravascular coagulation (DIC) secondary to massive soft-tissue trauma. Release of tissue thromboplastin from the injured tissue activates the extrinsic and intrinsic coagulation systems, leading to the formation of clots in the microvasculature. The consumption of fibrinogen, factors V and VIII, and platelets by the clots renders the patient anticoagulated, so bleeding occurs from all open wounds. Laboratory studies typically reveal the following:

- Decreased plasma fibrinogen
- Prolonged prothrombin and partial thromboplastin times (resulting from the consumption of fibrinogen, factors V and VIII)
- Thrombocytopenia
- Increased fibrinogen degradation products (i.e., fibrin) from activation of the fibrinolytic system

- Schistocytes in the peripheral blood from damage to the red blood cells by fibrin strands in the microthrombi

The best treatment for DIC is to treat the underlying cause. Fresh frozen plasma replaces all of the coagulation fractures. Cryoprecipitate replaces fibrinogen and factor VIII. Platelet concentrates raise the platelet count. Packed red blood cells are used if symptomatic anemia is present. Because heparin enhances antithrombin III activity, the neutralization of thrombin produced by the extrinsic and intrinsic pathways prevents clot formation; therefore, heparin is not generally recommended for treating DIC if the patient is bleeding.

Thrombotic thrombocytopenic purpura (TTP) is not associated with trauma. It is characterized by a pentad of fever, central nervous system (CNS) abnormalities, thrombocytopenia, hemolytic anemia, and renal failure. An unknown circulating plasma factor damages vascular endothelium resulting in platelet thrombi. There is no consumption of clotting factors, so the prothrombin and partial thromboplastin times are normal. Primary fibrinolysis is extremely rare. It is associated with primary activation of the fibrinolytic system, most commonly in the setting of open heart surgery and prostate surgery. Fat embolism syndrome is seen 1 to 3 days following trauma associated with multiple fractures of long bones, most commonly the femur. There is a debate as to whether the fat in the vessels comes from the marrow cavity or traumatized adipose tissue. Dyspnea is the first symptom and neurologic problems are the most common cause of death. Diffuse bleeding problems like those described in this patient are not usually part of this syndrome.

70. The answer is E. *(Obstetrics; cesarean delivery)*
One of the main benefits of a classic incision is minimal trauma risk to the fetus regardless of how abnormal the presentation or lie. It is also valuable when access to the lower uterine segment is restricted because of fibroids, adhesions, varicosities, or extreme immaturity. The first four

options are advantages of a transverse low segment incision, and they are disadvantages of a classic incision.

71. The answer is B. *(Nephrology; acute cystitis)*
The history of suprapubic pain, dysuria, and increased urinary frequency plus the urinary sediment findings of clumps of neutrophils (pyuria), scattered red blood cells (RBCs), and bacteria without the presence of casts is consistent with acute cystitis. The most common cause of pyuria is acute cystitis due to *Escherichia coli*. The absence of white blood cell (WBC) casts, fever, and costovertebral angle pain excludes acute pyelonephritis.

In pyuria, the dipstick nitrite is positive, because most of the common urinary pathogens (e.g., *E. coli*) are nitrate reducers. Leukocyte esterase is positive, because neutrophils contain esterase in their granules.

Excessive proteinuria is often associated with hyaline casts or fatty casts, if the patient has the nephrotic syndrome. Proteinuria is the most common urinary finding in renal disease.

A nephritic type of glomerulonephritis (e.g., poststreptococcal glomerulonephritis) is associated with hematuria, RBC casts, and mild-to-moderate proteinuria.

Patients with renal stones have colicky pain emanating from the costovertebral angle and extending anteriorly to the groin. The urinalysis reveals numerous RBCs and occasional WBCs.

72. The answer is C. *(Pediatrics; phenylketonuria)*
Phenylketonuria is caused by deficiency or absence of phenylalanine hydroxylase. Excess phenylalanine and other toxic metabolites are responsible for brain damage. Infants are normal at birth; but after a few months, mental retardation becomes evident, and it is eventually severe. Vomiting, often mistaken for pyloric stenosis, can occur. Physical examination shows these children to be fair, with blue eyes; some have a rash resembling eczema, which fades with age. They have a mousey or musty odor of phenylacetic acid. Hyperactive deep tendon reflexes are

found. Treatment consists of early diagnosis and dietary management.

73. The answer is D. *(Psychiatry; depression)*
Depression is characterized by a depressed mood, coupled with rumination and demoralization, trouble concentrating, and changes in circadian rhythms. Hypersomnia and hyposomnia are both fairly common. Mania and anxiety might also be associated with decreased sleep, but concurrent demoralization would be unusual. Somatization disorder involves complaints from multiple organ systems, but its long clinical course starts before age 30. Delirium would usually have a shorter course, with less clearly defined worries.

74. The answer is C. *(Pulmonary medicine; assisted ventilation)*
Minute volume is the ventilatory rate per minute times the tidal volume (V_T). This volume is the most important component of adequate ventilation. Increasing the minute volume blows off Pa_{CO_2} (respiratory alkalosis), whereas decreasing minute volume increases the Pa_{CO_2} (respiratory acidosis). Therefore, to answer this question, the minute volume that is smallest is the one most likely to result in the greatest retention of CO_2.

The patient's current minute volume is 16 breaths/min $\times$ 700 ml (V_T) = 11,200 ml. The addition of 150 ml of dead space (space where there is no gas exchange) decreases the minute volume to 11,050 ml (11,200 − 150 = 11,050 ml). Decreasing the ventilatory rate to 12 breaths/min produces a minute volume of 8400 ml (12 × 700 = 8400 ml). Reducing the ventilatory rate to 14 breaths/min and the V_T to 600 ml produces a minute volume of 8400 ml (14 × 600 = 8400 ml). Decreasing the V_T to 500 ml results in a minute volume of 8000 ml (16 × 500 = 8000 ml), which would produce the greatest retention of CO_2. This factor underscores the importance of changing V_T in the clearance of CO_2 in a patient on assisted ventilation.

75. The answer is B. *(Gynecology; reproductive endocrinology)*
Disorders of prolactin secretion can be mediated by many causes. All of the options listed, with the exception of Sheehan's syndrome, are associated with elevated prolactin levels. Sheehan's syndrome is the only clinical entity of significance characterized by lower than normal levels of serum prolactin. This syndrome results from hypoperfusion of the anterior pituitary gland, usually as a result of obstetric hemorrhage, and is associated with failure to lactate.

76. The answer is B. *(Pediatrics; pilocytic astrocytoma of the cerebellum)*
Brain tumors are the most common solid tumors in childhood and are second only to leukemia as the most prevalent malignancy. Infratentorial tumors are the most common in childhood, supratentorial in adults. Infants less than 2 years of age and adolescents approximate adults in location of tumors. Tumors can further be broken down into those of glial cells and those of primitive neuroectodermal origin. Astrocytomas, ependymomas, and glioblastoma multiforme make up the glial tumors. Neuroectodermal tumors include medulloblastoma and pineoblastoma. Cerebellar astrocytomas constitute the most common posterior fossa tumors of childhood. They also have the best prognosis, with a 90% 5-year survival rate. Medulloblastomas are the second most common posterior fossa tumors of childhood. Ependymomas are responsible for about 10% of tumors of the posterior fossa.

77. The answer is C. *(Psychiatry; mood disorder)*
The quality of mood distinguishes mania from schizophrenia. Manic moods include elation, expansiveness, and irritability. Depressive moods include dysphoria and loss of pleasure. In other ways, such as changes in activity levels and sleep problems, mania and depression may have a surprising resemblance.

78. The answer is D. *(Neurology; cluster headaches)*
This patient is suffering from cluster headaches, often striking young men in the nocturnal hours. Oxygen in a high concentration is a vasoconstrictor and can abort many cluster headaches. Both nitroglycerin and alcohol are vasodilators and may worsen vascular headaches. Exercise and a warm pack may distract the sufferer, but do nothing to end the underlying cluster attacks.

79. The answer is C. *(Pediatrics; intussusception)*
Intussusception is the most common cause of intestinal obstruction in children between 3 months and 6 years of age, but decreases in frequency after 3 years. The cause is unknown, but it has been associated with gastroenteritis, Meckel's diverticulum, polyps, and sarcoma. Patients have paroxysmal colicky abdominal pain. Bloody, currant-jelly stools are passed, and a sausage-shaped mass can be palpated in the abdomen. Barium enema reveals a coil-spring sign and may even be therapeutic. Otherwise, surgical reduction is necessary. Pyloric stenosis is characterized by nonbilious projectile vomiting in a 1 to 3 month old. Meckel's diverticulum, although common at 2 years of age, usually presents as painless rectal bleeding. Meconium ileus and necrotizing enterocolitis both present in the neonatal period.

80. The answer is B. *(Gynecology; ovarian cancer)*
Staging criteria generally use the best clinically available information from physical examination data and minimally invasive imaging or inspection techniques. Cervical, uterine, vaginal, and vulvar malignancies have readily available information from clinical examination or imaging methods. Ovarian cancer can be thoroughly evaluated by laparotomy only.

81. The answer is B. *(Psychiatry; somatoform disorder)*
Hypochrondriasis is characterized by unrealistic worry about the meaning of a symptom. The worry does not respond to physician reassurance even after an adequate workup. Conversion disorder usually involves a loss of sensory or motor function. Delusional disorder is characterized by bizarre beliefs. A patient with a somatization disorder has simultaneous compliants about many organ systems. In factitious disorder, patients voice false complaints.

82. The answer is B. *(Pulmonary medicine; adult respiratory distress syndrome)*
Adult respiratory distress syndrome (ARDS) is marked by the rapid onset of dyspnea, within 12 to 24 hours of an initiating event. Initiating events with an increased propensity for ARDS are sepsis (most common), aspiration of gastric contents (this patient), drug overdose, shock, burns, diffuse pneumonias, and oxygen toxicity, to name only a few.

The mechanism of injury is primarily a neutrophil-related event in the lungs, with the release of proteases, free radicals, and leukotrienes that produce pulmonary vasoconstriction and increased vessel permeability. The increased vessel permeability results in leaky capillaries that lose protein-rich fluid into the alveoli to produce hyaline membranes. Lymphocytes and monocytes release cytokines, which also contribute to the inflammatory process. Type I pneumonocytes are damaged, therefore decreasing the production of surfactant, which results in widespread atelectasis (alveolar collapse). Increased inflammation and edema in the interstitium of the lungs decrease compliance (ability of the lungs to expand). Damage to elastic tissue support decreases elasticity, or the recoil properties of the lung. Because atelectasis is a prominent feature of ARDS, the primary defect is intrapulmonary shunting of blood accompanied by profound hypoxemia. Ventilation and perfusion abnormalities plus diffusion abnormalities are also present. The pulmonary capillary wedge pressure is normal because the left ventricular end-diastolic pressure is normal.

Laboratory studies exhibit an initial respiratory alkalosis due to tachypnea and a profound hypoxemia with an increased alveolar–arterial gradient (A–a gradient). In this patient, the Pa_{CO_2} is 29 mm Hg, which is respiratory alkalosis; the

A = alveolar a = arterial.

interstitial → alveolar pattern.

bicarbonate is 21 mEq/L, which is metabolic acidosis; and the pH is alkaline (7.50). This combination is compatible with primary respiratory alkalosis and a mild compensatory metabolic acidosis. The A–a gradient, which is the difference between the alveolar and arterial oxygen concentration due to uneven ventilation and perfusion, is calculated as follows: The alveolar P_{O_2} (P_{AO_2}) = (% inspired air $\times$ 713 mm Hg) – ($P_{ACO_2}/0.8$). Therefore, the A–a gradient equals the P_{AO_2} – P_{aO_2}: This patient's A–a gradient is 0.21 (713) – 29/0.8 = 114 mm Hg; 114 – 40 = 74 mm Hg. A medically significant A–a gradient is any gradient over 30 mm Hg. An increased gradient always indicates a problem with ventilation, perfusion, and diffusion, either alone or in combination.

The chest x-ray in ARDS reveals diffuse or patchy bilateral infiltrates, with an initial interstitial pattern due to interstitial edema progressing into an alveolar pattern as protein-rich exudate emanates from leaky pulmonary capillaries. The costophrenic angles are characteristically clear. Air bronchograms secondary to peribronchiolar edema are present in 80% of patients.

The management of ARDS involves treatment of the underlying event plus tracheal intubation accompanying mechanical ventilation and oxygen therapy. Positive end-expiratory pressure (PEEP) at low pressures is combined with oxygen. Increased PEEP increases the positive intrathoracic pressure, which increases interstitial edema and decreases compliance; therefore, it must be used cautiously. Corticosteroids have not been shown to improve survival. The most common cause of death in ARDS is multi-organ failure.

Aspiration of gastric contents is particularly common in trauma patients who are unconscious, patients with strokes, pregnant women, or those recovering from anesthesia. The more acid the material, the worse the prognosis.

Clinically, patients present with an abrupt onset of severe dyspnea with cough, wheezing, and tachypnea. Rales are present at both lung bases. Arterial blood gases show severe hypoxemia. A chest x-ray shows patchy infiltrates at both lung bases. ARDS, as in this patient, is a common complication.

Antibiotics are given if secondary infection occurs, which is usually within 2 or 3 days. The use of corticosteroids is controversial. The mortality rate is 50%.

83. The answer is A. *(General surgery; superior vena caval syndrome)*
The patient has superior vena caval syndrome, which is most commonly secondary to extension of a primary lung cancer into the neck with obstruction of superior vena caval blood flow. Clinical findings consist of a puffiness and bluish discoloration of the face, arms, and shoulders, along with distention of the jugular veins. In addition, there are central nervous system (CNS) signs of dizziness, visual disturbances, and convulsions. Prompt administration of diuretics, fluid restriction, and radiation therapy are useful in restoring blood flow. Surgery is rarely indicated. The mean survival is 6 to 8 months.

Sclerosing mediastinitis is uncommon but most commonly results from histoplasmosis. A pericardial effusion distends the neck veins but would not be associated with the degree of venous engorgement noted in this case. Polycythemia rubra vera is associated with an increase in plasma volume and red blood cell mass, but does not produce the type of venous engorgement noted in this patient.

84. The answer is A. *(Gynecology; cervical cancer)*
Stage I cervical carcinoma has the best 5-year survival (90%). The rates for the other malignancies are as follows: vaginal (85%); endometrial (75%); ovarian (70%); and oviductal (60%).

85. The answer is C. *(Pediatrics; neonatal meningitis pathogen)*
Streptococcus agalactiae (group B streptococcus) is the most common cause of neonatal meningitis, followed by *Escherichia coli* and *Listeria*. Group B streptococcus is a common inhabitant of the maternal genitourinary tract. It is acquired by newborns via vertical transmission. Early-onset disease is associated with sepsis; late onset is associated with meningitis.

Streptococcus pneumoniae and *Neisseria meningitidis* are seen in older age-groups.

86. The answer is D. *(Biostatistics; chi-squared test)*
The question relates to assessing group differences of a categorical variable, in this question, Apgar scores. If the comparison were between two groups with a continuous variable, a Student's *t*-test would be correct. If the comparison were among three groups with a continuous variable, analysis of variance would be correct. A correlation coefficient assesses the strength of association, not differences between groups. Logistic regression is used to assess a categorical outcome for a continuous predictor.

87. The answer is C. *(Psychiatry; somatoform disorder)*
In malingering, a patient falsifies symptoms for obvious gains, sometimes referred to as secondary gains. These gains might include insurance payments or avoidance of military service. Factitious disorder offers no such clear gains. The presumption is that the patient complains as a way of dealing with intrapsychic conflict. The falsified symptoms may lead to detrimental consequences for the patient.

88. The answer is E. *(Pharmacology; antibiotics)*
In addition to skin lesions, the clinical picture suggests bacteremia in this patient, who may still be immunosuppressed. The likely causative organisms include gram-positive cocci and gram-negative bacteria. Note: The present infection may be nosocomial, in which case knowledge of the hospital pathogens would be helpful. Treatment should be initiated before the results of culture and susceptibility are available. Erythromycin is bacteriostatic, it would not cover for gram-negative rods, and its oral administration is not appropriate here. Ampicillin would not cover for staphylococci, which are overwhelmingly penicillinase-producing; and many bacteria are resistant to tetracycline, a bacteriostatic drug. The best choice for "coverage" is a first-generation cephalosporin plus an aminoglycoside, both

of which are bactericidal. However, this regimen would not handle anaerobes.

89. The answer is A. *(Psychiatry; somatoform disorder)*
This patient's symptoms suggest somatization disorder. Numerous studies have demonstrated that morbidity from this illness is significantly decreased with regularly scheduled follow-up medical appointments. The focus of such visits is general, and the physician should avoid arguments about the veracity of symptoms. Such an approach also decreases costs associated with overuse of emergency services.

90. The answer is D. *(General surgery; solitary coin lesions in the lung)*
The majority of solitary coin lesions in the lung are benign (60%) with the remaining causes representing primary lung cancer (35%) and metastatic lung cancer (5%). Of the 60% of benign causes, granulomas (e.g., histoplasmosis, tuberculosis) account for 55% and the remaining 5% are due to bronchial hamartomas or mixed tumors. The patient's midwestern origins strongly suggest histoplasmosis as the etiology for the calcified granuloma. Calcification of a coin lesion is more commonly seen in granulomas than in cancer. Absence of growth within a year, target or popcorn calcifications, or concentric calcifications strongly favor a benign process. Indistinct margins, increased growth rate when compared with previous films, flecks of calcium in the mass, and sizes greater than 3 cm in diameter favor malignancy.

91. The answer is C. *(Emergency medicine; carbon monoxide poisoning)*
Carbon monoxide (CO) poisoning is a common accidental injury or method of suicide. CO is a colorless, odorless gas produced by incomplete combustion of carbon-containing compounds. Because of its high affinity for hemoglobin, CO passes straight through the lungs and pulmonary capillaries and attaches to the heme group of the red blood cells (RBCs) without setting up any gradients in the alveoli or arterial blood. Therefore, both the alveolar and arterial P_{O_2} are

normal. However, the oxygen saturation is decreased, because it represents the percentage of heme groups occupied by oxygen. In the standard blood-gas laboratory, only the pH, $Paco_2$, and Pao_2 are directly measured. The oxygen saturation is calculated from the Pao_2, so it is normal in CO poisoning. Blood-gas analyzers that have a co-oximeter attachment directly measure the oxygen saturation, as well as oxygen content, CO level, and methemoglobin level.

Clinically, patients present with headache in mild forms of poisoning and with coma in severe exposure. The blood has a cherry-red color, which is often a good clue for the presence of CO.

The first step in the management of CO poisoning is the administration of 100% oxygen by nonrebreathing mask or endotracheal tube. The increased oxygen displaces the CO on the RBCs. Since the half-life of CO on RBCs is less than 1 hour when a patient is on 100% oxygen versus 5 to 6 hours when breathing room air, oxygen must be started immediately in order to prevent permanent neurologic damage.

Intravenous methylene-blue therapy is for methemoglobinemia. Methemoglobin refers to the presence of hemoglobin iron in the ferric state, which cannot bind with oxygen. Cyanosis is present. The blood has a chocolate-brown color. The arterial blood-gas findings are exactly the same as for CO, because the true oxygen saturation is not measured on standard blood-gas instruments. Methylene blue enhances the methemoglobin reductase system, which converts iron back into the ferrous state. Ascorbic acid, which is a reducing agent, is also used as an ancillary treatment.

Amyl nitrite, sodium nitrite, and sodium thiosulfate are used in the treatment of cyanide poisoning. Cyanide is a systemic asphyxiant that blocks cytochrome oxidase in the electron transport chain in the mitochondria. This blockade prevents the synthesis of adenosine triphosphate (ATP). The breath has a bitter almond smell. The arterial blood gases are normal. Nitrites in the treatment scheme oxidize hemoglobin into methemoglobin, which competes with cyanide for cytochrome oxidase. Cyanide combines with thiocyanate to form a nontoxic thiocyanate, which is excreted.

Activated charcoal has great adsorptive properties for orally administered poisons such as theophylline, phenytoin, salicylates, and phenobarbital. It is not useful in poisonings due to alcohols, potassium, lithium, and iron.

92. The answer is E. *(Gynecology; infertility)*
Up to 15% of couples experience infertility. In 40% of couples, multiple causes may be present. Of the factors listed, the incidence is as follows: ovulatory, 15%–20%; cervical, 5%–10%; uterine–tubal, 30%; male, 40%.

93. The answer is A. *(Pediatrics; Haemophilus influenzae type B in meningitis)*
Haemophilus influenzae type B is the most common cause of meningitis in this age-group. *Neisseria meningitidis* can occur in any age-group, but is less common in the others. *Escherichia coli* and group B streptococcus are more common pathogens in neonates. *Streptococcus pneumoniae* is seen more frequently after 5 years of age.

94. The answer is C. *(General surgery; acute appendicitis)*
The patient has acute appendicitis. Low grade fever with absolute neutrophilic leukocytosis and left shift, and pain beginning in the epigastric area, moving to the umbilicus, and finally to McBurney's point between the umbilicus and the anterior iliac spine, strongly suggest acute appendicitis. Other signs and symptoms include rebound tenderness at McBurney's point (Blumberg's sign); pain in the right lower quadrant on palpation of the left lower quadrant (Rovsing's sign); abdominal pain on extension of the right thigh with the patient on the left side (psoas sign); abdominal pain on internal rotation of the flexed right thigh with the patient supine; pain preceding nausea and vomiting. Facial flushing may occur in children due to the release of serotonin. Diarrhea is absent in all but retrocecal appendicitis. Complications include perforation with peritonitis; periappendiceal abscess; pyle-

phlebitis (inflammation of the portal vein); subphrenic abscess; and septicemia.

Ulcerative colitis presents with left lower quadrant pain and bloody diarrhea. Crohn's disease presents with crampy, right lower quadrant pain with diarrhea. Irritable bowel syndrome is associated with stress-induced diarrhea, constipation, or both, with mucus in the stools. Psychogenic pain is usually periumbilical.

95. The answer is B. *(Neurology; narcolepsy)*
The patient has narcolepsy, clinically described by the tetrad of daytime hypersomnolence, cataplexy, hypnagogic hallucinations, and sleep paralysis. Sleep studies will demonstrate sleep-onset rapid eye movement (REM). Obstructive sleep apnea and periodic leg movements are also sleep disorders, but are not associated with cataplexy. Delta wave sleep onset is not particularly associated with any sleep disorder.

96. The answer is C. *(Gynecology; cervical cancer)*
Cervical carcinoma has four subcategories in stage I, which are IA, IA$_1$, IA$_2$, and IB. Endometrial carcinoma has stage IA and IB only. All the others have no subdivisions of stage I.

97. The answer is C. *(Psychiatry; psychosis)*
Hallucinations are common in both delirium and schizophrenia. Social withdrawal and a family history of psychopathology are more common with schizophrenia. Memory impairment and rapid fluctuation of symptoms are more suggestive of delirium.

98. The answer is B. *(Pediatrics; metachromatic leukodystrophy)*
Metachromatic leukodystrophy is a disorder of myelin metabolism. Arylsulfatase A activity is deficient. The six disorders are based on age of onset and enzyme deficiency. All are characterized by gait disturbances that progress to complete inability to walk. The extremities become hypotonic, and deep tendon reflexes are lost. Speech becomes slurred; nystagmus is present. Feeding and swallowing are impaired, and death from bronchopneumonia occurs by 5 to 6 years

of age. Cerebrospinal fluid (CSF) shows elevated protein. Metachromatic granules in urine are very suggestive of metachromatic leukodystrophy. Infants with Krabbe's disease tend to be hypertonic. Globoid histiocytes are seen in the white matter. Fabry's disease is X-linked recessive, and manifestations occur at adolescence. Skin eruptions around the navel and buttocks are characteristic.

99. The answer is D. *(General medicine; Haemophilus influenzae meningitis)*
Sterile subdural effusions are so common in *Haemophilus influenzae* meningitis that many consider it to be a natural progression of the disease. The effusions are sometimes the cause of persistent fever in meningitis that is being treated appropriately. Diagnosis is confirmed by computed tomography (CT) scan. Aspiration is recommended only if the meningitis is symptomatic (increased intracranial pressure, depressed level of consciousness).

100. The answer is E. *(Psychiatry; somatoform disorder)*
Symptoms in conversion disorder are considered to be beyond the voluntary control of the patient. In factitious disorder, symptom production is deliberate. In both disorders, unconscious conflict and emotional distress may be underlying reasons for the pathology.

101. The answer is C. *(Gynecology; cervical cancer)*
Cervical malignancy of the squamous cell type is associated with human papillomavirus (HPV) types that are transmitted sexually. Therefore, it is considered an epidemiological venereal disease.

102. The answer is B. *(General surgery; dumping syndrome)*
The patient has dumping syndrome, which is a complication of a Billroth II procedure. In this procedure, the duodenum is closed at the pylorus (afferent limb) and a gastrojejunostomy (efferent limb) is performed. The dumping syndrome is characterized by palpitations, sweating, diarrhea,

and flushing of the face 30 minutes after eating secondary to reactive hypoglycemia, which precipitates the onset of adrenergic signs and symptoms. Dumping syndrome is least likely to occur with a superselective parietal cell vagotomy.

Afferent loop syndrome (blind loop syndrome) is another complication of a Billroth II procedure. It is characterized by postprandial epigastric fullness that is relieved by vomiting of bilious material that is free of ingesta; the ingesta has already passed into the efferent limb. Efferent loop syndrome can complicate a Billroth II procedure. It is characterized by postprandial epigastric fullness and pain that is relieved by immediate vomiting of food and bilious material. Gastroparesis, a problem with emptying of the stomach, is most often associated with autonomic neuropathy (e.g., diabetes mellitus).

103. The answer is A. *(Pharmacology; antibiotics)*
A drug for gonorrhea must include coverage for possible accompanying chlamydial infection. The incidence of gonococcal strains resistant to penicillin G, amoxicillin, and tetracycline is high; therefore, none of these drugs are considered first choice for gonorrhea. However, a tetracycline eradicates most strains of *Chlamydia trachomatis* causing urogenital infections. Spectinomycin is active only against gonococci, but resistant strains have emerged. Ceftriaxone is the drug of first choice in gonorrhea, and a single oral dose of the newer macrolide azithromycin is effective in chlamydial infections.

104. The answer is C. *(Biostatistics; validity)*
Validity describes how well a study measured what it was designed to measure. Association expresses the degree to which two things are related. Reliability implies that the results of a test can be reproduced. Relative risk measures the strength of a cause-and-effect relationship. A *p*-value is defined as the probability of obtaining a given result by chance.

105. The answer is E. *(Behavioral science; malpractice)*
Malpractice is generally defined as deviation from the normal standards of professional care, i.e., professional negligence. For a claim of malpractice, the patient must prove that the doctor was negligent, caused damages (not necessarily deliberately), and had a duty to the patient because of their professional relationship.

106. The answer is A. *(Gynecology; Pap smear)*
The Pap smear was designed to screen for preinvasive or early invasive cervical malignancy in asymptomatic women. Although the cause of vaginal infections or postmenopausal bleeding may be identified via the Pap smear, the rates of sensitivity and specificity are unacceptably low. Screening for ovarian malignancy is not accomplished through a Pap smear. Suspicious cervical lesions need to be evaluated through histology from a biopsy, not through cytology from a Pap smear.

107. The answer is B. *(Pediatrics; neurofibromatosis)*
Optic gliomas are present in approximately 15% of patients with neurofibromatosis-1, and they are one of the criteria used in diagnosing the disease. Most patients with optic gliomas are asymptomatic, but approximately 20% show signs of visual disturbances. Optic nerve gliomas present with decreased visual acuity and pale discs.

108. The answer is C. *(Psychiatry; personality disorder)*
The symptoms of schizotypal personality disorder and the residual symptoms of schizophrenia are very similar. However, the patient with schizotypal personality disorder has no history of psychosis. A history of psychosis is necessary for the diagnosis of schizophrenia. Both disorders include bizarre preoccupations and social impairment. Similar family histories for schizophrenia further suggest a close relationship between the two disorders. Generally, neither schizotypal personality disorder nor the residual symptoms of schizophrenia respond well to antipsychotic medications.

109–110. The answers are: 109-E, 110-C.
(Pharmacology; antibiotics)
Microbial overgrowths can occur with almost any antibiotic. Pseudomembranous colitis due to overgrowth of *Clostridium difficile* has been reported following use of ampicillin, clindamycin, tetracyclines, and cephalosporins—it has even occurred following use of vancomycin, the drug that is commonly used to treat such infections. In this patient, oral administration of vancomycin is effective, and few adverse effects would be anticipated because the drug is not absorbed systemically. Note: Fluid and electrolyte replacement is essential.

Allergic reactions have occurred following oral administration of vancomycin, and it would be prudent to avoid the drug in this patient because an alternative is available. Pseudomembranous colitis is life-threatening, and it is essential that treatment be initiated as soon as possible with a drug that is active against *C. difficile*. Of the alternatives listed, only metronidazole is appropriate, but it would also be possible to use bacitracin orally. Note: The antibacterial activity of metronidazole is restricted to anaerobes.

111. The answer is B. *(General surgery; perforated peptic ulcer)*
The patient has perforated the anterior wall of a duodenal ulcer. Duodenal ulcers are three times more common in men than women. Perforation of a peptic ulcer is characterized by the sudden onset of epigastric pain with radiation of the pain into the left shoulder, which results from irritation of the phrenic nerve (C4) by air underneath the diaphragm. Abdominal rigidity, rebound tenderness, and ileus occur as a result of chemical peritonitis. The first step in management is to obtain an upright and supine film of the abdomen, which shows air beneath the diaphragm in 85% of cases. An upper gastrointestinal series is indicated if air is not present beneath the diaphragm. Intravenous cefazolin is given as prophylaxis against infection. Surgical intervention is necessary. The mortality rate is greater with a perforated gastric ulcer (10% to 40%) than with a perforated duodenal ulcer (5% to 15%). Peritoneal lavage is usually indicated in the workup of intraabdominal bleeds. Antacids are not indicated in the treatment of peptic ulcer perforation.

112. The answer is B. *(Gynecology; ovarian cancer)*
Each tumor listed is associated with measurable tumor markers. Dysgerminomas are the only ones that have lactate dehydrogenase (LDH) associated with them and also lack both alpha-fetoprotein (AFP) and human chorionic gonadotropin (hCG). Endodermal sinus tumor, embryonal cell carcinoma, and immature teratoma can produce AFP. Embryonal cell carcinoma, choriocarcinoma, and immature teratoma can produce hCG.

113. The answer is A. *(Psychiatry; oppositional defiant disorder)*
Oppositional defiant disorder involves problems in relating to authority figures. Generally, such children get along well with peers and have no other problems of conduct or development. Unlike conduct disorder, oppositional defiant disorder is rarely associated with mental retardation or attention-deficit disorders. Childhood disintegrative disorders involve the development of psychopathology in various areas following a period of normal development.

114. The answer is C. *(Pediatrics; sinusitis)*
Cavernous sinus thrombosis is a complication of sinusitis. Sinusitis also can be complicated by meningitis, epidural or subdural abscesses, optic neuritis, periorbital and orbital cellulitis and abscess, and osteomyelitis of surrounding bones. Complications occur secondary to local extension of the infection.

115. The answer is C. *(Gynecology; cancer in women)*
Breast cancer was the number one cancer killer in women until recently, when it was overtaken by lung cancer, probably owing to the increase in cigarette smoking among women.

116–117. The answers are: 116-B, 117-C.
(Pharmacology; antibiotics)
Antimicrobial prophylaxis is indicated in surgery when the postoperative infection rate is 5% or greater under optimal conditions. In this case, the patient may be immunosuppressed from cancer chemotherapy and be at special risk. Cephalosporins are the most frequently used drugs in this setting. Cefoxitin is slightly less active against gram-positive cocci than are first-generation cephalosporins, but cefoxitin is more active against strains of *Proteus, Serratia,* and other penicillinase-producing gram-negative rods. It is very unlikely that this reaction would have been avoided with a lower dose of cefoxitin, but it might have been less severe. Erythromycin (bacteriostatic) and penicillin G would not have provided coverage.

This classic type I (immediate) IgE-mediated allergic reaction commonly includes urticaria, anaphylaxis, and angioedema. Such reactions are more likely with penicillins than with cephalosporins. Note: Some cross-allergenicity (< 10%) exists between these two groups of β-lactam antibiotics. Hypoxia due to bronchoconstriction is likely to have been responsible for the cardiovascular effects, especially if the patient had ischemic heart disease. Although skin tests may be useful, they often give false-negative results; therefore, drug hypersensitivity may not be revealed by such tests in all patients. However, the severity of the reaction could have been attenuated if a test dose of cefoxitin had been administered 10 minutes before the full dose.

118. The answer is E. *(Behavioral science; surgical consent for minors)*
In the case of an emancipated minor such as this 16-year-old boy, parental consent is not required; he can give consent for the procedure himself. Married or self-supporting minor children generally are considered emancipated minors and have the rights of adults.

119. The answer is D. *(General surgery; distal splenorenal shunt for portal hypertension)*
The distal splenorenal shunt is considered the most physiologic of the shunts used to reduce portal pressure in cirrhosis. This shunt maintains portal blood flow, selectively decompresses esophageal varices, and controls bleeding from varices in 90% of patients. The 5-year survival rate is improved to 60%.

Total portosystemic shunts reduce portal pressure but deprive the liver of portal blood flow, thus exacerbating hepatic encephalopathy and increasing serum ammonia levels (because the ammonia cannot be metabolized in the urea cycle). The end-to-side (portal vein–inferior vena cava) shunt is most commonly used as an emergency procedure for active esophageal bleeding that is uncontrolled by other methods. The side-to-side (portal vein–inferior vena cava) shunt decompresses sinusoidal pressure in the liver and relieves ascites in most patients. The "H" shunts include anastomoses between the superior mesenteric vein and vena cava (i.e., mesocaval shunts), the portal vein and vena cava, and the mesenteric vein and renal vein. In general, these shunts decompress esophageal veins, control ascites, and have a high rate of patency.

120. The answer is D. *(Gynecology; osteoporosis prevention)*
Estrogen is thought to work by decreasing bone resorption. It is less effective in reversing bone loss than in preventing it.

121. The answer is A. *(Biostatistics; measurement bias in double-blind study)*
The practice of double-blinding investigators is directed at preventing identification of study subjects from control subjects. This control prevents bias in measuring the outcome from one subject to the next (i.e., measurement bias). It should not be expected to impact selection of subjects, which is selection bias, and analysis of the data, which is analysis bias. Due to the prospective nature of the study design, recall bias and ascertainment bias are irrelevant.

122. The answer is E. *(Psychiatry; depression)*
The greatest risk for suicide occurs after partial response to antidepressants. Usually, energy and motivation return before a subjective improvement in mood. A patient who has been too apa-

thetic to act on suicidal rumination may, at this point, attempt suicide.

123. The answer is D. *(Gynecology; osteoporosis prevention)*
Cigarette smoking is associated with the development of osteoporosis. The other options protect against osteoporosis.

124. The answer is C. *(Psychiatry; cognitive disorder)*
This patient's condition is most suggestive of delirium, possibly caused by analgesics or sedative hypnotics. This reaction is not uncommon in the elderly. In addition to treatment for the underlying cause, she should receive supportive measures such as frequent interaction and help with orientation. Darkness and restraint often further agitate delirious patients. Benzodiazepines can increase confusion, especially in the elderly. Cognitive approaches, such as guided imagery, are usually nonproductive in delirium.

125. The answer is A. *(General surgery; acute cholecystitis)*
The patient has acute cholecystitis, which most commonly results from a stone impacted in the cystic duct (90%). Ischemic damage to the gallbladder mucosa and secondary invasion by bacteria, most commonly *Escherichia coli,* result from the impacted stone. Right upper quadrant pain usually occurs within 15 to 30 minutes after eating. Vomiting does not relieve the pain. The pain is steady and aching in quality and often radiates to the right scapula. Right upper quadrant tenderness on palpation after deep inspiration is called Murphy's sign. The gallbladder is palpable in 30% to 40% of patients. The patients are usually febrile. Jaundice occurs in 20% of patients. Absolute neutrophilic leukocytosis with a shift to the left is usually present. A HIDA nuclear scan (i.e., a nuclear scan following an intravenous injection of iminodiacetic acid) is the study of choice to identify the stone in the cystic duct. Assuming that the patient is in otherwise good health, most surgeons recommend surgery within the first 72 hours, in order to reduce overall morbidity. Other surgeons manage the patient expec-

tantly, since the majority of acute attacks (60%) resolve when the stone disengages from the cystic duct.

Chemically induced inflammation of the gallbladder is more commonly associated with chronic, rather than acute, cholecystitis. A stone in the common bile duct most commonly presents with an obstructive jaundice. Biliary dyskinesia presents with right upper quadrant pain in the absence of stones. It results from abnormal motor function of the gallbladder musculature.

126. The answer is B. *(Behavioral science; power of attorney)*
In a durable power of attorney, an individual designates a legal representative to make decisions concerning health care in the event that the individual can no longer do so. In a living will, the patient directs what future health care will be when the patient is no longer competent to determine this care. If a patient is unable to give consent in a critical care situation, family members and providers must determine what the patient would have done if competent.

127. The answer is B. *(Gynecology; menopausal endocrinology)*
Estrogen levels are decreased; therefore, only options B, C, and D are worth considering. Follicle-stimulating hormone (FSH) levels are increased; therefore, option D is rejected. Options B and C are identical except for the direction of gonadotropin-releasing hormone (GnRH). Because menopause is associated with increased GnRH levels, option C is rejected.

128. The answer is B. *(Cardiovascular surgery; dissecting aortic aneurysm)*
The patient has Marfan syndrome complicated by a dissecting aortic aneurysm. In the aorta, cystic medial necrosis (characterized by elastic tissue fragmentation, mucoid degeneration, or both) affects the middle and outer layers of the tunica media. Hypertension is thought to apply shearing force to the intimal surface that results in an intimal tear, usually within 10 cm of the aortic valve. Under arterial pressure, blood dissects through the areas of weakness in the aorta and progresses

superiorly, inferiorly, or in both directions. Eventual sites of egress of the blood include rupture into the pericardial sac (the most common cause of death), mediastinum, or peritoneum, or reentry through another tear to create a "double-barreled" aorta. Patients present with an acute onset of severe retrosternal chest pain that is often described as "tearing." Pain often radiates into the back.

Marfan syndrome is an autosomal dominant disease with a defect in fibrillin in the connective tissue, which weakens collagen. Eunuchoid proportions (i.e., span greater than height), arachnodactyly, lens dislocation, and a predisposition for dissecting aortic aneurysms (the most common cause of death in these patients) round out the clinical picture. Dissecting aortic aneurysms in general are more common in men and occur at a mean age of 60–65 years. Hypertension is the most common predisposing event. Other predisposing causes for dissection include a congenitally malformed bicuspid aortic valve, Ehlers-Danlos syndrome, pregnancy, copper deficiency (cofactor in lysyl oxidase), coarctation of the aorta, and trauma.

Eighty percent of the time, the diagnosis is established by noting an increased aortic diameter on chest x-ray. Retrograde arteriography is considered the gold standard for making the diagnosis. Type A dissections involve the ascending aorta, whereas type B dissections begin below the subclavian artery. Treatment consists of employing immediate hypertensive measures (e.g., nitroprusside) in order to decrease the rate of dissection. This is followed by surgery and insertion of a graft. The overall long-term survival rate is 60%.

Atherosclerosis is the most common cause of abdominal aortic aneurysms. Syphilitic aortitis involves the arch of the aorta. It produces a vasculitis of the vasa vasorum with ischemic damage to the aortic wall resulting in aneurysmal dilatation and leading to aortic regurgitation. Granulomatous inflammation involving the aorta (Takayasu's arteritis) can predispose to a dissection, but this is uncommon.

129. The answer is C. *(Psychiatry; autism)*
The hallmark of autism is a qualitative disturbance in development, as opposed to merely a retardation of development. Although autistic individuals may have normal intelligence, or even areas of giftedness, most have concurrent mental retardation. The prognosis for autism is most severe when associated with mental retardation or failure to speak by age 5.

130. The answer is A. *(Obstetrics; postpartum hemorrhage)*
It usually occurs in the immediate postpartum period but can occur slowly over the first 24 hours. The overdistention of her uterus with a large baby is the most likely cause of her uterine atony. Her parity, length of labor, duration of oxytocin, and age are probably not contributors.

131. The answer is E. *(Psychiatry; psychodynamics)*
Psychodynamic psychotherapy is often effective for patients with the chronic depression seen in dysthymia. The response rate for antidepressants in this disorder is only about 30%. Social phobia, enuresis, and obsessive-compulsive disorder seem to respond best to behavioral therapies and certain psychotropic medications. Schizophrenia usually requires antipsychotic medication and social therapies.

132. The answer is A. *(Gynecology; risks of menopause)*
Osteoporosis, genital atrophy, urinary tract atrophy, depression, and cardiovascular disease are all health hazards to the postmenopausal woman. However, the one that presents the greatest mortality risk is development of osteoporosis, resulting in an increase in hip fractures with subsequent deep vein thrombosis and embolic sequelae.

133. The answer is D. *(General surgery; acute ascending cholangitis)*
The patient has ascending cholangitis, which results from concurrent biliary tract infection and obstruction (e.g., by a stone, stricture, or neoplasm). The classic Charcot triad is colicky right

upper quadrant pain, fever, and jaundice. Laboratory studies reveal an absolute neutrophilic leukocytosis, a direct hyperbilirubinemia, and elevation of alkaline phosphatase and γ-glutamyltransferase, which are increased in obstructive jaundice. Septicemia resulting from *Escherichia coli* is frequently present as infected bile regurgitates into the liver and the liver sinusoids. Ascending cholangitis is the most common cause of liver abscesses, because the infection extends into the portal triads. The initial treatment is with intravenous cefazolin. If the inflammation does not subside, then surgery is indicated to decompress the common bile duct and remove the source of obstruction. The mortality rate approaches 90% in untreated patients.

Acute hepatitis is not associated with colicky pain and has a mixed indirect and direct hyperbilirubinemia. Acute pancreatitis presents with a steady, boring, midepigastric pain, with radiation into the back or periumbilical area. Jaundice is unusual. An amebic liver abscess does not present with colicky pain or jaundice. The organisms drain into the liver via the portal vein from a primary site of infection in the cecum.

134. The answer is B. *(Behavioral science; rape)*
Rape is frequently associated with the use of weapons. About half of all rapists are white, half are black, most are younger than 25 years, and they generally rape women of the same race. The emotional results of rape, the "rape trauma syndrome," often last for 1 year or longer.

135–136. The answers are: 135-B, 136-C. *(Pediatrics; epiglottitis, Haemophilus influenzae type B)*
This child has acute epiglottitis, caused by *Haemophilus influenzae* B. This situation is an emergency, and an airway is the most important part of management. Acute epiglottitis is most common in the 3- to 7-year age-group and presents with sudden onset of high fever, sore throat, drooling, inspiratory stridor, and respiratory distress. A brassy, croupy cough is uncommon. Lateral soft-tissue x-ray of the neck reveals a swollen epiglottis (thumbprint sign), but is not

recommended if airway compromise is imminent. The patient should be escorted to the radiology area by a physician, and equipment to establish an airway should be nearby. A throat swab for culture and Gram's stain often shows *H. influenzae* B, but is not the first step in management. Arterial blood gases should be obtained only after diagnosis and establishment of an airway. In fact, the child should be disturbed as little as possible so as not to precipitate sudden closure of the airway by an inflamed, cherry-red epiglottis. After an airway is established, treatment consists of appropriate antibiotics. The prognosis is good.

Haemophilus influenzae type B is the most common cause of acute epiglottitis. In this situation, the patient develops high serum antibody titers against *H. influenzae* B; however, this is not the case in meningitis, which may also be caused by this pathogen. Group A *Streptococcus, Staphylococcus,* and pneumococcus are less common causes of epiglottitis. Respiratory syncytial virus is a common cause of bronchiolitis, whereas parainfluenza virus is the most common cause of croup.

137–138. The answers are: 137-D, 138-A. *(Laboratory medicine; effect of prevalence on predictive value of a positive test result)*
A laboratory test has inherent operating characteristics that describe how often it is positive in patients who have a disease, which is called the sensitivity of the test ("positivity in disease") and how often it is negative (normal) in people who do not have the disease, which is called the specificity of the test ("negativity in health"). When a test is performed on people with a disease, it can return with a positive or negative test result. A positive test result is called a true-positive (TP), whereas a negative test result is called a false-negative (FN). An FN misclassifies the patient as normal. Similarly, when a test is performed on a normal person, it can return with a negative or positive test result. A negative test result is called true-negative (TN), whereas a positive test result is called a false-positive (FP). An FP misclassifies the person as having disease.

Because the sensitivity of the test is established by performing the test only on patients with known disease, who may have positive (TP) or negative (FN) test results, it is calculated with the following formula:

$$\text{Sensitivity} = \text{TP}/(\text{TP} + \text{FN}) \times 100$$

If a test has 100% sensitivity, there are no FNs. This result means that every person in the known disease population has a positive test. Therefore, if this test is performed on any patient in an office or hospital setting, a negative (normal) test result must be a TN rather than an FN, because there are no FNs using this test. This test then qualifies as useful in screening for disease, because normal test results exclude disease. However, a positive test result may represent a TP or an FP; therefore, another test must be used to decide whether it is a TP or an FP. Note that the formula for sensitivity says nothing about the FP rate, because it deals only with the disease population and not with the normal population.

Because the specificity of a test applies only to normal people, who can have negative (TN) or positive (FP) test results, it is calculated with the following formula:

$$\text{Specificity} = \text{TN}/(\text{TN} + \text{FP}) \times 100$$

A test with 100% specificity has no FPs. This result means that the test is always normal in normal people. Therefore, if this test is used in a clinical setting on a patient, when the test returns positive, it must be a TP. However, a normal test result could represent a TN or an FN, because nothing in the formula relates to findings in the diseased population (e.g., the FN rate). A test with 100% specificity qualifies as being useful to confirm disease, because a positive test result must be a TP and not an FP.

Once the sensitivity and specificity of a test are established, they remain the same because they are established under controlled conditions involving a known disease population and control population. However, when the test is applied in the clinical arena, the prevalence of disease in the general population or hospital setting does affect how the test is interpreted. In a low-prevalence situation, a negative (normal) test is more likely to represent a TN than an FN, whereas a positive test result is more likely to represent an FP than a

TP. In a high-prevalence situation, a positive test result is more likely to represent a TP than an FP, and a negative test result is more likely to be an FN than a TN.

When a test result returns positive, the question to ask is whether it represents a TP or an FP. This response is called the predictive value of a positive test (PV +test) and is calculated as follows: TP/(TP + FP) × 100. Note: If the FP of the test is 0, as in a test with 100% specificity, the PV +test indicating a TP is always 100%. This result underscores why tests with 100% specificity are used to confirm disease. If the test result returns negative, then the question is whether it represents a TN or an FN. This determination is called the predictive value of a negative test (PV −test). It is calculated with the following formula: TN/(TN + FN) × 100. Note: If the FN rate of the test is 0, as in a test with 100% sensitivity, then the PV −test indicating a TN is 100%. This result underscores why tests with 100% sensitivity are used to screen for disease.

The first part of the question is asking for the predictive value of a positive test result when the prevalence of disease in the total population of 200 people studied is 50% (100 people with SLE/200 people total). To simplify the calculation, the information is best placed into the following format.

	+Test result		−Test result	
Patients with SLE	TP	60	FN	40
Control population	FP	20	TN	80
Totals		80		120

The PV +test in this patient is TP/(TP + FP) × 100 = 60/80 × 100 = 75%. In this population of 200 people, when the prevalence of disease is 50%, a positive test result has a 75% chance of being a TP and a 25% chance of being an FP. The sensitivity of the test is 60% [60/(60 + 40) × 100], the specificity is 80% [80/(80 + 20) × 100], and the PV −test is 66% [80/(80 + 40) × 100].

The second part of the question is changing the prevalence of SLE to 10% and asking what percent probability does a positive test result have of indicating that the patient has SLE. First, the prevalence must be converted to the number of diseased and normal people in a population. Using 1000 people as an arbitrary population of people, a prevalence of 10% means that 100 people have SLE and 900 people are normal. Because the sensitivity of test X is 60%, then 60 out of the 100 people in this population will have a TP and 40 an FN test result. Because the specificity of test X is 80%, then 720 of the 900 people will have a TN and 180 an FP test result.

	+Test result		−Test result	
Patients with SLE	TP	60	FN	40
Normal population	FP	180	TN	720
Totals		240		760

The PV +test result is 25% [60/(60 + 180) × 100]. Note: The PV +test result changed between the two questions. When prevalence is 50%, the PV +test result is 75%; but when the prevalence is only 10%, it drops to 25%. The PV −test result changes in a similar manner. When prevalence is 50%, the PV −test is 66%; but when it drops to 10%, the PV −test result is 95% [720/(720 + 40) × 100].

In summary, these two questions demonstrate that the PV +test result is highest when the prevalence of disease is highest, because TPs outnumber FPs; and the PV −test result is highest when the prevalence of disease is lowest, because TNs outnumber FNs.

139–140. The answers are: 139-B, 140-C. *(Psychiatry; personality disorder)*
Passive–aggressiveness is described as covert aggression expressed through passivity, masochism, and self-defeating behavior. Such an individual often is angry—and often angers others. The usual result is further deterioration of the interaction, with even greater anger and passive–aggressiveness.

The most effective way to deal with covert communication is to bring it into the open and deal with it. This technique is called "identifying the process." Threats and expressions of anger or hurt are generally not useful. Since personality traits are generally stable in various environments, it is unlikely that a different clinician

would be spared this patient's passive–aggressiveness.

141. The answer is D. *(Gynecology; endometrial cancer)*
Endometrial cancer is staged by the thickness of myometrial invasion after hysterectomy. The other malignancies listed are staged clinically before surgery.

142. The answer is C. *(General surgery; acute pancreatitis)*
The patient has acute pancreatitis. Approximately 70% of cases are related to alcohol abuse or biliary tract disease. Other etiologies include metabolic conditions (hypertriglyceridemia, uremia, and hypercalcemia), drugs (azathioprine, sulfasalazine, corticosteroids, thiazides, L-asparaginase, sulfonamides, and estrogen preparations), a penetrating posterior duodenal ulcer, and infection (usually viral—e.g., coxsackie, mumps).

Patients present with an acute onset of midepigastric pain that is described as steady and boring. The pain radiates into the back or periumbilical area. Leaning forward often relieves the pain, whereas vomiting aggravates it. Physical examination reveals abdominal tenderness without guarding or rebound. Diminished bowel sounds result from a localized ileus, which corresponds with a dilated sentinel loop on x-ray. Low-grade fever is present in 70% to 85% of patients. Shock resulting from loss of isotonic fluid from the peripancreatic third space is present in 20% to 40% of patients. Turner's sign (purplish discoloration of the flank) and Cullen's sign (purplish discoloration around the umbilicus) indicate a hemorrhagic pancreatitis. A left-sided pleural effusion rich in amylase is noted in 10% of patients.

The serum amylase is elevated in 95% of acute attacks during the first 12 to 24 hours. It increases within 2 to 6 hours after the onset of pain, peaks within 12 to 30 hours, and declines after 2 to 4 days as the glomerular filtration rate increases and clears the enzyme. A urine amylase is most useful when the serum amylase is normal after 2 to 4 days, because it remains elevated for 7 to 10 days after the onset of pain. Serum lipase is slightly more sensitive and specific than amylase. Ultrasound is also an excellent screen for pancreatitis. Stippled calcification in the pancreas results from enzymatic fat necrosis. Abdominal x-ray reveals a localized ileus (sentinel loop) in the small bowel next to the pancreas. Upper gastrointestinal series, HIDA nuclear scans, oral cholecystogram, and endoscopy are not usually part of the workup of acute pancreatitis.

143. The answer is A. *(Biostatistics; cohort study)*
The use of the words random and prospective alone are not an indication of the study design. A study group for any research design can be selected at random from a population, but that practice does not make the study a randomized controlled trial. Such a trial requires selecting the study and control groups at random. Because the random sample in this question became a cohort that was followed over a period of time, the design is a cohort study.

144. The answer is E. *(Psychiatry; separation anxiety)*
Separation anxiety disorder is characterized by worry about being separated from caregivers, severe protest on impending separation, or severe anxiety after separation. Such worry often takes the form of fantasies about how the separation will occur. Homesickness is another form of this disorder.

145. The answer is A. *(Gynecology; endometrial cancer)*
The best prognosis is associated with the straightforward secretory type of endometrial carcinoma, which implies a low-grade type of carcinoma. Grade III, adenosquamous, clear cell, and papillary serous carcinomas have a worse outcome by comparison.

146. The answer is E. *(General medicine; bronchogenic carcinoma)*
Patients with a smoking history, weight loss, clubbing of the fingers, hemoptysis, and hilar adenopathy are strongly suspect for a primary bronchogenic carcinoma, particularly squamous

cell carcinoma and small cell carcinoma (oat cell carcinoma). Cough is the most common presenting symptom of lung cancer (75%), followed by weight loss (40%) and hemoptysis (25%–30%).

The physical findings indicate chronic obstructive lung disease. The bronchitic component consists of productive cough, rhonchi, wheezes, and dilated tubular shadows representing thickened bronchial walls. The emphysematous component is represented by an increased anteroposterior diameter, distant heart sounds, and flattened diaphragms.

Cytology is the gold standard test for bronchogenic carcinoma and has its highest diagnostic yield in centrally located cancers such as squamous and small cell carcinoma. The sputum cytology using the Papanicolaou stain reports eosinophilic staining cells with irregular nuclei. Because keratin stains bright red with this stain, the patient most likely has a primary squamous cell carcinoma. Small cell carcinomas have small, lymphocyte-sized, basophilic staining cells in cytology smears.

Tuberculosis, bronchiectasis, and pulmonary embolism can all be associated with hemoptysis but would have a different clinical presentation and absence of neoplastic cells in sputum.

147. The answer is E. *(Gynecology; ovarian cancer)*
Ovarian carcinoma is the only gynecologic malignancy that has subcategories a, b, and c for stages I through III.

148. The answer is E. *(Psychiatry; personality disorder)*
A neglect of the basic rights of others is most characteristic of antisocial personality disorder. A history of earlier abuse during childhood, and other childhood psychopathology, is often found in patients with several types of adult psychopathology. A belief in violence does not necessarily indicate antisocial personality disorder. Dismissal of most people and idealization of a few famous figures are characteristic of narcissistic personality disorder.

149. The answer is B. *(General surgery; pancreatic pseudocyst)*
The patient has a pancreatic pseudocyst, which is a cystic collection of tissue, fluid, and necrotic debris surrounding the pancreas. Pancreatic pseudocysts do not have a true epithelial lining and are most commonly associated with chronic pancreatitis, but may also be seen in acute pancreatitis. They present as an abdominal mass with a persistent hyperamylasemia, because enzyme-rich fluids continue to leak into the circulation. Ultrasound is the best test to identify pseudocysts. If the pseudocyst persists beyond 4 to 6 weeks or continues to enlarge, surgical decompression is indicated. The cyst fluid is drained into the stomach or bowel (not to the skin surface).

Pancreatic cystadenomas are rare and are not related to chronic pancreatitis. Pancreatic carcinoma can be associated with chronic pancreatitis, but rarely presents as a palpable mass with persistent hyperamylasemia. Pancreatic abscesses are a feature of acute pancreatitis.

150. The answer is E. *(Geriatric medicine; normal laboratory values)*
In elderly men, the gonadotropins are increased because of decreased production of testosterone by Leydig cells [i.e., luteinizing hormone (LH) is increased] and decreased production of inhibin from Sertoli cells in the seminiferous tubules [i.e., follicle-stimulating hormone (FSH) is increased]. Hemoglobin drops into adult female ranges, because the testosterone level is decreased, and testosterone normally stimulates erythropoiesis. The arterial oxygen partial pressure (PaO_2) normally decreases as ventilation and perfusion become less evenly matched in the lungs. Albumin decreases because of increased protein catabolism and decreased liver synthesis of albumin. The level of alkaline phosphatase increases because of degenerative bone disease (e.g., osteoarthritis) and reactive bone formation.

151. The answer is B. *(Pediatrics; vitamin-D–resistant rickets)*
Vitamin-D–resistant rickets (familial, X-linked hypophosphatemia) is the most common form of rickets. It is X-linked dominant, so some mothers may have clinical manifestations of the disease. Defects in the proximal renal tubular reabsorption of phosphate account for the hypophosphatemia. Bowing of the legs is a common presentation. Calcium levels in blood are normal. Treatment consists of phosphate supplementation.

152. The answer is B. *(Psychiatry; anxiety)*
Phobia is characterized by fear of an object or situation, efforts to avoid it, and a feeling that the fear is irrational. The object or degree of danger is not relevant to a diagnosis of phobia. It is difficult to determine that a particular fear has no symbolism.

153. The answer is B. *(Gynecology; DES exposure in utero)*
Koilocytic cervical dysplasia has not been linked to prenatal diethylstilbestrol (DES) exposure. Although colposcopically the immature metaplastic squamous epithelium of the cervix resembles dysplasia with a mosaic and punctate appearance, histologically this epithelium is benign. Numerous nonneoplastic uterine and vaginal anomalies have been reported in young women exposed in utero to DES. Spontaneous abortion and clear cell vaginal adenocarcinoma are associated with DES exposure as well.

154. The answer is D. *(Pediatrics; child abuse)*
Bruised knees are commonly seen in children of this age and are not specific evidence of child abuse. Specific evidence of child abuse includes old healed fractures, belt marks, bruises on the buttocks or lower back (areas where the child is unlikely to harm himself), subdural hematomas, and rupture of internal organs. Evidence of sexual abuse includes genital or anal trauma, sexually transmitted diseases, and urinary tract infection.

155. The answer is D. *(Gynecology; menopause)*
Although metromenorrhagia may precede menopause, it is absent when menopause is present. Menopause is characterized by depletion of ovarian follicles and the decreasing estrogen levels

that result. Elevated gonadotropins, hot flashes, night sweats, and decreased vaginal secretions are a consequence of estrogen deficiency and are present with menopause.

156. The answer is A. *(Psychiatry; psychosis)*
Schizoid personality disorder, by definition, has no associated peculiarities of thought. It is characterized by a detachment from social relationships and a restricted emotional life. Major depression, cocaine delirium, bipolar disorder (manic), and Alzheimer's dementia can all present with psychosis.

157. The answer is C. *(Laboratory medicine; laboratory differences between men and women)*
Adult males and females have slightly different normal values in certain laboratory parameters. The level of serum creatinine, a metabolic product of creatine in muscle, parallels the muscle mass of an individual. Because women have less muscle mass than men, their serum creatinine level is slightly lower. The hemoglobin in women is 1 to 2 g/dl lower than that in men, because women lose blood on a monthly basis and also have lower testosterone levels than men. Testosterone stimulates erythropoiesis in the bone marrow. Iron stores are decreased in women because of the menstrual cycle and pregnancy. Estradiol is the main female hormone, which is analogous to testosterone in men.

158. The answer is D. *(Pediatrics; genetic disease)*
The urinary abnormality in maple syrup urine disease is the presence of high concentrations of branched-chain amino acids—leucine, isoleucine, and valine. The addition of 2,4-DNPH will cause their ketoacids to precipitate. The urine, skin, or hair has a characteristic smell of maple syrup or caramel. Infants present with symptoms 3 to 5 days after birth, with feeding difficulties, hypoglycemia, seizures, opisthotonos, and muscular rigidity with or without intermittent flaccidity. Cortical atrophy is seen on computed tomography (CT) or magnetic resonance imaging (MRI) scan. Dietary management of intake of branched-chain amino acids is the cornerstone of

therapy. However, most patients have already suffered permanent brain damage by the time diagnosis is made and treatment initiated.

159. The answer is A. *(Psychiatry; psychopharmacology, lithium)*
Lithium has no demonstrated hepatotoxicity but tremor, hypothyroidism, polyuria, and leukocytosis are common complications of lithium therapy. These untoward effects necessitate monitoring. A complete blood count (CBC) should be taken, and renal function, thyroid function, and electrolyte balance should be monitored. A baseline electrocardiogram (ECG) is also indicated because of lithium's nonspecific effect on tracings.

160. The answer is C. *(Gynecology; endometrial cancer)*
Late, rather than early, menopause is a risk factor for endometrial cancer. Obesity, diabetes mellitus, a history of breast cancer, and unopposed estrogen are also predisposing factors. Cancer of the endometrium is the most common gynecologic malignancy in the United States, being twice as common as carcinoma of the cervix.

161. The answer is D. *(Pediatrics; neonatal meningitis)*
Nuchal rigidity is not as common as a full or bulging fontanelle in neonatal meningitis. Clinical manifestations of meningitis in infants are usually nonspecific. Lethargy, jaundice, and feeding difficulties are common presenting signs. Fever may or may not be present, and sometimes hypothermia or temperature instability is the only sign. Grunting and respiratory distress are frequently seen.

162. The answer is B. *(Behavioral science; homosexuality)*
Transsexual individuals seek sex-change surgery. Homosexual (lesbian) individuals, like this patient, are content with their biologic sex. There is some evidence for a genetic and prenatal hormonal basis for homosexuality; but in adulthood, homosexual individuals have normal sex hormone levels. Homosexual individuals often have

experienced heterosexual sex and many have had children.

163. The answer is E. *(Gastroenterology; diseases presenting with obstruction)*
Bowel obstruction presents with nausea and vomiting, obstipation (absence of bowel movements), and physical findings of abdominal distention, visible peristalsis (late finding), and diffuse pain without rebound tenderness. Abdominal x-rays frequently show dilated loops of bowel with air–fluid levels in a stepladder pattern. In some patients, the cause of the obstruction is obvious on physical examination. For example, strangulated bowel can be present in the scrotal sac of an indirect hernia. In other patients, a previous history of abdominal surgery suggests the presence of adhesions, which are the most common cause of bowel obstruction.

Angiodysplasia is not associated with bowel obstruction. It is an acquired disease of the elderly characterized by the presence of dilated submucosal vessels that open into the bowel lumen, most commonly the cecum and right colon. Both angiodysplasia and diverticulosis are common causes of massive lower gastrointestinal bleeds in the elderly. Mesenteric angiography is the most sensitive diagnostic test to locate the abnormal vessels for diagnosis and surgical treatment. On occasion, they can be seen on colonoscopy. There is an unexplained association between aortic stenosis and von Willebrand's disease.

Carcinoid tumors are neuroendocrine tumors of neural crest origin that contain neurosecretory granules. All carcinoid tumors, regardless of location, are potentially malignant. The size of the tumor is most closely related to its ability to metastasize. Approximately 80% of tumors over 2 cm have already metastasized, whereas those less than 2 cm rarely metastasize. Although the tip of the appendix is the most common site for these tumors (40%), their small size keeps them confined to the appendix. However, those tumors that are located in the small bowel (25%) tend to be over 2 cm and behave in a more malignant fashion. The tumors produce serotonin, which has the ability to stimulate fibrogenesis, thus causing kinking of the small bowel and obstruc-

tion. The serotonin produced by the tumor is drained via the portal vein to the liver, where it is metabolized to 5-hydroxyindoleacetic acid (5-HIAA). However, if the tumor metastasizes to the liver, the serotonin and other secretion products such as bradykinin empty into the hepatic vein, producing systemic signs of the carcinoid syndrome, particularly flushing and diarrhea.

Intussusception refers to the telescoping of one segment of proximal bowel into the distal bowel. It is predominantly seen in children between 3 months and 3 years of age, but is also seen in adults. In children, there is a positive correlation of adenovirus infections and hyperplasia of Peyer's patches in the terminal ileum, which serves as a nidus for intussusception. The leading edge of a peristaltic wave coming down the terminal ileum hits the elevated mound of tissue, causing the terminal ileum to evert into the secum. This eversion produces a sudden onset of colicky pain in the abdomen, abdominal distention resulting from obstruction, and "currant-jelly" stools resulting from ischemic damage to the bowel mucosa. Frequently, intussusceptions spontaneously reduce or can be reduced by a gentle barium enema. In adults, intussusceptions more commonly occur in the large bowel, where polyps or cancer commonly serve as the nidus for intussusception.

Volvulus refers to twisting of bowel around the mesenteric root. It is most commonly seen in the elderly population. The sigmoid colon (65%) is the most common site, followed by the cecum. Volvulus produces a combination of obstruction and bleeding in association with infarction of bowel.

Hirschsprung's disease (congenital megacolon) refers to bowel obstruction secondary to the absence of ganglion cells in Meissner's submucosal plexus and Auerbach's myenteric plexus. It is most commonly localized in the rectum (90%). Symptoms almost always occur shortly after birth, when the newborn is unable to pass meconium. The peristaltic wave cannot pass beyond the area involved, so the fecal material remains stationary at that point, resulting in obstruction associated with proximal dilatation of the bowel. An important physical finding is the absence of stool in the rectal vault on rectal examination. There is an association of Hirschsprung's disease with Down syndrome and Chagas' disease. The diagnosis of Hirschsprung's disease is made by biopsy of the rectum and notation of the absence of ganglion cells. Enterocolitis is the most common cause of death.

164. The answer is E. *(Gynecology; breast cancer)*
A history of oral contraceptive use is not associated with breast cancer; however, a history of endometrial carcinoma, a low-fiber diet, a first-degree relative with breast cancer, and a previous history of contralateral breast cancer are all risk factors. Breast cancer is the second most common female malignancy, lung cancer being first.

165. The answer is B. *(Psychiatry; developmental disorder)*
Patients with behavioral disturbances and learning difficulties have not shown improvement by avoiding foods that provoke allergies. Lead poisoning, impaired hearing, family stress, and IQ have all been clearly associated with behavioral disturbances. Thus, early detection of these four problems is important in minimizing morbidity.

166. The answer is D. *(Pediatrics; heroin addiction in newborns)*
Generalized hypotonia is not a sign of heroin addiction in the newborn. Approximately 50% of heroin-addicted newborns are low–birth-weight infants. Heroin addicts also experience a higher incidence of premature births and stillbirths. Withdrawal occurs in 50% to 75% of infants, usually within 48 hours of birth. Symptoms include jitters and tremors, hyperirritability, high-pitched and excessive crying, and restlessness. Low–birth-weight heroin-addicted infants show a lower incidence of respiratory distress syndrome and jaundice.

167. The answer is B. *(Behavioral science; diabetes and sexual problems)*
One-fourth to one-half of diabetic men suffer from erectile dysfunction; orgasm and ejaculation are less likely to be affected than erection.

Microscopic nerve damage and vascular changes as well as psychological factors influence the erectile problems associated with diabetes. Poor metabolic control of diabetes is associated with increased incidence of sexual problems.

168. The answer is D. *(Rheumatology; polyarthritis)*
Gout most commonly presents with involvement of a single joint, usually the first metatarsophalangeal joint (75%). Its onset is described as explosive and often occurs at night. Inflammation in the joint is secondary to the deposition of needle-shaped, monosodium urate crystals in the synovial fluid. The negative charge of the monosodium urate crystals adsorbs immunoglobulin G (IgG) onto their surface. Neutrophils and mononuclear phagocytes with Fc receptors for IgG phagocytose the crystals causing the release of lysosomal enzymes and free radicals into the joint space, where they initiate an inflammatory reaction in the synovial tissue. Diffuse periarticular inflammation is so intense that it is often confused with a cellulitis.

Polyarthritis is one of the Jones' criteria for the diagnosis of acute rheumatic fever. It is also the most common presenting symptom (75%). The knees and wrists are the most commonly affected joints.

Wilson's disease is an autosomal recessive disease characterized by impaired biliary excretion of copper. The accumulation of copper in the hepatocytes produces an aggressive chronic hepatitis, which often progresses into cirrhosis. Chronic liver disease, in turn, results in a decreased synthesis of ceruloplasmin, which is the carrier protein for copper in the blood. This change in synthesis lowers the total copper level, because ceruloplasmin is decreased. However, the free-copper level in the blood is increased. The excess copper is deposited in many different tissues. Deposition in the lenticular nuclei of the brain produces resting and intention tremors. Excess copper in Descemet's membrane in the cornea results in the classic Kayser-Fleischer ring. Accumulation of copper in the renal tubules is associated with renal tubular acidosis. Deposition in the joints produces a degenerative arthritis. The spine and large joints such as the knees, wrists, and hips are most commonly involved.

Whipple's disease is a multi-organ systemic disease caused by a bacillus, which has been identified as a gram-positive actinomycete called *Tropheryma whippeli*. It is most commonly seen in white middle-aged men. Whipple's disease presents with emaciation, polyarthritis (75%), fever, lymphadenopathy, a peculiar gray–brown pigmentation of skin due to excess melanin deposition, and malabsorption. The latter complication is secondary to the accumulation of macrophages in the lamina propria of the villi in the small intestine. The macrophages contain periodic acid-Schiff–positive inclusions, which, on electron microscopy, represent the bacteria. These same inclusions are noted in synovial tissue and host the inflammatory response associated with polyarthritis. The disease responds to the trimethoprim–sulfamethoxazole combination or procaine penicillin.

The polyarticular variant accounts for 40% of cases of juvenile rheumatoid arthritis. Girls are more frequently affected than boys. It presents with low-grade fever, growth retardation, generalized lymphadenopathy, vasculitis, anemia, and arthritis. The primary joints involved are the cervical spine, wrists, knees, and ankles. Patients who are positive for rheumatoid factor (15%) have a worse prognosis, with more disabling arthritis, more vasculitis, and more rheumatoid nodules than seronegative patients.

169. The answer is D. (*Gynecology; menopause management*)
Active liver diseases such as hepatitis may be exacerbated by estrogen supplementation. Cystocele, urethritis, and osteoporosis may be improved by estrogen therapy.

170. The answer is C. (*Gynecology; menopause*)
Libido is not related to ovarian estrogen production, and sexual interest is unchanged after menopause. The loss of ovarian estrogen production that occurs with menopause results in hot flashes and reduced vaginal lubrication and thinning of the vaginal mucosa, which may lead to painful intercourse. These symptoms can be reversed with estrogen replacement therapy.

171. The answer is C. (*Clinical endocrinology; acromegaly*)
The patient has acromegaly secondary to a benign pituitary adenoma with excess secretion of growth hormone (GH) and somatomedins from the liver. If the condition occurs prior to fusion of the epiphyses, gigantism occurs.

Clinical findings of acromegaly include:

- Generalized enlargement of bone, cartilage, and soft tissue, resulting in large hands and feet, frontal bossing, a prominent jaw, an increase in hat size, spaces between the teeth, and hypertrophy of the left ventricle
- Cardiomyopathy with congestive heart failure (the most common cause of death)
- Diastolic hypertension
- Muscle weakness
- Peripheral neuropathies
- Diabetes mellitus from the gluconeogenic properties of GH
- Headaches and visual field defects from encroachment on the optic chiasm
- Hypopituitarism due to the expanding adenoma
- Degenerative arthritis

The laboratory findings include:

- Hyperglycemia (40%)
- Inability to suppress glucose with an oral glucose tolerance test
- A paradoxical increase in GH with thyrotropin-releasing hormone (TRH)
- No stimulation of GH release with L-dopa (normal people have an increase in GH)
- Increased serum phosphate associated with growth spurts
- Enlargement of the sella turcica in more than 90% of patients

Treatment consists of transsphenoidal surgery or the use of a somatostatin analogue called octreotide, which produces clinical improvement in 70% of cases.

172. The answer is B. *(Behavioral science; sexual dysfunction)*
Primary erectile dysfunction, in which a man has never been able to sustain an erection sufficient for penetration of the vagina, occurs in only 1% of men. Secondary erectile dysfunction occurs in 10% to 20% of men. Premature ejaculation is most common, comprising up to 35% of male sexual disorders. Delayed or absent orgasm and ejaculation occur in approximately 5% of men.

173–174. The answers are: 173-B, 174-A. *(Pediatrics; Friedreich's ataxia)*
Mental retardation is not associated with Friedreich's ataxia. Friedreich's ataxia can be autosomal recessive or dominant. Skeletal abnormalities include kyphoscoliosis, hammer toes, and high-arched feet (pes cavus). Ataxia occurs before 10 years of age and is slowly progressive. The lower extremities are more affected and the Romberg test is positive. Deep tendon reflexes are lost. Speech is explosive and dysarthric. Nystagmus is present. Most patients die from congestive heart failure secondary to hypertrophic cardiomyopathy.

175. The answer is A. *(Behavioral science; sexual activity in the elderly)*
People continue to have sexual interest into old age. However, reduced intensity of ejaculation, slower erection, a longer refractory period, illness, and lack of a partner due to death all contribute to decreased sexual activity in the elderly.

176. The answer is A. *(Clinical endocrinology; Graves' disease)*
A patient with exophthalmos and lid retraction has Graves' disease, which is the most common cause of hyperthyroidism. It is a female-dominant autoimmune disease with a characteristic triad of exophthalmos, a diffuse goiter, and hyperthyroidism. Other features that are unique to Graves' disease are pretibial myxedema (nonpitting) and immunoglobulin G (IgG) thyroid-stimulating autoantibodies against the thyroid-stimulating hormone (TSH) receptor that continually stimulate the gland without any negative feedback. Nodular toxic goiters produce hyperthyroidism but do not have the features unique to Graves' disease.

The treatment of Graves' disease is varied. Antithyroid medications, for example, methimazole and propylthiouracil, are used to block hormone synthesis, but there are problems with skin rashes, agranulocytosis, and recurrent disease. Radioactive iodine (^{131}I) is used to ablate the gland and is the treatment of choice for patients over 25 years of age. A subtotal thyroidectomy has a high success rate, but there is a risk for hypoparathyroidism. Beta blocking agents are useful for blocking adrenergic symptoms associated with the disease.

177. The answer is A. *(Pediatrics; twin-to-twin transfusion syndrome)*
Fetal transfusion syndrome, or twin-to-twin transfusion, occurs when an artery from one twin delivers blood to the vein of the other. Such placental vascular anastomoses occur with high frequency only in monochorionic twins. Because the recipient twin receives much more blood and becomes plethoric, that twin is therefore at higher risk than the donor twin for hyperbilirubinemia. Owing to the increased volume, the recipient twin also can develop heart failure. The donor twin, who has lost blood, is anemic and small. A difference of 20% in body weight and 15% hematocrit (5% hemoglobin) establishes the diagnosis. Maternal polyhydramnios in a twin pregnancy should arouse suspicion.

178. The answer is E. *(General medicine; obstructive sleep apnea)*
Obstructive sleep apnea is characterized by shallow, rapid respirations. Hypoxemia results, and respiratory acidosis can be expected. The chronic hypoxia can lead to failure to thrive and pulmonary hypertension with right ventricular hypertrophy. If upper airway obstruction is the cause, such as in hypertrophied tonsils and adenoids, mouth-breathing, snoring, and dental malocclusion can be described. Pectus excavatum is associated with upper airway obstruction.

179. The answer is D. *(Pediatrics; cyanotic congenital heart disease)*
Hemoglobin F is gradually replaced by adult hemoglobin regardless of whether congenital heart disease is present. In cyanotic disease, persistent hypoxia results in stimulation of erythrocyte production and a secondary polycythemia. Extreme polcythemia can cause cerebral thrombosis, usually in the cerebral veins. Brain abscess is less common than thrombosis and usually occurs in patients older than 2 years. A patent ductus arteriosus, although not a cyanotic lesion, can occur in association with cyanotic heart disease because the chronic hypoxia prevents closure of the ductus.

180. The answer is C. *(Pediatrics; caput succedaneum)*
Caput succedaneum is a diffuse swelling of the soft tissues of the scalp. It extends across suture lines, and the edema starts to resolve over the first few days. Underlying skull fractures, not seen in caput succedaneum, are occasionally associated with cephalhematomas. These hemorrhages are subperiosteal; therefore, they are limited to one bone and do not cross suture lines. Cephalhematomas tend to increase in size over the first few days and resorb in approximately 3 months.

181. The answer is B. *(Pulmonary medicine; pulmonary function studies in restrictive and obstructive lung disease)*
Pulmonary function studies are very important in differentiating restrictive from obstructive lung diseases. Restrictive diseases, such as sarcoidosis, have decreased compliance of the lungs (i.e., difficulty in expanding the alveoli) owing to interstitial fibrosis, but increased elasticity (good recoil once they are expanded). Obstructive diseases, such as emphysema, have increased compliance (ease in expanding the alveoli), but decreased elasticity (poor recoil), owing to destruction of elastic tissue in the supporting structures. Therefore, on expiration, air becomes trapped in the lungs behind the collapsed distal airways that lack elastic tissue support.

Spirometry is used to determine volumes (e.g., tidal volume) and capacities [two or more volumes, e.g., total lung capacity (TLC)] in the lung as well as measurements of flow rate of air out of the lungs [e.g., forced expiratory volume in 1 second (FEV_1)]. In restrictive lung disease, the poor compliance affects all volumes and capacities equally, so they are all decreased. In obstructive lung disease, the inability to eliminate all of the air on expiration increases the residual volume (RV, i.e., the air left in the lung after maximal expiration), which ultimately increases the TLC (sum of all the lung volumes) and expands the chest cavity to produce an increased anteroposterior diameter (barrel chest) and flattened diaphragms. Limited expansion of the rigid chest wall accompanied by an ever-expanding RV eventually decreases the other lung volumes and capacities such as tidal volume (i.e., the volume of air entering or leaving the lungs in quiet inspiration or expiration, respectively) and vital capacity (i.e., the maximal amount of air exhaled from the lungs after full inspiration).

Regarding flow studies, an FEV_1 refers to the amount of air that is forcibly expelled in 1 second after maximal inspiration. Normally, a person expels 4 liters of air in 1 second. The forced vital capacity (FVC) is the total amount of air expelled after maximal inspiration. Normally, the FVC is 5 liters. When expressed as a ratio, FEV_1/FVC is 80% (4 liters/5 liters). In both restrictive and obstructive lung disease, the FEV_1 is decreased; however, the magnitude of the decrease is less in restrictive (e.g., 3 liters) than in obstructive (e.g., 2 liters) lung disease, owing to the greater problem in expelling air in the latter disease. In restrictive lung disease, the FEV_1 and the FVC are almost identical, because of the increased elasticity in the lungs, which quickly expresses air out of the lung in 1 second. Therefore, the FEV_1/FVC ratio is increased (e.g., 3 liters/3 liters = 100%). In obstructive lung disease, however, the FVC is usually 3 liters or less, so the ratio of FEV_1/FVC is usually decreased (e.g., 2 liters/3 liters = 66%). The $Paco_2$ is usually increased in obstructive lung disease (respiratory acidosis), because CO_2 remains behind in the lung on expiration. In restrictive disease, the $Paco_2$ is either normal or decreased, since the patient must breathe more frequently for adequate ventilation of lungs that do not expand well on inspiration.

Comparison Between Restrictive and Obstructive Lung Disease

Parameter	Obstructive	Restrictive
TLC	Increased	Decreased
RV	Increased	Decreased
Tidal volume	Decreased	Decreased
Vital capacity	Decreased	Decreased
FEV_1	Decreased (++)	Decreased (+)
FVC	Decreased (+++)	Decreased (+)
FEV_1/FVC	Decreased	Increased
$Paco_2$	Increased	Normal to decreased

Number of + signs indicates magnitude of change.

FEV_1 = forced expiratory volume in 1 second; FVC = forced vital capacity; $Paco_2$ = arterial CO_2 tension; RV = residual volume; TLC = total lung capacity.

182. The answer is D. *(Pediatrics; respiratory distress syndrome)*
Pulmonary infarction is not associated with respiratory distress in the newborn. Respiratory distress syndrome in newborns results from a deficiency in lung surfactant, and its complications are many. Delayed closure of the ductus arteriosus most likely occurs secondary to the hypoxia, acidosis, local release of prostaglandins, and other complications associated with respiratory distress syndrome in newborns. Respiratory distress syndrome also predisposes infants to intraventricular hemorrhage. Necrotizing enterocolitis is often seen, probably related to gut ischemia. Bronchopulmonary dysplasia is a common complication of respiratory distress syndrome. Barotrauma from the ventilator and oxygen toxicity have both been implicated.

183. The answer is E. *(Pediatrics; tumors in children)*
Chondrosarcoma is rare in children. It occurs most commonly in the pelvis. Metastasis is usually by local extension. Osteosarcoma is the most common malignant bone tumor of children. Ewing's sarcoma most commonly presents during the teen years. Astrocytoma is the most common brain tumor in children. Rhabdomyosarcoma has two age peaks— before 5 years of age and at 15 to 19 years. Embryonal rhabdomyosarcomas account for 60% of all rhabdomyosarcomas.

184–186. The answers are: 184-M, 185-L, 186-E. *(Pharmacology; anesthesia and analgesia)*
Nalbuphine, a drug used parenterally, is classified as a mixed agonist–antagonist opioid analgesic. Although its analgesic actions are mainly exerted at the spinal level, the drug has high efficacy. Nalbuphine does not activate μ receptors, which may explain its reduced tendency to depress respiratory function or to cause dependence with chronic use when compared with morphine. However, if respiratory failure does occur in overdose, it is not always readily reversed with naloxone, a μ-receptor antagonist.

Flumazenil is a benzodiazepine receptor antagonist with clinical application to reversing the central nervous system (CNS) actions of such drugs when overdose occurs or when they have been used in anesthesia combinations (e.g., diazepam, midazolam). Although benzodiazepines have a flatter dose/response curve than barbiturates in terms of CNS depressant actions, at high doses they depress both respiratory and cardiac functions. Intravenous (IV) flumazenil is an effective antagonist, but has a short half-life so that relapse may occur in benzodiazepine overdose. Flumazenil will not reverse CNS depressant actions of other drugs such as ethanol, barbiturates, or opioids.

Ketamine is a structural congener of the psychoactive drug phencyclidine (PCP). IV administration produces "dissociative anesthesia," characterized by catatonia, amnesia, and short-term analgesia. Unlike most other anesthetics, ketamine is a cardiovascular stimulant. Although postoperative emergence reactions can be reduced by preoperative diazepam, in the United States, ketamine is mainly used in outpatient anesthesia and for short painful procedures (e.g., changing burn dressings in children).

187–189. The answers are: 187-D, 188-A, 189-C. (*Endocrinology; adjusting NPH and regular insulin in patients on a split-dose mixed-insulin program*)
Most insulin-dependent type I diabetics are best managed on a split-dose mixed-insulin regimen using NPH and regular insulin. The total dose of insulin is calculated with the following formula—0.7 units/kg body weight. Two-thirds of this dose is given in the A.M. and one-third in the P.M. Two-thirds of the A.M. dose is NPH and one-third is regular insulin, and the P.M. dose is divided into one-half to two-thirds NPH and one-third to one-half regular insulin. Insulin is given 30 minutes before breakfast and dinner. The following example is a calculation for a 68-kg insulin-dependent diabetic:

Total dose = 68 kg × 0.7 unit/kg = 48 units/day

A.M. dose = 2/3 × 48 = 32 units:
NPH 2/3 × 32 = 22 units; regular = 10 units

P.M. dose = 1/3 × 48 = 16 units:
NPH 2/3 × 16 = 10 units; regular = 6 units

Interpretation of the blood-sugar values at different time intervals uses the following strategy:

7 A.M. glucose correlates with the P.M. NPH insulin.
12 P.M. glucose correlates with the A.M. regular insulin.
5 P.M. glucose correlates with the A.M. NPH insulin.
9 P.M. glucose correlates with the P.M. regular insulin.

Two- to five-unit increments should be used when changing the doses of insulin.

In patient D, who shows a 12 P.M. glucose of 200 mg/dl, the dose of regular insulin should be increased in the morning.

Patient A, with a 10 P.M. glucose of 90 mg/dl, a 3 A.M. glucose of 40 mg/dl, and a 7 A.M. glucose of 200 mg/dl has the Somogyi effect. The nocturnal hypoglycemia at 3 A.M. is a reactive hypoglycemia precipitated by too much NPH at dinnertime. The treatment is to decrease the NPH dose at dinnertime, give a portion of it at bedtime, or give more food at bedtime.

Patient C, with a 10 P.M. glucose of 110 mg/dl, a 3 A.M. glucose of 160 mg/dl, and a 7 A.M. glucose of 220 mg/dl, has the waning effect. This patient does not take enough NPH insulin at dinnertime. The treatment is to increase the NPH at dinnertime or to give the NPH at bedtime.

Patient B, with a 10 P.M. glucose of 110 mg/dl, a 3 A.M. glucose of 110 mg/dl, and a 7 A.M. glucose of 150 mg/dl, has the dawn phenomenon. This phenomenon is secondary to increased growth hormone release between 5 A.M. and 8 A.M. Growth hormone antagonizes insulin, therefore causing the early A.M. hyperglycemia. The treatment is to divide the NPH dose between dinner and bedtime.

Patient E, with a 5 P.M. glucose of 220 mg/dl, requires an increase in the A.M. dose of NPH.

Patient F, with a 9 P.M. glucose of 200 mg/dl, requires an increase in regular insulin at dinnertime.

190–192. The answers are: 190-K, 191-I, 192-B. (*Pharmacology; cardiac drugs*)
The nonselective β-adrenoceptor blocker propranolol is the standard against which other β blockers are compared. Its additional clinical uses include treatment of both cardiac arrhythmias and certain neurologic and psychiatric disorders. Predictable consequences of β blockade include worsening of asthma and other obstructive pulmonary disease and exacerbation of hypoglycemia in insulin-dependent diabetic patients. β blockers may also mask signs of developing hyperthyroidism.

Only two catecholamines are listed: epinephrine and dobutamine. Epinephrine is naturally occurring and activates both α and β₂ adrenoceptors in addition to its direct actions on the heart (β₁). Because dobutamine is less effective in activating vasodilator β₂ receptors, less reflex tachycardia occurs than with nonselective β activators such as isoproterenol (not listed). Although tolerance with chronic use is a problem with any sympathomimetic drug, dobutamine appears to be useful on an acute basis in some patients with congestive heart failure or cardiogenic shock.

Thiazide diuretics are related chemically to sulfonamides, but so is the loop diuretic furosemide (not ethacrynic acid). Thiazides inhibit the NaCl cotransporter in the distal tubule and also cause peripheral vasodilation, which contributes to their antihypertensive actions. Furosemide and other loop diuretics are used in volume overload states including refractory edemas, in renal failure to eliminate a pigment load, and in hypercalcemic states (thiazides decrease calcium excretion). Adverse effects of loop diuretics include predictable hypokalemic metabolic alkalosis and dose-related ototoxicity.

193–194. The answers are: 193-C, 194-A.
(Psychiatry; child development)
Erik Erikson described psychosocial development as a set of stages. During each stage, a particular "task" must be successfully mastered. These tasks are characterized by polarities. Trust/mistrust, autonomy/shame, initiative/guilt, and industry/inferiority are the first four stages, but Erikson described other, later stages of psychosocial development as well.

Jean Piaget described stages of cognitive development (i.e., sensory–motor, preoperational–operational, formal operational). Each stage is mastered through "assimilation" and "accommodation" and requires a reorganization of the thinking process.

Paranoid—schizoid position, depressive position is a developmental scheme of Melanie Klein.

Autism, symbiosis, differentiation is a developmental scheme of Margaret Mahler.

Oral, anal, phallic, genital is a developmental scheme of Sigmund Freud.

195–197. The answers are: 195-C, 196-E, 197-C. *(Pharmacology; anti-inflammatory drugs)*
Chronic use of inhaled corticosteroids, such as triamcinolone, reduces symptoms and improves pulmonary function in patients with mild asthma. A reduction in bronchial reactivity usually becomes apparent after 3 to 4 weeks, but may be delayed considerably in some patients. Systemic toxicity is negligible compared to that following the chronic use of oral steroids, but oropharyngeal fungal overgrowths may occur.

Aminophylline is the most commonly used theophylline preparation. The precise mechanism of bronchodilating action of the methylxanthines is unclear, but effects on cyclic adenosine monophosphate (cAMP) and adenosine have both been proposed. At plasma levels only two to three times those in the therapeutic range (10–20 mg/L), theophylline may cause severe adverse effects, including seizures and cardiac arrhythmias. Monitoring of plasma theophylline levels is particularly advised in patients with hepatic dysfunction or cardiac disease.

In addition to the chronic use of glucocorticoids in asthma, such drugs are also useful (along with inhalational sympathomimetics) in alleviating symptoms of an acute asthmatic attack. This symptom alleviation is due in part to their inhibition of phospholipase A_2–mediated hydrolysis of membrane lipids, which results in decreased formation of prostaglandins and leukotrienes. The use of high-dose glucocorticoids for prolonged periods may cause severe adverse effects, including weight gain, fat deposition, diabetes, osteoporosis, peptic ulcers, and suppression of the pituitary–adrenal axis. Cromolyn also acts at site 1, but it is only prophylactic in asthma and will not reverse acute responses such as bronchospasm.

198–200. The answers are: 198-C, 199-E, 200-A. *(Behavioral science; health care delivery systems)*
In a Preferred provider organization (PPO), a third-party payer, such as an insurance company or union trust fund, contracts with physicians and hospitals to provide medical care to its subscribers.

An intermediate-care facility is a nursing home that provides only limited nursing care, typically restorative nursing and assistance with self-care.

In a Health maintenance organization (HMO), physicians are paid a yearly salary to provide medical services to a group of people who have voluntarily enrolled and paid a yearly premium in advance.

Test IV

QUESTIONS

DIRECTIONS: Each of the numbered items or incomplete statements in this section is followed by answers or by completions of the statement. Select the ONE lettered answer or completion that is BEST in each case.

1. The prognostic factor that is most often associated with a poor prognosis in breast cancer is

(A) diploidy status on DNA flow cytometry
(B) location of the tumor
(C) lymph node metastasis
(D) a negative estrogen and progesterone receptor assay
(E) size of the tumor

2. A 4-year-old child suddenly develops a high fever and no other physical findings. On the third day, the fever rapidly declines and a maculopapular rash develops on the trunk, spreading to the extremities. The most likely diagnosis is

(A) erythema infectiosum
(B) roseola
(C) rubella
(D) rubeola
(E) an echovirus infection

3. A 35-year-old man has diastolic hypertension and hematuria. There is a positive family history of hypertension in his father, who is on renal dialysis, and in his paternal grandmother, who died of a stroke. He complains of discomfort in the abdomen. His serum creatinine level is normal. An ultrasound of the kidney reveals numerous black spaces in both kidneys. The most likely diagnosis in this patient is

(A) immunoglobulin A (IgA) nephropathy
(B) Goodpasture's syndrome
(C) staghorn calculus
(D) Alport's syndrome
(E) polycystic kidney disease

4. A 3-year-old girl presents with fever, rash, arthritis, hepatosplenomegaly, a pericardial effusion, an elevated erythrocyte sedimentation rate (ESR), and an absolute neutrophilic leukocytosis. The most likely diagnosis in this patient is

(A) acute rheumatic fever
(B) systemic lupus erythematosus (SLE)
(C) juvenile rheumatoid arthritis
(D) Lyme disease
(E) ankylosing spondylitis

5. Gender identity is generally established by age

(A) 1
(B) 2
(C) 3
(D) 4
(E) 5

6. Which statement about dysfunctional uterine bleeding is true?

(A) It results from unopposed estrogen stimulation
(B) Pelvic pathology is frequently noted
(C) It is seldom found in adolescent women
(D) Treatment of choice is dilation and curettage (D and C)
(E) Regular ovulation is common

7. A 23-year-old woman presents with low-grade fever, weight loss, crampy left lower quadrant pain, bloody diarrhea, and a history of tenesmus. Flexible sigmoidoscopy reveals a granular, hyperemic, and friable rectal mucosa that bleeds easily on minimal contact. The most likely diagnosis is

(A) ulcerative colitis
(B) Crohn's disease
(C) an anal fissure
(D) ischemic bowel disease

8. Thirty days after bone marrow transplantation, a lung biopsy is performed on a febrile patient with dyspnea. The chest radiograph reveals a predominantly interstitial pattern. The hematoxylin-eosin–stained lung biopsy reveals basophilic-staining intranuclear inclusions in alveolar cells. The most likely pathogen is

(A) *Pneumocystis carinii*
(B) cytomegalovirus (CMV)
(C) *Cryptococcus neoformans*
(D) *Blastomyces dermatitidis*
(E) *Candida albicans*

9. Which factor brings the most increased risk for ectopic pregnancy?

(A) History of diethylstilbestrol (DES) exposure in utero
(B) Intrauterine device (IUD) in place
(C) Previous ectopic pregnancy
(D) History of pelvic inflammatory disease (PID)
(E) Tubal ligation in the last 2 years

10. A study is proposed to determine whether a single 60-mg dose of aspirin, compared to placebo, reduces preeclampsia in primigravid women. Subjects would be recruited and randomized to study and control groups. Placebo and aspirin doses would be administered in identical unmarked capsules. What is the study design?

(A) Cohort study
(B) Case–control study
(C) Randomized controlled trial
(D) Cross-sectional study
(E) Crossover prospective study

11. Which statement about antisocial behavior in young men is true?

(A) It usually has its onset after age 15
(B) It is associated with rigid family upbringing
(C) It tends to fluctuate in intensity over a lifetime
(D) It is often accompanied by periods of extreme remorse
(E) It decreases markedly after age 40

12. Electromyography (EMG) and a nerve conduction velocity (NCV) study would be appropriately used in which of the following conditions?

(A) Severe low-back pain, leg weakness, and bladder control loss of 2 days' duration
(B) Diffuse joint pain
(C) Suspected spinal cord involvement in multiple sclerosis (MS)
(D) Ulnar neuropathy of 1 month's duration
(E) Right footdrop of 1 month's duration associated with a known large L5 disk

13. During a rectal examination, a physician discovers that a 71-year-old man has a suspicious mass in his prostate. Blood drawn prior to his rectal examination reveals a serum prostatic acid phosphatase of 2.5 ng/ml (normal is < 3.7 ng/ml) and a serum prostate-specific antigen of 11.2 ng/ml (normal is < 4.0 ng/ml). Transrectal ultrasonography reveals three suspicious areas. Biopsies from each of these areas reveals prostate adenocarcinoma with a Gleason score of four. A radical prostatectomy is performed and reveals cancer limited to the left lobe of the prostate. There is no capsular invasion or invasion of the seminal vesicles. This patient is stage

(A) A1
(B) A2
(C) B1
(D) B2
(E) C1

14. Which condition is the most common cause of intracranial hemorrhage in children?

(A) Hypertension
(B) Ruptured berry aneurysm
(C) Arteriovenous malformation
(D) Trauma
(E) Hypoxia

15. Which statement about polycystic ovary disease is true?

(A) A clinical feature is low body mass index
(B) Signs of virilization are frequently seen
(C) A major site of androgen production is the adrenals
(D) Mechanism is hypothalamic–pituitary axis miscommunication
(E) Menarche is usually delayed

16. A 65-year-old man presents with a sudden onset of abdominal pain and abdominal distention associated with bloody diarrhea. There is no rebound tenderness present. Bowel sounds are absent. Laboratory data reveal an absolute neutrophilic leukocytosis and left shift plus elevation of serum amylase. The most likely diagnosis is

(A) acute ulcerative colitis
(B) hemorrhagic pancreatitis
(C) aortoenteric fistula
(D) small bowel infarction

17. A 3-year-old child with a long history of sinopulmonary disease is noted to have ataxia and dilated vessels in the conjunctiva and skin. A chest x-ray reveals an absent thymic shadow. Pertinent laboratory data reveal elevated alpha-fetoprotein levels, normal serum immunoglobulin G (IgG) levels, and low IgA and IgE levels. What is the most likely diagnosis in this child?

(A) Wiskott-Aldrich syndrome
(B) Ataxia–telangiectasia
(C) Rendu-Osler-Weber disease
(D) Friedreich's ataxia
(E) Cerebral palsy

18. Cognitive psychotherapy is well documented for its effectiveness in

(A) major depression, single episode, without psychosis
(B) psychogenic amnesia, after other conditions are ruled out
(C) substance abuse and dependence, without acute intoxication
(D) dementia caused by neurodegenerative disease
(E) borderline personality disorder

19. A 60-year-old woman has acute onset of right-arm and -leg weakness, with normal sensation and speech. Her initial computed tomography (CT) scan is normal. What is likely to be the best long-term treatment?

(A) Warfarin

(B) Aspirin

(C) Left carotid endarterectomy

(D) Treatment of underlying heart disease

(E) Control of hypertension and diabetes

20. Which statement about adenomyosis is true?

(A) Endometrial glands are found within the myometrium

(B) Age at diagnosis is usually in the early reproductive years

(C) Medical therapy is often highly successful

(D) Menstrual flow is frequently diminished

(E) The diagnosis is usually made by pelvic examination

21. Natural and man-made disasters are most closely associated with an increase in the frequency of

(A) psychosomatic symptoms

(B) factitious symptoms

(C) dissociative symptoms

(D) vegetative symptoms

(E) psychotic symptoms

22. A 2-year-old girl has recurrent sinopulmonary infections and otitis media associated with *Haemophilus influenzae* and *Streptococcus pneumoniae*. Quantitative immunoglobulins for immunoglobulin G (IgG), IgA, IgM, and IgE are normal. Complement studies are normal. The complete blood count (CBC) is normal. Which disorder best explains this patient's disease?

(A) Chédiak-Higashi syndrome

(B) Chronic granulomatous disease (CGD) of childhood

(C) Job syndrome

(D) IgG$_2$ subclass deficiency

(E) Wiskott-Aldrich syndrome

23. A 50-year-old man is hospitalized after experiencing racing thoughts, insomnia, increasing impulsivity, and grandiosity for 1 month. A 1-month trial of lithium, with a blood level of 1.3 mEq/L, fails to ameliorate his symptoms. Assuming no contraindications, the next step should be

(A) a trial of imipramine

(B) a trial of carbamazepine

(C) an increase in the dose of lithium

(D) the addition of haloperidol

(E) a trial of thioridazine

24. The photograph shows an 8-month-old female infant with ambiguous genitalia. Her urinary 17-ketosteroids (17-KS) and pregnanetriol levels are twice normal, testosterone levels are four times normal, and the urinary 17-hydroxy-corticosteroids are decreased. Her brother has a similar disorder. This patient most likely has

(A) 21-hydroxylase deficiency
(B) 17-hydroxylase deficiency
(C) 11-hydroxylase deficiency
(D) adrenal Cushing's syndrome
(E) a masculinizing ovarian tumor

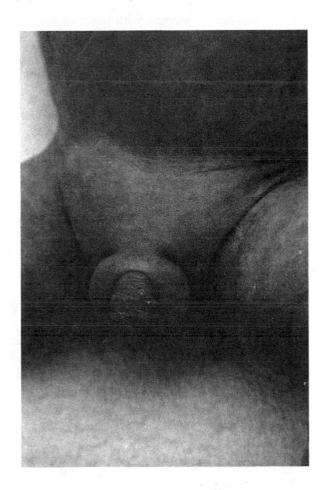

25. Which urodynamic profile is characteristic in urinary stress incontinence?

	Voiding Flow Rate	Residual Volume	Bladder Compliance
(A)	Increased	Increased	Decreased
(B)	Decreased	Normal	Normal
(C)	Normal	Decreased	Increased
(D)	Increased	Decreased	Increased
(E)	Normal	Normal	Normal

26. A patient has severe rectal pain related to defecation. The stool is coated with bright red blood. A sentinel pile is noted on physical examination. The patient most likely has

(A) internal hemorrhoids
(B) external hemorrhoids
(C) an anal fissure
(D) a solitary rectal ulcer

27. An afebrile 12-week-old infant presents with bilateral conjunctivitis, cough, tachypnea, inspiratory rales, and scattered expiratory wheezing. A complete blood count (CBC) reveals eosinophilia. The chest x-ray shows hyperinflation and patchy interstitial infiltrates bilaterally. The most likely diagnosis is

(A) respiratory syncytial viral pneumonia
(B) bronchiolitis
(C) chlamydial pneumonitis
(D) cystic fibrosis
(E) the larval phase of ascariasis

28. The most important initial step in lowering cholesterol is

(A) drug therapy
(B) decreasing intake of carbohydrate
(C) a low-fat diet
(D) decreasing stress

29. After recovery from his third episode of psychosis, a 22-year-old man returns home to live with his parents and younger siblings. The family asks what they can do to improve his adjustment. The best advice would be to

(A) insist that the patient abstain from social interaction

(B) keep family stresses and overt conflicts to a minimum

(C) encourage animated discussions at dinner, with an emphasis on exploring areas of friction among family members

(D) keep the patient at home as much as possible

(E) strongly encourage the patient to return to school or get a job

30. A 50-year-old man who does house repair presents with acute onset of right wristdrop consistent with radial nerve palsy. His complete blood count (CBC) shows anemia, but his iron level is normal. Which diagnostic test would be appropriate?

(A) Nerve conduction velocity (NCV) study of the right arm

(B) X-ray of the right arm and wrist

(C) Magnetic resonance imaging (MRI) scan of the right arm and wrist

(D) Urine screen for heavy metals (lead, mercury, arsenic)

(E) Screening for diabetes

31. A 60-year-old man complains of pain and numbness in the left leg when walking. The pain is relieved by resting. He also complains of impotence. Physical examination reveals atrophy of the left leg muscles, normal reflexes, and a bruit over the femoral artery. The patient most likely has

(A) the Leriche syndrome

(B) a herniated lumbar disc

(C) osteoarthritis of the hip

(D) phlegmasia alba dolens

32. A 34-year-old woman with onset of a severe depressive episode has responded very well to 250 mg of imipramine daily for 1 month. Since the woman has no significant untoward effects, she should now be advised to

(A) stop the imipramine immediately

(B) switch to fluoxetine

(C) continue the imipramine for 6 months

(D) continue the imipramine indefinitely

(E) decrease the imipramine by 50 mg every week until she is medication-free, unless depression recurs

33. In the workup of an infertile couple, the husband's semen analysis reveals the following: a sperm count of 59 million/ml; motility of 60%; volume of 4 ml; normal morphology of 40%; and a pH of 7.3. The parameter that is outside normal values is

(A) sperm count

(B) motility

(C) volume

(D) morphology

(E) pH

34. A 24-year-old male HIV-positive patient has been maintained on low-dose zidovudine (100 mg 5 times daily) for several months with only minor gastrointestinal distress. Until recently, he has remained asymptomatic and has not suffered from opportunistic superinfections. His CD4 lymphocyte count has remained above 250 cells/mm^3 during the period of treatment with zidovudine. For the last couple of weeks, he has had spiking fevers (temperature greater than 100°F), and on examination he has a mild case of oropharyngeal candidiasis. His present CD4 cell count is 240 cells/mm^3. What is the most appropriate course of action?

(A) Double the dose of zidovudine

(B) Prescribe trimethoprim–sulfamethoxazole for daily use

(C) Make no changes in drug treatment, but monitor CD4 counts closely

(D) Prescribe oral ketoconazole, and tell the patient to take aspirin for fever

(E) Halve the dose of zidovudine

35. What is the correct association of visual field deficit and pathology?

(A) Left superior quadrantanopia—right parietal lesion

(B) Right homonymous hemianopsia—right occipital lesion

(C) Superior bitemporal quadrantanopia—chiasmal lesion

(D) Enlarged blind spot—low intracranial pressure

(E) Blindness in the left eye—right occipital lesion

36. A 40-year-old man worries about so many things in his life that he has become "paralyzed" at work and feels "nervous" all the time. He has been taking diazepam by mouth at 10 mg twice a day for 2 weeks, with mild but incomplete relief. However, he now complains of feeling "mentally dulled" and does not want to take it anymore. The best pharmacologic intervention at this point would be to

(A) lower the dose of diazepam to 5 mg by mouth twice a day

(B) taper off medication entirely over several weeks and concentrate on relaxation training

(C) switch to alprazolam

(D) switch to buspirone

(E) switch to propranolol

37. A 40-year-old man develops dizziness and other neurologic signs and symptoms after exercising his arms. A bruit is heard in the right supraclavicular region. The right radial pulse is weaker than the left, and there is a significant difference in blood pressure readings as well. The femoral pulse and blood pressure are normal. These findings are most compatible with

(A) a coarctation of the aorta

(B) subclavian steal syndrome

(C) thoracic outlet syndrome

(D) cervical disk disease

38. Which location of uterine leiomyomata is associated with abnormal bleeding?

(A) Submucosal

(B) Subserosal

(C) Intramural

(D) Intraligamentous

(E) Pedunculated

39. The distribution of age in a population is positively skewed. The option that arranges the three main indexes of central tendency in increasing order of magnitude is

(A) mean, mode, median
(B) mode, median, mean
(C) median, mean, mode
(D) median, mode, mean
(E) mode, mean, median

40. A 5-year-old boy presents with a long history of recurrent infections, eczema, and thrombocytopenia. Immunoglobulin E (IgE) levels are markedly elevated, and mitogen assays are abnormal. Which diagnosis is most likely in this patient?

(A) Atopic dermatitis
(B) Common variable immune deficiency
(C) Acquired immune deficiency syndrome (AIDS)
(D) Wiskott-Aldrich syndrome
(E) Nezelof syndrome

41. Which type of degenerative change within uterine leiomyomata is most associated with pain?

(A) Hyaline
(B) Carneous
(C) Calcareous
(D) Cystic
(E) Myxomatous

42. Which statement about using methadone to treat heroin abuse is true?

(A) It cannot be undertaken except through federally licensed programs
(B) Patients must be warned that concurrent use of methadone and heroin can result in severe physical distress
(C) It is generally appropriate only if a patient has no psychosocial resources that can be used instead
(D) It can be considered as prophylaxis for groups at high risk for heroin dependence
(E) It has been shown to improve social or occupational function of patients with a significant history of heroin abuse

43. Trimethoprim–sulfamethoxazole is effective against which organism responsible for opportunistic superinfections in the acquired immune deficiency syndrome (AIDS) patient?

(A) *Cryptococcus*
(B) Cytomegalovirus (CMV)
(C) *Nocardia*
(D) Herpes simplex virus (HSV)
(E) Enterobacteriaceae

44. A 50-year-old man with normal-appearing tympanic membranes has a conductive hearing loss in the right ear. This is most likely due to

(A) presbycusis
(B) chronic otitis media
(C) otosclerosis
(D) a cholesteatoma

45. In women, the leading causes of cancer death in the United States in descending order are

(A) breast, lung, colorectal
(B) breast, uterine, lung
(C) lung, breast, colorectal
(D) uterine, breast, colorectal
(E) lung, breast, uterine

46. Which treatment is most appropriate for cervical ectropion?

(A) Cryotherapy
(B) Podophyllin
(C) Electrocautery
(D) Acetic acid
(E) Observation

47. A 1-month-old infant is treated with chloramphenicol for a bacterial meningitis of unknown origin. After a few days, the child becomes hypothermic, hypotensive, lethargic, and bradycardic; the skin is ashen. A repeat cerebrospinal fluid (CSF) tap shows some improvement over the previous tap. The most likely diagnosis is

(A) an intraventricular hemorrhage
(B) exacerbation of meningitis
(C) endotoxic shock
(D) the gray syndrome
(E) a sterile subdural effusion

48. The best example of a tertiary prevention strategy for alcohol dependence would be

(A) disulfiram
(B) chlorpromazine
(C) imipramine
(D) chlordiazepoxide
(E) school-based drug education

49. The family of a 63-year-old man with Alzheimer's disease seeks treatment with tacrine. The most accurate statement about this treatment is that

(A) it has been remarkably effective in reversing cognitive decline in some patients
(B) it increases levels of dopamine in the hippocampal region
(C) it has been somewhat effective in reducing symptomatology in mildly affected individuals
(D) it is somewhat effective in individuals with severe memory impairment
(E) it is contraindicated in patients with renal disease

50. The bone most commonly fractured in the wrist and the bone most commonly associated with avascular necrosis is the

(A) scaphoid
(B) lunate
(C) triquetrum
(D) hamate
(E) capitate

51. The most effective way to prevent adolescent substance abuse is to

(A) provide the facts about drugs
(B) create alternative activities
(C) create psychological wellness programs
(D) provide warnings
(E) teach social resistance skills

Questions 52–53

A 5-year-old boy, who is to undergo surgery for strabismus correction, is anesthetized with an intravenous bolus of thiopental and is maintained via inhalation of a nitrous oxide and halothane gas mixture. Intravenous atropine and a small bolus dose of midazolam are also given. Before the procedure can be completed, the child shows signs and symptoms of a crisis, including tachycardia, labile blood pressure, hypercapnea, muscle rigidity, and an elevated body temperature. The presumptive diagnosis is malignant hyperthermia. The anesthetics and other drugs are discontinued, the patient is ventilated with 100% oxygen, and measures are taken to reduce body temperature.

52. The mainstay of therapy of a malignant hyperthermic crisis is the immediate intravenous administration of

(A) haloperidol
(B) physostigmine
(C) dantrolene
(D) phenytoin
(E) diazepam

53. The drug most likely to have precipitated a malignant hyperthermic crisis in this particular patient is

(A) atropine
(B) halothane
(C) midazolam
(D) nitrous oxide
(E) thiopental

54. Which statement about endometriosis is true?

(A) The most common site is the uterosacral ligaments
(B) Medical treatment is seldom curative
(C) The average age of onset is older than 35 years
(D) The chance of malignant transformation is significant

55. A competent 57-year-old patient refuses to have his gangrenous leg amputated. The first step the physician should take is to

(A) remove herself from the case
(B) tell the patient the consequences of refusing the amputation
(C) transfer the patient to another hospital
(D) obtain permission for the amputation from the patient's wife
(E) obtain permission for the amputation from the hospital board of directors

56. A 3-year-old afebrile child develops unilateral, nontender anterior cervical nodes that have been enlarging over the past few weeks. A lymph node biopsy reveals microabscesses with neutrophils. Culture is pending. A Mantoux skin test exhibits only 7-mm induration after 48 hours. What is the most likely diagnosis in this patient?

(A) *Mycobacterium tuberculosis* infection
(B) *M. scrofulaceum* infection
(C) *M. bovis* infection
(D) Cat-scratch disease

57. A 23-year-old woman has tearing and moderate pain in her left eye. Her pupillary light reflex is normal. She recently was placed on topical corticosteroids for suspected allergic conjunctivitis. A Gram stain and Giemsa stain are negative for organisms. A fluorescein stain of the eye exhibits a shallow ulcer with a dendritic appearance and irregular borders. The treatment for this lesion would be topical

(A) ketoconazole
(B) idoxuridine
(C) phenylephrine
(D) erythromycin
(E) sulfacetamide

58. A 29-year-old man complains of extreme anxiety when in social situations. As a result, he avoids parties and lunches, feels lonely, and is not being promoted in his job. In general, the treatment of choice for this problem would be

(A) assertiveness training and phenelzine
(B) implosion therapy and low-dose lorazepam
(C) psychodynamic psychotherapy and an antidepressant
(D) lorazepam alone
(E) systematic desensitization alone

59. Among elderly patients hospitalized for medical conditions, the incidence of concurrent psychiatric conditions is closest to

(A) 10%
(B) 25%
(C) 50%
(D) 75%
(E) 90%

60. Which benign ovarian tumor has the highest malignant potential?

(A) Serous
(B) Mucinous
(C) Endometrioid
(D) Brenner's
(E) Teratoma

61. A 29-year-old woman is in the seventh month of pregnancy when she is hospitalized with appendicitis. Which anesthesia regimen is most appropriate for this patient?

(A) Spinal anesthesia provided via intrathecal injection of lidocaine
(B) Intravenous ketamine by infusion as the sole anesthetic agent
(C) Thiopental induction followed by a halothane and nitrous oxide gas mixture and succinylcholine
(D) Lumbar epidural infiltration with lidocaine, plus oral diazepam
(E) Propofol induction with methoxyflurane by inhalation

62. The most widely accepted indications for psychodynamic psychotherapy include

(A) personality and adjustment disorders
(B) substance abuse
(C) schizophrenia and schizophreniform disorders
(D) obsessive-compulsive disorder and simple phobias
(E) social phobia

63. Which association is correct?

(A) Ash-leaf spot—neurofibromatosis
(B) Cherry-red spot in the macula—phenylketonuria
(C) Mees lines—lead poisoning
(D) Port-wine staining—Sturge-Weber disease
(E) Pseudohypertrophy of the calves—Charcot-Marie-Tooth disease

64. A 9-year-old boy presents with a limp in his right leg and groin pain. Physical examination reveals that his right leg is shorter than his left leg. A radiograph exhibits increased density of the femoral head. These findings are most compatible with

(A) osteoarthritis
(B) osteomyelitis
(C) Legg-Calvé-Perthes disease
(D) a slipped capital femoral epiphysis
(E) osteogenic sarcoma

65. Which type of hospital provides most of the population with medical care?

(A) Investor-owned
(B) For-profit
(C) Voluntary
(D) Federally owned
(E) State-owned

66. Using the progesterone challenge test in a patient with amenorrhea can

(A) assess whether the patient is pregnant
(B) indicate that the patient is producing estrogen
(C) differentiate primary from secondary amenorrhea
(D) rule out a pituitary adenoma
(E) provide no help if the response is spotting

67. A 6-year-old child develops fever, arthralgias, and a confluent rash on the cheeks, with a "slapped face" appearance. Which diagnosis is most likely in this child?

(A) Erythema infectiosum
(B) Roseola
(C) German measles
(D) Measles
(E) Echovirus infection

68. In 1993 in one town, there were 2100 live births and 100 stillbirths (≥ 20 weeks' gestation). Five infants died in the first 28 days of life; 11 deaths occurred in the first year of life. There were 25 sets of twins and 3 sets of triplets. Two mothers died. What was the infant mortality rate in this town in 1993?

(A) 5/2200
(B) 11/2200
(C) 16/2100
(D) 5/2100
(E) 11/2100

69. Behavioral therapy is most effective for

(A) social phobia and drug abuse
(B) dementia caused by neurodegenerative diseases
(C) adjustment and personality disorders
(D) conversion and dissociative disorders
(E) schizophrenia and bipolar disorder

70. A military recruit complains of pain in the right forefoot that is accentuated by walking. A radiograph reveals new bone formation along the periosteum of the second and third metatarsals. These findings are most compatible with

(A) a greenstick fracture

(B) a stress fracture

(C) osteochondritis

(D) a sprain

71. Which endocrinologically active ovarian tumor is associated most with precocious puberty in girls?

(A) Granulosa cell tumor

(B) Fibrothecoma

(C) Sertoli-Leydig cell tumor

(D) Hilar cell tumor

(E) Gynandroblastoma

72. A 4-year-old child presents with fever, conjunctivitis, photophobia, posterior cervical adenopathy, and coryza. Red lesions with a white center are present on the buccal mucosa. A generalized, blanching, erythematous rash is also noted. The most likely diagnosis is

(A) Kawasaki disease

(B) rubella

(C) adenovirus infection

(D) rubeola

(E) Still's disease

73. Which statement about adoptees is true?

(A) Changed family environments rarely raise IQ scores in such individuals

(B) About 50% of adoptions are considered successful

(C) Their relationships with their adoptive parents are no more troubled than nonadoptees' relationships with their biologic parents

(D) Narcissistic injury is a significant psychological issue with such individuals

(E) Rates of psychopathology among adopted individuals are comparable to rates among individuals reared by their biologic parents

74. A 12-year-old girl exhibits paraspinus prominence on her right side when she bends forward. This physical finding is most consistent with

(A) ankylosing spondylitis

(B) Pott's disease of the spine

(C) idiopathic scoliosis

(D) osteomyelitis

75. Which statement about attachment theory is true?

(A) A secure attachment improves survival, but later makes it difficult for the adult to practice altruistic behavior

(B) Secure attachment retards the development of basic trust

(C) Infant survival is predicated on making a successful transition from attachment to the mother to independence

(D) Improper attachment is generally caused by developmental psychopathology

(E) Early insecure attachments to caregivers cause later personality disorders

76. Which finding is characteristic of dysmaturity syndrome?

(A) Excessive fundal height
(B) Thick placenta
(C) Polyhydramnios
(D) Fetal macrosomatia
(E) Decreased Wharton's jelly

77. Which description about sensitivity of a screening test is true?

(A) Ability to include persons with a disease
(B) Ability to exclude persons with a disease
(C) Ability to include persons free of disease
(D) Ability to exclude persons free of disease
(E) Ability to diagnose persons with a disease

78. The first-line drug for the treatment of status epilepticus is

(A) intravenous phenytoin
(B) intravenous diazepam or lorazepam
(C) paraldehyde
(D) intravenous lidocaine
(E) intravenous pentobarbital

79. A 10-year-old girl is on summer vacation with her parents on Long Island, New York. She presents with fever, generalized lymphadenopathy, and an expanding, annular, erythematous papular rash on the trunk. The right knee is painful and slightly swollen. The mother remembers having picked a few ticks off the girl over the past few weeks. Which diagnosis is the most likely in this child?

(A) Rocky Mountain spotted fever
(B) Babesiosis
(C) Colorado tick fever
(D) Lyme disease
(E) Juvenile rheumatoid arthritis

80. The concept that refers to the requisite environment for the development of emotionally healthy children is

(A) "as if personality"
(B) "lock and key"
(C) "goodness of fit"
(D) "good-enough mothering"
(E) "emerging competencies"

81. A 9-year-old child is having difficulty swallowing. There is a painless mass located in the midline at the base of the tongue. There is no cervical adenopathy. Which of the following would be most useful in confirming your diagnosis?

(A) Needle biopsy
(B) Excisional biopsy
(C) Iodine-131 (^{131}I) uptake
(D) Throat culture

82. A 19-year-old woman comes to the physician's office stating that she has never had a menstrual period. Physical examination reveals normal breast development, but no uterus can be palpated on pelvic examination. Which of the following tests for serum levels would be most helpful in identifying the cause of her amenorrhea?

(A) Follicle-stimulating hormone (FSH)

(B) Luteinizing hormone (LH)

(C) Prolactin

(D) Testosterone

(E) Progesterone

83. A 13-year-old girl presents with a low-grade fever, painful postauricular and posterior occipital lymphadenopathy, and a maculopapular rash that began on the face and spread to the trunk. She also complains of pain in both wrists and her right knee. Splenomegaly is present on examination. Which diagnosis is the most likely in this patient?

(A) Measles

(B) Infectious mononucleosis

(C) German measles

(D) Erythema infectiosum

(E) Roseola

84. A 47-year-old homeless male alcoholic presents with a fever and expectoration of foul-smelling sputum. His dental hygiene is poor. A chest radiograph reveals a cavitary lesion with a fluid layer in the superior segment of the right lower lobe. A Gram's stain of sputum would be expected to show

(A) predominantly gram-positive diplococci

(B) predominantly gram-positive rods

(C) gram-positive cocci and variable gram-positive and gram-negative rods with tapered ends

(D) gram-positive filamentous and branching bacteria

85. If the blood glucose cutoff point on a screening test for gestational diabetes is lowered from 140 mg/dl to 135 mg/dl, what effect would the change have on the following four parameters?

	Sensitivity	Specificity	False-positive Rate	False-negative Rate
(A)	Increased	Decreased	Decreased	Increased
(B)	Increased	Decreased	Increased	Decreased
(C)	Decreased	Increased	Increased	Decreased
(D)	Decreased	Decreased	Increased	Increased
(E)	Increased	Increased	Decreased	Decreased

86. A 40-year-old woman, with diabetes mellitus, comes to the office complaining of pruritic, whitish, cheesy vaginal discharge. Which diagnostic test is most cost-effective for identifying the cause of this condition?

(A) Wet prep

(B) Gram's stain

(C) pH

(D) Culture

(E) Potassium hydroxide (KOH) prep

87. A biopsy of a posterior cervical lymph node in a 45-year-old, nonsmoking, Chinese woman reveals a poorly differentiated carcinoma. A chest radiograph, indirect laryngoscopy, and oral examination are normal. The next step in the management of this patient should be

(A) a sputum cytology

(B) a blind biopsy of the nasopharynx

(C) radiographic tomography of the lung

(D) an iodine-131 (^{131}I) scan of the thyroid

88. An HIV-positive patient presents with fever, dyspnea, tachypnea, and peripheral cyanosis. The chest x-ray reveals extensive "ground-glass" opacities in the lower zones of both lungs. The physician would expect

(A) the organism to respond to amphotericin B

(B) the organism to respond to erythromycin

(C) granulomas in the bone marrow

(D) the organism to respond to trimethoprim–sulfamethoxazole

89. A 9-month-old infant presents with a bloody vaginal discharge. Vaginoscopic examination shows a grape-like necrotic mass in the vaginal vault. Which diagnosis is the most likely in this child?

(A) Clear cell adenocarcinoma

(B) Embryonal rhabdomyosarcoma

(C) Leiomyosarcoma

(D) Granular cell myoblastoma

(E) Squamous cell carcinoma

90. Which anatomic site is the most likely location for an ectopic pregnancy?

(A) Isthmus of the oviduct

(B) Uterine cornu

(C) Ampullae of the oviduct

(D) Ovary

(E) Infundibulum of the oviduct

91. A 12-year-old Boy Scout, who went on a summer camping trip in Oklahoma 1 week ago, presents with fever, lethargy, headache, and abdominal pain. Petechial lesions are noted on the palms of the hand. The vector most likely responsible for this disease is a

(A) virus

(B) bacteria

(C) mite

(D) cat

(E) tick

92. A 25-year-old man received a basilar skull fracture in a motorcycle accident. Clear fluid exudes from his ear. The physician suspects that it is cerebrospinal fluid (CSF). Chemical analysis of the fluid when compared with serum would be expected to show

(A) a higher protein concentration than serum

(B) a higher chloride concentration than serum

(C) a higher glucose concentration than serum

(D) more white blood cells in the CSF than in serum

93. Which combination of maternal, paternal, and fetal red blood cell (RBC) antigens places the pregnant woman at risk for isoimmunization?

	Maternal	Paternal	Fetal
(A)	Negative	Negative	Negative
(B)	Positive	Positive	Positive
(C)	Positive	Negative	Positive
(D)	Positive	Negative	Negative
(E)	Negative	Positive	Positive

94. A 65-year-old woman developed fever and watery diarrhea while on ampicillin for a urinary tract infection. A colonoscopic examination reveals yellow–white plaques surrounded by hemorrhagic borders on the mucosal surface of the colon. The test of choice for this patient's disease is a

(A) Gram's stain of the yellowish material

(B) culture of the yellowish material

(C) toxin assay of liquid stool

(D) blood culture

(E) stool sample examination for ova and parasites

95. In what order are the top five causes of death in the United States (in order of decreasing frequency)?

1. Accidents
2. Chronic obstructive pulmonary disease (COPD)
3. Heart disease
4. Cerebrovascular disease
5. Cancer

(A) 2-3-5-1-4

(B) 3-5-4-1-2

(C) 5-3-1-2-4

(D) 3-4-5-2-1

(E) 4-3-5-2-1

96. Which statement about cytomegalovirus (CMV) in pregnancy is true?

(A) No specific effective treatment exists

(B) Cesarean delivery is recommended

(C) Risk of fetal infection is highest during the first trimester

(D) Gamma globulin is useful prophylaxis after exposure

97. Test X has a reference interval from 0 to 7 mg/dl. Changing the reference interval to 0 to 3 mg/dl would

(A) increase the test's specificity

(B) decrease the number of false-positive results

(C) increase the number of false-negative results

(D) increase the sensitivity of the test

98. A referral patient presents with intermittent neurologic abnormalities associated with hypoglycemia. The patient experiences an attack in the office, and the physician draws blood for serum insulin, C peptide, and glucose. The attack is relieved by giving the patient glucose. One week later, the following laboratory results return:

Serum glucose:	Low
Serum insulin:	High
Serum C peptide:	Low

Which condition best explains the clinical and laboratory findings?

(A) Insulinoma
(B) Reactive hypoglycemia from eating
(C) Glucagonoma
(D) Insulin taken surreptitiously
(E) Somatostatinoma

99. A 28-year-old woman has a painless right cervical lymph node, which reveals well-differentiated branching structures and blue-staining concretions. The source of this lesion is most likely the

(A) vocal cord
(B) parotid gland
(C) thyroid gland
(D) lung
(E) breast

100. Which statement about Venereal Disease Research Laboratories (VDRL) testing for syphilis is true?

(A) A positive test is conclusive for syphilis
(B) In primary syphilis, the test is positive
(C) Recent immunizations can give a false-positive result
(D) The fluorescent treponemal antibody absorption (FTA-ABS) test does not provide additional information
(E) The test is negative when condylomata lata are seen

101. A door-to-door survey takes place at 250 randomly selected homes in one town to determine whether the use of air conditioning is associated with a decrease in asthma attacks. What is the study design?

(A) Cohort study
(B) Case-control study
(C) Randomized controlled trial
(D) Cross-sectional study
(E) Crossover prospective study

Questions 102–105

A 20-year-old male college student is hospitalized after assaulting a girlfriend whom he accuses of using "radar" to place bizarre thoughts in his mind, just after she broke off her relationship with him. He has been increasingly withdrawn and preoccupied over the last year, but has no history of substance abuse or other physical problems. Mental status examination reveals an alert, anxious, and oriented male, with dysphoria, suspiciousness, constricted affect, mildly tangential thinking, bizarre ideation, and no memory impairment.

102. This patient's most significant psychiatric syndrome is

(A) delirium
(B) psychosis
(C) depression
(D) anxiety
(E) mania

103. The most likely diagnosis is

(A) schizophrenia
(B) bipolar disorder
(C) cocaine-induced psychosis
(D) major depression with psychosis
(E) shared psychotic disorder

104. The most diagnostically significant feature of the past history would be

(A) a family history of psychiatric hospitalizations in several relatives
(B) a history of early childhood conflicts with parents
(C) a recent painful breakup with a girlfriend
(D) a history of anxiety when speaking in public
(E) a history of LSD ingestion 2 years ago

105. A brief reactive psychosis is unlikely because

(A) a period of increasing social withdrawal occurred before the breakup with his girlfriend
(B) dysphoria is present
(C) ideation is bizarre
(D) the condition lasted more than a few hours
(E) the patient is attending college

Questions 106–107

106. A 5-year-old child develops abdominal pain, nausea and vomiting, bloody diarrhea, headache, confusion, ataxia, and renal failure after drinking an unknown liquid. Which metallic element did the liquid most likely contain?

(A) Arsenic
(B) Lead
(C) Mercury
(D) Iron
(E) Cadmium

107. Which therapy would be best for the child?

(A) Ethylenediaminetetraacetic acid (EDTA)
(B) Penicillamine
(C) Deferoxamine
(D) British antilewisite (BAL, dimercaprol)
(E) EDTA and BAL

108. A patient has a prosthetic aortic valve and a normocytic anemia with an increased reticulocyte count and schistocytes present in the peripheral blood. Which protein would be most useful for following the severity of this patient's intravascular hemolytic anemia?

(A) Ceruloplasmin
(B) Albumin
(C) C-reactive protein
(D) Transferrin
(E) Haptoglobin

109. A 75-year-old woman with Alzheimer's disease falls in the nursing home and hits her head. No fractures are noted on a skull radiograph. She has fluctuating levels of consciousness and complains of a severe headache on the left side of her head. Mydriasis is noted in the left pupil. The most likely diagnosis in this patient is

(A) epidural hematoma
(B) subdural hematoma
(C) subarachnoid hemorrhage
(D) intracerebral hemorrhage
(E) hemorrhagic infarction of the brain

110. Which condition is most likely to be a cause of urinary stress incontinence?

(A) Multiple sclerosis
(B) Grand multiparity
(C) Bladder tumor
(D) Interstitial cystitis
(E) Detrusor instability

Questions 111–112

A 65-year-old woman develops compression fractures of the vertebrae in the spinal column. An x-ray of the spine shows generalized osteopenia and narrowing of the disc spaces. The serum calcium and phosphorus levels are normal.

111. The mechanism responsible for this patient's x-ray findings is

(A) increased osteoclastic activity
(B) decreased osteoblastic activity
(C) an imbalance between osteoclastic and osteoblastic activity
(D) secretion of osteoclast activating factor by macrophages
(E) increased secretion of parathormone

112. All of the following treatments could have prevented the patient's problems EXCEPT

(A) estrogen replacement therapy at the time of menopause
(B) vitamin D supplements
(C) weight-bearing exercises
(D) progesterone therapy
(E) calcium supplementation

113. An 8-year-old child develops scarlet fever and recovers uneventfully. Approximately 3 weeks later, the child develops a smoke-colored urine and puffiness beneath the eyes. Physical examination reveals mild hypertension. Urinalysis shows hematuria and red blood cell (RBC) casts. The most likely diagnosis is

(A) minimal change disease
(B) idiopathic membranous glomerulonephritis
(C) Henoch-Schönlein glomerulonephritis
(D) systemic lupus glomerulonephritis
(E) poststreptococcal glomerulonephritis

114. Which of the following statements best describes the primary usefulness of mammography?

(A) Detects nonpalpable breast masses
(B) Assigns a clinical stage for breast cancer
(C) Distinguishes benign from malignant breast cancer
(D) Reduces the role of excisional biopsy in diagnosing breast cancer

115. Which recommendation is appropriate for management of a woman who is rubella-susceptible?

(A) Provide gamma globulin for prophylaxis after exposure
(B) Administer rubella vaccine in the third trimester
(C) Avoid breast-feeding after postpartum maternal vaccination
(D) Avoid pregnancy for 3 months after maternal vaccination
(E) Offer genetic amniocentesis for amniotic fluid culture

116. A 6-month-old black infant presents with low-grade fever and acute onset of painful swelling of the hands and feet. Radiographs taken at the onset of symptoms reveal soft tissue swelling, and the peripheral smear is shown below. The findings in this infant most likely correlate with

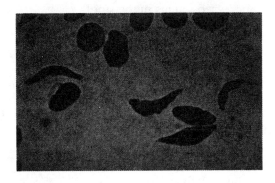

(A) deficiency of glucose-6-phosphate dehydrogenase (G6PD)
(B) *Salmonella* osteomyelitis
(C) a decrease in hemoglobin F (Hgb F) concentration
(D) a coxsackievirus infection
(E) a deletion of a chromosome

117. The prevalence of serious major depression in the general population of elderly individuals is closest to

(A) 10%
(B) 33%
(C) 66%
(D) 75%
(E) over 90%

118. A perianal cellophane-type preparation from a 3-year-old child would most likely be performed because of

(A) rectal bleeding
(B) pain on defecation
(C) constipation
(D) anal pruritus
(E) increased mucus in the stool

119. A 60-year-old man, who is an alcoholic, complains of difficulty in swallowing solids. In addition, he has progressive weight loss and weakness. The most likely diagnosis is

(A) diffuse esophageal spasm
(B) Zenker's diverticulum
(C) achalasia
(D) esophageal carcinoma

120. In addition to its use in the management of moderate to severe pain states associated with malignant disease or terminal illness, morphine (at high dose) is also used intravenously in anesthesia for situations in which cardiovascular reserve is limited or may be compromised during surgery. Morphine is also clinically important in

(A) relief of the pain of wisdom tooth extraction
(B) management of pulmonary edema
(C) decreasing inflammation in rheumatoid arthritis
(D) closure of the ductus arteriosus
(E) anesthesia for patients with head injuries

121. A 25-year-old woman complains of a pruritic, painful vaginal discharge. A wet mount of vaginal secretions reveals a highly motile protozoan. Which pharmacologic agent would be the most appropriate treatment?

(A) Metronidazole
(B) Clotrimazole
(C) Miconazole
(D) Acyclovir
(E) Spectinomycin

122. The sensitivity for the results of the following test is

<u>**True Diagnosis**</u>

	Disease Present (D+)	Disease Absent (D−)	Totals
Test positive (T+)	40	60	100
Test negative (T−)	80	20	100
Totals	120	80	200

(A) 20%
(B) 33%
(C) 40%
(D) 67%
(E) 89%

123. "Masked depression" usually refers to

(A) the presentation of seemingly cognitive problems, which actually result from poor concentration due to depression
(B) the presence of mood-incongruent psychosis, which obscures underlying depressive symptomatology
(C) the denial of depression and adoption of stoicism
(D) the use of manic defenses to hide depressive symptomatology
(E) the presentation of depression as multiple somatic complaints instead of subjective complaints of mood change

124. A 6-year-old boy presents with café-au-lait macules on his right lower abdomen. His mother also has similar skin lesions. The most likely diagnosis is

(A) dysplastic nevus syndrome

(B) Sturge-Weber disease

(C) tuberous sclerosis

(D) neurofibromatosis

(E) tinea versicolor

125. Which contraceptive method has the highest failure rate?

(A) Spermicides

(B) Intrauterine device (IUD)

(C) Postcoital douche

(D) Diaphragm

(E) Oral contraceptives

126. Which statement is true for the majority of adults with mental retardation?

(A) They need a full range of psychosocial services to function

(B) They engage in substance abuse

(C) They have recurrent psychiatric hospitalizations

(D) They live and work in the community

(E) They are at significant risk for bearing mentally retarded children

127. Scabies in infants differs from adult scabies in that the former

(A) has no burrows

(B) is not limited to the intertriginous areas

(C) often presents with red-brown nodules in the axillae and groin

(D) spares the face and scalp

128. A 15-year-old presents to the emergency room with a swollen left eye and respiratory difficulty. She gives a history of falling asleep while sunbathing on the grass in her backyard then waking up suddenly with pain and swelling in her face and trouble breathing. Physical examination reveals expiratory wheezes. There is no inspiratory stridor or swelling of the oropharyngeal mucosa present. The first step in the management of this patient is to

(A) administer intravenous hydrocortisone

(B) treat the patient with nebulized albuterol sulfate

(C) administer intravenous aminophylline

(D) administer subcutaneous epinephrine 1:1000

(E) administer intravenous epinephrine 1:10,000

129. According to many studies, the percentage of the homeless population with chronic and severe mental illness is closest to

(A) 10%

(B) 35%

(C) 50%

(D) 65%

(E) 90%

130. A 67-year-old woman presents with intense pruritus of the vulva. On examination, the vaginal introitus is stenotic, with the skin appearing thin, wrinkled, and parchment-like. Which treatment is most appropriate?

(A) 5-Fluorouracil

(B) Testosterone cream

(C) Fluorinated corticosteroids

(D) Miconazole

(E) Estrogen cream

131. A 10-year-old boy has progressive ataxia. Examination shows very poor proprioception and vibratory sensation, as well as a clubfoot and scoliosis. He is areflexic. Which condition might also be associated?

(A) Sick sinus syndrome
(B) Diabetes
(C) Mental retardation
(D) Rapid blindness
(E) Seizures

132. Five days after an operation for a perforated appendix, a 62-year-old man presents with shaking chills, high fever, and jaundice. A radiograph of the abdomen reveals air in the portal system. These findings are most consistent with

(A) gallstone ileus
(B) Budd-Chiari syndrome
(C) ascending cholangitis
(D) pylephlebitis

133. In the United States, the mortality rate for black infants is

(A) 20% higher than the rate for white infants
(B) 40% higher than the rate for white infants
(C) 50% higher than the rate for white infants
(D) 80% higher than the rate for white infants
(E) equal to the rate for white infants

134. An 80-year-old woman comes to the physician's office with numerous white skin lesions on her vulva. Which statement about diagnosis through biopsy is true?

(A) Colposcopy will not help in the identification of biopsy sites
(B) Toluidine blue staining should be avoided because it may alter histologic appearance
(C) A large lesion should be biopsied from the central area of the lesion
(D) The definitive diagnosis rests on clinical rather than histologic findings
(E) More than one biopsy may be needed to assess the condition adequately

135. An agitated woman is brought in by the police because she has threatened suicide. Her risk of actually committing suicide is greatest if

(A) she is married to an abusive spouse
(B) she is under 30
(C) she is unhappy at her job
(D) she has schizophrenia
(E) she is lesbian

136. The most common complication associated with recurrent otitis media in children is

(A) hearing loss
(B) cerebral abscess
(C) cholesteatoma
(D) thrombosis of the dural sinuses
(E) acute mastoiditis

137. A 14-year-old boy was hit hard on the side of the head with a baseball bat during practice. A laceration with palpable bone fragments was present in the wound when he was examined in the emergency room. Approximately 5 hours after receiving the injury, the boy died. The initial event that most likely caused the death of the patient is

(A) a hemorrhagic infarction of the brain
(B) a subarachnoid hemorrhage
(C) an epidural hematoma
(D) a subdural hematoma
(E) an intracerebral hemorrhage

138. Which characteristic best describes primary dysmenorrhea?

(A) Onset after 20 years of age
(B) Postmenstrual continuation
(C) Normal gross pelvic anatomy
(D) Associated with abnormal bleeding
(E) Best treated surgically

139. The specificity for this test is

| | True Diagnosis | | |
	Disease Present (D+)	Disease Absent (D−)	Totals
Test positive (T+)	30	20	50
Test negative (T−)	10	40	50
Totals	40	60	100

(A) 20%
(B) 33%
(C) 40%
(D) 67%
(E) 80%

140. The vessel that is most commonly injured during a cholecystectomy is the

(A) right hepatic artery
(B) portal vein
(C) inferior vena cava
(D) right gastroepiploic artery

141. The psychiatric disorder most often cited as a specific sequel of child sexual abuse is

(A) schizophrenia
(B) autism
(C) antisocial personality disorder
(D) somatization disorder
(E) multiple personality disorder

142. The most common cause of permanent loss of visual acuity in the elderly is

(A) macular degeneration
(B) trauma
(C) cataract surgery
(D) optic neuritis
(E) diabetic retinopathy

143. A 55-year-old white woman complains of pelvic pressure symptoms and a mass at her vaginal opening. It has been 3 years since her last menstrual period. She is not taking estrogen replacement therapy. She has difficulty in stool evacuation. She has a chronic cough from a 30 pack-year history of smoking. She had three vaginal deliveries, the largest infant weighing 4500 g. Her postvoiding residual was 60 cc. The most likely physical finding on pelvic examination would be

(A) rectocele
(B) cystocele
(C) enterocele
(D) urethrocele
(E) vaginocele

144. A 45-year-old Vietnam veteran complains of a 20-year history of nightmares about horrific events that he witnessed during the war. He also feels emotionally distant from other people and anxious in their presence. He now says that he feels rejected by "society" and wants to seek out other veterans with similar experiences in an attempt to "relate." He would be best advised to

(A) consider meeting with Vietnamese–Americans to heal anger and guilt
(B) cognitively reframe his experiences and focus on the present
(C) initiate a combination of clonazepam and paroxetine
(D) initially avoid unstructured meetings or recollections of Vietnam, then consider psychodynamic psychotherapy to explore feelings of guilt about his experiences
(E) join a peer support group

145. After a deadly automobile accident that kills her child but leaves her with only minor cuts, the mother seems oddly calm and says that she has no emotion. Which psychodynamic defense is the mother using?

(A) Isolation
(B) Depersonalization
(C) Disorientation
(D) Intellectualization
(E) Derealization

146. A 28-year-old woman is bitten on the hand by a stray cat in the neighborhood. Twenty-four hours later, the hand is swollen, and there is swelling and warmth around the puncture sites of the bite. The organism most likely responsible for these findings is

(A) *Afipia felis*
(B) *Pasteurella multocida*
(C) *Staphylococcus aureus*
(D) group A streptococci

147. An aspirate from one of four pustular lesions on the wrist of a 25-year-old sexually active woman with fever and pain in the wrist joint reveals neutrophils with gram-negative, coffee-bean–shaped diplococci. These lesions can be associated with

(A) deficiency of immunoglobulin G2 (IgG2) and IgG4 subclasses
(B) Still's disease
(C) C6 through C8 complement deficiencies
(D) Reiter's syndrome

148. The most common major medication used to treat androgen excess is

(A) prednisone
(B) dexamethasone
(C) progestogen
(D) estrogen
(E) spironolactone

149. The cell depicted in this peripheral smear is representative of the majority of cells in an afebrile 75-year-old male with generalized, non-painful lymphadenopathy, hepatosplenomegaly, and petechiae and ecchymoses scattered over his body. His complete blood count (CBC) shows a hemoglobin of 9.0 g/dl (normal is 13.5–17.5 g/dl), normal red blood cell indices, a leukocyte count of 90,000 cells/μl (normal is 4500–11,000 cells/μl), and a platelet count of 70,000 cells/μl (normal is 150,000–400,000 cells/μl). Which one of the following scenarios should be expected?

(A) The leukocytes have a positive tartrate-resistant acid phosphatase stain

(B) The patient's disease progresses into an acute myelogenous leukemia

(C) The leukocytes have Auer rods

(D) Lymphocyte marker studies indicate a T-cell malignancy

(E) Diffuse bone marrow and lymph node infiltration by the cells represented in the peripheral smear

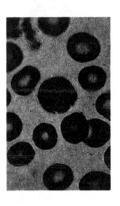

DIRECTIONS: Each of the numbered items or incomplete statements in this section is negatively phrased, as indicated by a capitalized word such as NOT, LEAST, or EXCEPT. Select the ONE lettered answer or completion that is BEST in each case.

150. Major criteria for the diagnosis of acute rheumatic fever include all of the following EXCEPT

(A) increased anti–streptolysin O (ASO) titer
(B) carditis
(C) chorea
(D) polyarthritis
(E) subcutaneous nodules

151. A 25-year-old woman with an acute erythematous rash on the face also complains of morning stiffness of her hands and left-sided chest pain that increases with inspiration. Physical examination reveals symmetric, fusiform swelling of the metacarpophalangeal and proximal interphalangeal joints and dullness to percussion at the left lung base. There is no calf tenderness. A chest x-ray shows a small pleural effusion in the left pleural cavity. Which of the following findings would LEAST likely be expected in this patient?

(A) Transudate in the left pleural effusion
(B) Positive serum antinuclear antibody test
(C) Low complement C4 and a normal factor B level
(D) Positive band fluorescence test in a biopsy of grossly normal skin
(E) Increased erythrocyte sedimentation rate

152. The clinical features of poor-prognosis metastatic gestational trophoblastic neoplasia include all of the following EXCEPT

(A) disease present less than 4 months from antecedent pregnancy
(B) serum human chorionic gonadotropin (hCG) greater than 40,000 IU
(C) metastasis to the brain or liver
(D) failure to respond to single-agent chemotherapy
(E) choriocarcinoma following a full-term delivery

153. All of the following characteristics differentiate minimal change disease from acute poststreptococcal glomerulonephritis in children EXCEPT

(A) serum albumin
(B) red blood cell (RBC) casts
(C) fatty casts
(D) hypertension
(E) edema

154. Which procedure is NOT considered appropriate for staging cervical carcinoma?

(A) Physical examination
(B) Cystoscopy
(C) Sigmoidoscopy
(D) Laparoscopy
(E) Colposcopy

155. All of the following characteristics are significant risk factors for substance abuse EXCEPT

(A) peer drug use
(B) iatrogenic exposure to psychostimulants or opiates
(C) social isolation
(D) involvement in drug trafficking
(E) academic difficulties

156. Complications associated with chickenpox include all of the following EXCEPT

(A) bloody diarrhea
(B) hemorrhagic vesicles
(C) cerebellar inflammation
(D) pneumonitis
(E) Reye's syndrome

157. All of the following features characterize hospice care EXCEPT

(A) grief counseling
(B) support groups
(C) inpatient supportive care
(D) outpatient supportive care
(E) restricted use of pain medication

158. All of the following conditions are a sign or symptom of battering in women EXCEPT

(A) pelvic pain
(B) insomnia
(C) urinary tract infection
(D) substance abuse
(E) gastrointestinal symptoms

159. Cerebrospinal fluid (CSF) findings that characterize a viral, rather than a bacterial, meningitis include all of the following EXCEPT

(A) normal glucose
(B) substantially increased protein concentration
(C) negative Gram stain
(D) lymphocyte-predominant differential after 48 hours
(E) normal lactate concentration

160. The peripheral smear shown below is from a 65-year-old man who complains of tiredness and generalized weakness. A complete blood count (CBC) reveals a hemoglobin of 7.0 g/dl (normal is 13.5–17.5 g/dl), a mean corpuscular volume of 62 μm³ (normal is 80–100 μm³), a red cell distribution width of 20 (normal is 10 +/– 5), a leukocyte count of 8500 cells/μl (normal is 1500–11,000 cells/μl), and a platelet count of 650,000 cells/μl (normal is 150,000–450,000 cells/μl). The leukocyte differential is unremarkable except for the presence of absolute monocytosis. The serum alkaline phosphatase concentration is 225 U/L (normal is 20–70 U/L), the gamma glutamyltransferase is 175 U/L (normal is 6–35 U/L), and the lactate dehydrogenase concentration is 250 U/L (normal is 45–90 U/L). The total bilirubin and transaminase levels are normal. In the course of the patient's workup, a barium enema reveals a polypoid mass in the ascending colon. Laboratory studies on this patient should reveal all of the following EXCEPT

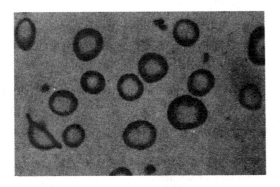

(A) low serum ferritin concentration
(B) positive stool guaiac
(C) metastatic lesions to bone
(D) increased total iron-binding capacity
(E) biopsy evidence of an adenocarcinoma

161. All of the following teratogen and developmental defect relationships are correct EXCEPT

(A) phenytoin—hypoplasia of the distal phalanges and growth retardation
(B) isotretinoin—microtia and cardiac defects
(C) diethylstilbestrol (DES)—vaginal adenosis and cervical incompetence
(D) valproate—microcephaly
(E) smoking—small-for-gestational-age infant

162. The left index finger from a febrile 28-year-old male intravenous drug abuser reveals a painful, erythematous nodule on the finger pad and a linear hemorrhage beneath the fingernail. Cardiac examination reveals a grade II high-pitched diastolic murmur heard best along the second and third right intercostal space. Which condition would be LEAST expected as a potential complication in this patient?

(A) Cardiac tamponade
(B) Immune complex glomerulonephritis
(C) Embolic stroke
(D) Positive blood culture
(E) Roth's spots

163. All of the following developmental defects are associated with the fetal alcohol syndrome EXCEPT

(A) hydrocephaly
(B) atrial septal defect
(C) hypoglycemia
(D) maxillary hypoplasia
(E) mental retardation

164. Which condition is NOT an indication for cervical conization?

(A) Neoplasia on biopsy with unsatisfactory colposcopy
(B) Neoplasia on endocervical curettage with unsatisfactory colposcopy
(C) Significant discrepancy between Pap smear and biopsy
(D) Microinvasive squamous cell carcinoma on biopsy
(E) Stage IA_2 carcinoma on biopsy

165. Tobacco substantially contributes to death in all of the following patients EXCEPT

(A) those with pancreatic cancer
(B) those with liver disease
(C) those with pneumonia
(D) those with stroke
(E) low–birth-weight infants

166. Diet substantially contributes to the actual cause of death in all of the following diseases EXCEPT

(A) coronary artery disease
(B) hypertension
(C) colon cancer
(D) chronic obstructive pulmonary disease (COPD)
(E) diabetes mellitus

167. All of the following conditions characterize pseudohypoparathyroidism EXCEPT

(A) mental retardation
(B) decreased serum parathormone
(C) decreased serum calcium
(D) increased serum phosphate
(E) calcification of the basal ganglia

168. All of the following statements about the drugs used in the treatment of metastatic choriocarcinoma are accurate EXCEPT

(A) saline hydration alone or with mannitol reduces nephrotoxicity due to cisplatin
(B) etoposide is a cell cycle–specific anticancer drug
(C) antibacterial sulfonamides should be avoided in a patient on methotrexate
(D) a major advantage of etoposide is that it has minimal hematotoxicity
(E) when used in combination drug regimens, cisplatin frequently enhances tumor cell kill

169. All of the following tests are commonly utilized in the workup of patients with an allergic diathesis EXCEPT

(A) radioallergosorbent test (RAST)
(B) Coombs' test
(C) nasal smear for eosinophils
(D) scratch testing
(E) immunoglobulin E (IgE) levels

170. In comparison to men, women are LESS likely to

(A) smoke cigarettes
(B) abuse alcohol
(C) visit doctors
(D) be hospitalized
(E) suffer from unipolar depression

171. An innocent heart murmur in children includes all of the following characteristics EXCEPT

(A) best heard in the second left intercostal space
(B) common in children 3 to 7 years old
(C) intensifies with fever or excitement
(D) best heard with the patient lying on the left side
(E) systolic ejection murmur grade 1 to 2 out of a possible 6

172. An elevated erythrocyte sedimentation rate (ESR) is expected in all of the following disorders EXCEPT

(A) multiple myeloma
(B) anemia
(C) rheumatoid arthritis
(D) sickle cell anemia

173. A 55-year-old man has a 10-year history of ulnar deviation of both hands, enlarged joints, and nodules down both forearms. In addition, he has an ulcer on his lower leg. This patient would be expected to have all of the following signs EXCEPT

(A) a positive rheumatoid factor
(B) polyclonal gammopathy on a serum protein electrophoresis
(C) rheumatoid vasculitis
(D) osteophytes at the margins to the joints
(E) anemia of chronic disease

174. All of the following statements concerning acquired immune deficiency syndrome (AIDS) in the newborn are true EXCEPT

(A) most commonly AIDS is contracted from an infected mother who is an intravenous drug abuser
(B) the newborn has a 90% chance of contracting AIDS if the mother is infected
(C) all infants of mothers with AIDS are human immunodeficiency virus (HIV)-positive whether or not the infants develop AIDS
(D) chronic mucocutaneous candidiasis is a common manifestation
(E) Kaposi's sarcoma tends to be less common and less aggressive than in adults

175. For informed consent, a patient must do all of the following EXCEPT

(A) sign a document consenting to the procedure
(B) understand what will happen if consent is not given
(C) understand the diagnosis
(D) understand the benefits of the procedure
(E) understand that consent can be withdrawn at any time

176. Characteristics of a generalized tonic–clonic (grand mal) seizure include all of the following EXCEPT

(A) tonic rigidity of all extremities, followed by 15 to 30 seconds of tremors
(B) urinary incontinence
(C) tongue- and/or cheek-biting
(D) clonic jerking for 1 to 2 minutes, followed by normal consciousness
(E) no localized onset in the primary form of the disease

177. Bile salt deficiency with subsequent malabsorption could be secondary to all of the following disorders EXCEPT

(A) cirrhosis of the liver
(B) Crohn's disease
(C) diverticular disease of the small bowel
(D) pancreatic insufficiency
(E) hyperlipidemia treated with cholestyramine

178. Characteristics of Wilms' tumor include all of the following EXCEPT

(A) hypertension
(B) unilateral palpable abdominal mass
(C) less than a 5% five-year survival rate
(D) propensity for lung metastasis
(E) association with chromosome-11 abnormalities

179. A 75-year-old obese woman with a 30 pack-year history of smoking presents with a 2-week history of fatigue and shortness of breath, particularly when she exerts herself or climbs stairs. She complains of nighttime episodes of difficulty breathing that require standing up and opening a window for air. Physical examination shows rales at both lung bases and a third heart sound. There is no evidence of peripheral pitting edema or neck vein distention. Which therapy would be LEAST indicated in this patient?

(A) Dietary salt restriction
(B) Weight loss
(C) Bed rest
(D) Furosemide
(E) Captopril

180. All of the following viruses are associated with congenital abnormalities EXCEPT

(A) varicella
(B) rubeola
(C) rubella
(D) cytomegalovirus (CMV)
(E) herpes simplex

181. Which patient is LEAST likely to be committed for involuntary treatment?

(A) A depressed man who expresses the intent to commit suicide
(B) A schizophrenic man who has threatened to kill his parents
(C) A borderline patient who has threatened to kill his psychiatrist
(D) An Alzheimer's patient who regularly starts fires in his apartment
(E) A homeless schizophrenic man

182. All of the following statements regarding febrile seizures are true EXCEPT

(A) they are tonic–clonic in nature and can last from a few seconds to 10 minutes
(B) they are uncommon before 9 months or after 5 years of age
(C) they may be associated with a family history
(D) they may be associated with upper respiratory infections, roseola, or acute otitis media
(E) they progress to epilepsy in 30% of patients

183. All of the following statements about childhood sexual abuse are true EXCEPT

(A) increased involvement of fathers in raising children decreases the risk of sexual abuse
(B) mothers who sexually abuse children are often lonely and emotionally deprived
(C) the majority of abused children are abused by fathers or stepfathers
(D) more women than men have a history of being abused
(E) more traditional, less democratic families are associated with an increased risk of abuse

184. All of the following characteristics are associated with child abuse EXCEPT

(A) environmental stresses (e.g., poverty)
(B) emotional immaturity in the adult
(C) single parenthood
(D) teenaged parents
(E) unwanted pregnancy

185. All of the following characteristics are consistent with menopause EXCEPT

(A) absence of menses for 1 year or more
(B) increased levels of follicle-stimulating hormone (FSH)
(C) atrophy of vaginal epithelium
(D) development of a cystocele
(E) enlargement of uterine leiomyomata

186. The Apgar score includes all of the following assessments EXCEPT

(A) blood pressure
(B) heart rate
(C) muscle tone
(D) respiratory effort
(E) respiratory catheter response in the nose

DIRECTIONS: Each set of matching questions in this section consists of a list of four to twenty-six lettered options (some of which may be in figures) followed by several numbered items. For each numbered item, select the ONE lettered option that is most closely associated with it. To avoid spending too much time on matching sets with large numbers of options, it is generally advisable to begin each set by reading the list of options. Then, for each item in the set, try to generate the correct answer and locate it in the option list, rather than evaluating each option individually. Each lettered option may be selected once, more than once, or not at all.

Questions 187–190

Match each clinical presentation with the location of the causative lesion.

(A) Nondominant frontal lobe
(B) Dominant frontal lobe
(C) Nondominant temporal lobe
(D) Dominant temporal lobe
(E) Nondominant parietal lobe
(F) Dominant parietal lobe
(G) Occipital lobes
(H) Temporal–occipital–parietal junction

187. A 65-year-old stroke patient cannot tell his right hand from his left hand

188. A 45-year-old stroke patient clearly can understand what someone says to him but he is unable to respond verbally to that person

189. Although he can repeat phrases, the speech of a 52-year-old stroke patient is impaired, and he has difficulty understanding what someone says to him

190. A well-educated stroke patient cannot add a column of four single-digit numbers

Questions 191–192

Match each description with the agent it best describes.

(A) Tissue plasminogen activator
(B) Warfarin
(C) Anistreplase
(D) Heparin
(E) Aspirin

191. The fibrinolytic action of this agent is confined to the formed thrombus. It is not antigenic in humans, and its action may be reversed by aminocaproic acid.

192. Some clinical studies have concluded that this agent, which irreversibly inhibits tissue cyclooxygenases, decreases the incidence of myocardial infarction.

Questions 193–195

Match each scenario with the test best suited for it.

(A) Minnesota Multiphasic Personality Inventory (MMPI)
(B) Rorschach Test
(C) Thematic Apperception Test (TAT)
(D) Sentence Completion Test (SCT)
(E) Halstead-Reitan Battery (HRB)
(F) Stanford-Binet Scale
(G) Wide-Range Achievement Test (WRAT)

193. Used by a primary care physician to evaluate depression in a 25-year-old patient

194. Used to evaluate the spelling skills of a 30-year-old patient

195. Used to localize the injured area in the brain of a patient who has been involved in a car accident

Questions 196–198

The lipoprotein cycle provides a framework for identification of the primary sites of action of drugs used in the treatment of atherosclerotic disease. Match each description with the agent that it best describes.

(A) Lovastatin
(B) Nicotinic acid (niacin)
(C) Cholestyramine
(D) Probucol
(E) Gemfibrozil

196. This drug increases the clearance of triglyceride-rich lipoproteins through the activation of lipoprotein lipases

197. Use of this drug requires monitoring plasma levels of transaminases and creatine kinase

198. Use of this drug leads to increases in the high-affinity low-density lipoprotein (LDL) and to increases in the liver catabolism of cholesterol

Questions 199–200

Match each disorder with the associated graph.

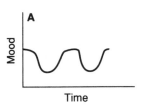
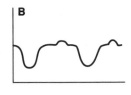
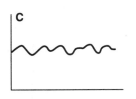
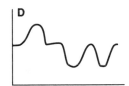
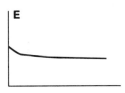

199. Cyclothymia

200. Bipolar II disorder

ANSWER KEY

1-C	31-A	61-A	91-E	121-A
2-B	32-C	62-A	92-B	122-B
3-E	33-D	63-D	93-E	123-E
4-C	34-B	64-C	94-C	124-D
5-C	35-C	65-C	95-B	125-C
6-A	36-D	66-B	96-A	126-D
7-A	37-B	67-A	97-D	127-A
8-B	38-A	68-E	98-D	128-D
9-D	39-B	69-A	99-C	129-B
10-C	40-D	70-B	100-C	130-B
11-E	41-B	71-A	101-D	131-A
12-D	42-A	72-D	102-B	132-D
13-C	43-C	73-D	103-A	133-C
14-D	44-C	74-C	104-A	134-E
15-D	45-C	75-E	105-A	135-D
16-D	46-E	76-E	106-C	136-A
17-B	47-D	77-A	107-D	137-C
18-A	48-A	78-B	108-E	138-C
19-E	49-C	79-D	109-B	139-D
20-A	50-A	80-D	110-B	140-A
21-C	51-E	81-C	111-C	141-E
22-D	52-C	82-D	112-D	142-A
23-B	53-B	83-C	113-E	143-A
24-A	54-B	84-C	114-A	144-E
25-E	55-B	85-B	115-D	145-A
26-C	56-B	86-E	116-C	146-B
27-C	57-B	87-B	117-A	147-C
28-C	58-A	88-D	118-D	148-E
29-B	59-C	89-B	119-D	149-E
30-D	60-C	90-C	120-B	150-A

151-A	161-D	171-D	181-E	191-A
152-A	162-A	172-D	182-E	192-E
153-E	163-A	173-E	183-C	193-A
154-D	164-E	174-B	184-C	194-G
155-B	165-B	175-A	185-E	195-E
156-A	166-D	176-D	186-A	196-E
157-E	167-B	177-D	187-F	197-A
158-C	168-D	178-C	188-B	198-C
159-B	169-B	179-C	189-H	199-C
160-C	170-B	180-B	190-F	200-B

ANSWERS AND EXPLANATIONS

1. The answer is C. *(General surgery; prognostic factors in breast cancer)*
The single most important prognostic factor in breast cancer is the lymph node status of the patient. For example, patients with no nodal involvement have an 80% 5-year survival rate; with one to three nodes involved, a 50% 5-year survival rate; and with four or more nodes involved, a 20% 5-year survival rate. Other prognostic factors in breast cancer include:

- Size of the tumor (Tumors smaller than 2 cm have a favorable prognosis.)
- The primary site (An axillary location is the worst, followed by the upper outer quadrant.)
- The histologic grade of the tumor (Patients with high-grade cancers do poorly.)
- The histologic type of cancer (Inflammatory carcinoma has the worst prognosis; tubular carcinoma has a good prognosis.)
- The presence or absence of estrogen/progesterone (ERA/PRA) receptors [Patients who are ERA/PRA receptor–positive appear to have a better remission rate (60% to 80% response rate), particularly if an endocrine-ablative treatment (e.g., tamoxifen) is administered, an antiestrogen agent is administered, or if the ovaries or adrenals have been ablated.]
- DNA ploidy (Diploidy indicates a normal multiple of 23 chromosomes and has a good prognosis; aneuploidy is an uneven multiple of 23 chromosomes and connotes a bad prognosis.)
- S phase fraction, which reflects the percentage of cells in the proliferating pool (A low S phase fraction is better than a high S phase fraction.)
- The cleanness of the surgical margins
- The presence or absence of activated c-*erb*2 (*neu* or HER-2) oncogene (Its presence indicates a poor prognosis.)

2. The answer is B. *(Pediatrics; roseola)*
Roseola infantum, also known as exanthema subitum, is a viral disease attributed to human herpesvirus type 6. The disease is most common between 6 months and 2 years of age, although patients described have been as old as 14 years. The fever is of sudden onset, with few physical findings, although there may be slight cold symptoms. Occasionally a febrile seizure may occur; otherwise the child looks quite well. The temperature is as high as 103°F to 106°F (39.4°C to 41.2°C). The fever falls by the third or fourth day, and a macular to maculopapular rash erupts, starting on the trunk and extending to the extremities, with only slight involvement of the face.

In contrast, the rash of measles occurs with the fever, starting on the neck and cheeks and spreading downward. As it reaches the feet, the rash starts fading on the face, proceeding downward. Desquamation occurs. The rash of erythema infectiosum begins as marked erythema of the cheeks ("slapped cheek" appearance), progresses to an erythematous maculopapular rash that invades the arms and spreads to the trunk and legs, and then lingers for 2 to 3 weeks, fluctuating in severity with environmental changes.

3. The answer is E. *(Nephrology; adult polycystic kidney disease)*
This patient has adult polycystic kidney disease, which shows up on the ultrasound as black spaces in the kidney parenchyma. Hematuria and hypertension are common presenting complaints. The disease has an autosomal-dominant inheritance pattern.

Patients with polycystic kidney disease do not have cysts present at birth. Renal function is usually retained until the third or fourth decade. There is an association with cysts in the liver (30%), berry aneurysms of the circle of Willis (10%–15%), and diverticulosis. The grandmother's stroke may have been secondary to a subarachnoid hemorrhage from a ruptured berry aneurysm.

Discomfort in the abdomen in this patient could be due to a ruptured cyst, bleeding into a cyst, or an infected cyst.

Long-term hemodialysis or renal transplantation is the recommended treatment for these patients.

Immunoglobulin A (IgA) nephropathy is the most common glomerulonephritis associated with hematuria. It commonly occurs in young men, who manifest microscopic hematuria a few days after an upper respiratory infection. Serum IgA levels are increased in 40% of patients. Immunofluorescent stains of glomeruli are strongly positive for IgA located predominantly in the mesangium. Approximately 50% of patients have a nephritic pattern, with hematuria, red blood cell (RBC) casts, and mild-to-moderate proteinuria; and the remainder present with a nephrotic pattern characterized by proteinuria greater than 3.5 g/24 hours. Corticosteroids are not useful in therapy. Approximately 75% of patients are well after 20 years.

Goodpasture's syndrome occurs most commonly in young men. Antibasement antibodies against pulmonary and glomerular capillaries are present. The disease initially presents with hemoptysis from pulmonary hemorrhage. Renal failure develops shortly thereafter. Glomerular biopsies show crescentic glomerulonephritis and a linear pattern of immunofluorescence. Plasmapheresis is useful in removing the antibodies. Cyclophosphamide is used to suppress antibody synthesis. Kidney transplantation is most successful when the antibasement membrane antibodies are not present.

A staghorn calculus is made up of magnesium ammonium phosphate (struvite). These calculi are commonly associated with urease-splitting organisms, such as *Proteus,* and production of an alkaline pH that favors stone formation.

Alport's syndrome is a genetic disease with varied patterns of inheritance and is particularly common in Mormons. It tends to be more common and more severe in boys than in girls, who frequently have a normal lifespan. It consists of nerve deafness and glomerulonephritis. Men usually die of renal failure by 40 years of age.

4. The answer is C. *(Pediatrics; juvenile rheumatoid arthritis)*
Juvenile rheumatoid arthritis is an autoimmune inflammatory disease that causes chronic synovitis as well as other extra-articular manifestations. This arthritis is divided into subgroups depending on presentation and laboratory findings. Systemic juvenile rheumatoid arthritis occurs in approximately one-fifth of patients and is associated with high fevers, rash, hepatosplenomegaly, pleural and pericardial effusions, leukocytosis, and anemia of chronic disease. The erythrocyte sedimentation rate (ESR) is elevated during active disease. Acute rheumatic fever can be differentiated from juvenile rheumatoid arthritis by the evidence of carditis and its transient migratory arthritis. Systemic lupus erythematosus (SLE) usually has milder joint manifestations and a characteristic malar rash. Lyme disease should be considered in the differential diagnosis. A careful history and physical examination, searching for tick bites and characteristic rash of erythema chronicum migrans, should be performed. Ankylosing spondylitis can be mistaken for juvenile rheumatoid arthritis until spine involvement is seen. Its onset is later in life and it is much more common in men.

5. The answer is C. *(Health maintenance/promotion; gender identity disorder)*
A sense of maleness or femaleness is generally established between age 2 and 3 years. Both genetic and social influences have been described in this process. Failure to develop accurate gender identity has been correlated with intersex physical abnormalities and with confusing rearing by caregivers.

6. The answer is A. *(Gynecology; menorrhagia)*
Dysfunctional uterine bleeding results from unopposed estrogen stimulation. The characteristic findings are anovulatory cycles, a normal pelvic examination, and often extremes of reproductive age. Hormonal manipulation, not surgery, is the treatment of choice.

7. The answer is A. (*General surgery; ulcerative colitis*)

The patient has ulcerative colitis, which is a chronic relapsing ulceroinflammatory disease primarily involving the rectum and left colon. Its etiology is unknown. There is a slightly increased incidence in females over males.

The clinical presentation is that of a young adult with fever, left-sided abdominal pain, bloody diarrhea with mucus, and rectal bleeding. Approximately 5% to 10% of patients may never have another attack after the initial episode but most have intermittent attacks often precipitated by stress.

The disease primarily involves the rectum, where it is confined in up to 50% of cases. The rectal mucosa is friable and bleeds easily. Ulcerative colitis can also involve the left colon in continuous fashion (i.e., no skip lesions) or the entire colon.

The treatment for ulcerative colitis is sulfasalazine, aminosalicylate enemas, and corticosteroid enemas (intravenous in very severe attacks). Surgery is indicated if there is a failure to respond to medications or if dysplasia or carcinoma is noted on biopsies. Surgery for extensive disease is mucosal proltectomy with anastomosis to the terminal ileum, thus preserving anal function.

Crohn's disease is an ulceroconstrictive inflammatory bowel disease that presents with right lower quadrant pain, fever, diarrhea, and perianal involvement. Ischemic bowel disease presents with diffuse abdominal pain and bloody diarrhea. Anal fissures produce severe rectal pain on defecation, bleeding, and anal tenderness.

8. The answer is B. (*Infectious disease; cytomegalovirus pneumonitis*)

The patient has the classic basophilic intranuclear inclusion of cytomegalovirus (CMV). CMV pneumonitis is particularly common in organ transplantation patients, especially bone marrow allograft recipients (10%–15%) and those with AIDS. CMV hyperimmune globulin given to seronegative bone marrow recipients provides some protection from contracting the infection. Ganciclovir is sometimes given to patients prior to transplantation as a preventive measure. It can

also be used in treatment of CMV. The mortality rate is 85%.

Pneumocystis carinii is not visualized with standard hematoxylin-eosin stains. Methenamine silver, Giemsa stains, and direct immunofluorescent stains are useful in identifying organisms in bronchial lavage specimens or biopsies of lung. The organisms look like crushed Ping-Pong balls.

Cryptococcus neoformans is the most common systemic fungal infection in the immunocompromised host. In tissue, it is an encapsulated yeast with narrow-based buds.

Blastomyces dermatitidis is a systemic fungal infection, which, in tissue, is a yeast with broad-based buds.

Candida albicans is a systemic fungal infection with yeast forms and pseudohyphae, the latter indicating the invasiveness of the organism.

Pneumocystis, Cryptococcus, Blastomyces, and *Candida* do not produce intranuclear inclusions.

9. The answer is D. (*Gynecology; ectopic pregnancy*)

In utero exposure to diethylstilbestrol (DES), a previous ectopic pregnancy, an implanted intrauterine device (IUD), and a tubal ligation within the past 2 years are all risk factors for ectopic pregnancy. However, the highest increase in risk (eightfold increase) is experienced by women with a history of pelvic inflammatory disease (PID).

10. The answer is C. (*Biostatistics; randomized controlled trial*)

The key elements in this study include randomization of study and control groups and the double-blind use of placebo and aspirin. These factors are the hallmarks of the randomized controlled trial.

11. The answer is E. (*Health maintenance/promotion; antisocial behavior*)

Antisocial behavior is most prevalent in young men, and it decreases greatly after age 40. The onset of antisocial behavior is often before midadolescence. It is associated with chaotic family settings, it tends to remain as a constant personality trait for a prolonged period, and it is characterized by a lack of guilt.

12. The answer is D. *(Neurology; ulnar neuropathy)*

The diagnosis of neuropathy can be confirmed and localized by both nerve conduction velocity (NCV) studies and electromyography (EMG).

Although a 2-day history of severe low-back pain, leg weakness, and loss of bladder control indicates severe nerve damage, EMG is of very limited use in a process of less than 3 weeks' duration, and the severe deficit would argue instead for an emergent imaging study [e.g., magnetic resonance imaging (MRI) or myelography]. Joint pain would be unlikely to have a neurogenic basis. Myelitis associated with multiple sclerosis would not likely involve the nerve roots. Finally, if a neurologic deficit is known and demonstrated by another test, EMG would add little to the diagnosis, and it would be best to begin appropriate therapy.

13. The answer is C. *(Urology; prostate cancer staging)*

The patient has a low-grade prostate cancer (Gleason score of four) and is stage B1, since the tumor was palpable on rectal examination and was confined to one lobe.

Prostate cancer is the most common cancer in men and is the second most common cause of death. The lifetime risk for an American man to develop clinically evident prostate cancer is 10%. It seldom occurs before age 50, but the incidence increases from 10% of men in their fifties to 70% of men in their eighties. The most important risk factor is age. Men who have an affected first-degree relative (brother or father) or an affected second-degree relative (uncle or grandfather) have an eightfold increase in risk. Blacks have a higher incidence of prostate cancer, which is androgen induced, because they have slightly higher testosterone levels.

Most prostate cancers are located in the posterior lobe, thus making them amenable to diagnosis by rectal examination. Approximately 50% of palpable nodules are confirmed as being cancerous. Prostate cancers grow peripherally through the capsule and frequently invade the seminal vesicles and the neck of the bladder. Much of the spread of prostate cancer is through perineural

spaces. Metastatic spread is both lymphatic and hematogenous, the former affecting the obturator and iliac nodes first, whereas the latter route is generally to bone, where it produces osteoblastic metastases. Osteoblastic metastases elevate the serum alkaline phosphatase level. Lymph node metastases occur earlier than bone metastases.

Approximately 60% of patients have localized cancer when first diagnosed. Most patients are asymptomatic or have symptoms of lower urinary tract obstruction. Patients with advanced disease present with bladder outlet obstruction with azotemia and urinary retention, anemia, or bone pain.

Screening tests include serum prostatic acid phosphatase (PAP), prostate-specific antigen (PSA), and rectal examination. A positive PAP, PSA, or rectal examination should be evaluated with transrectal ultrasound examination and core needle biopsies of suspicious lesions.

There is an excellent correlation between prognosis and the grade of prostate cancer. The Gleason scoring system is generally utilized. It is based on patterns, which are given a score; two is the lowest score and lowest grade, and ten is the highest score and highest grade. Staging of prostate cancer is as follows:

Stage A: Clinically unsuspected or incidental cancer:
  A1: Tumor involves < 5% of the curettings.
  A2: Tumor involves > 5% of the curettings.
Stage B: Tumor palpable on rectal examination:
  B1: Tumor is confined to one lobe.
  B2: Tumor is present in both lobes.
Stage C: Tumor extends outside the confines of the prostate but is not metastatic:
  C1: Tumor does not involve seminal vesicles.
  C2: Tumor involves seminal vesicles and periprostatic tissue.
Stage D: Metastasis present:
  D1: Tumor is thought to be at one of the above stages clinically but lymph nodes are involved at surgery.
  D2: There is evidence of spread to bone or elsewhere.

Radical prostatectomy is an option for patients with stages A2, B1, and B2 who are considered to be candidates for surgical cure. The nerve-sparing operation of Walsh preserves potency in a majority of patients. Pelvic lymphadenectomy has not been determined to be of therapeutic value but allows for more precise staging. Radiotherapy is effective in treating pain due to metastatic bone disease. Hormonal therapy is generally used for the treatment of metastatic disease. Orchiectomy or the administration of estrogens removes 90% to 95% of the circulating testosterone. Luteinizing hormone–releasing hormone (LHRH)-agonists (e.g., leuprolide) are as effective as orchiectomy or estrogen therapy. Flutamide is a nonsteroidal antiandrogen agent that can be used with an LHRH agonist. It blocks the uptake and nuclear binding of androgens in the target tissues.

The 15-year survival rate for patients with radical prostatectomies for cure is equivalent to age or matched control population. Recently, the use of radical prostatectomy for cure has been challenged.

14. The answer is D. *(Pediatrics; intracranial hemorrhage)*
Trauma is the most common cause of intracranial hemorrhage in children. In infants, intracranial hemorrhage can result from trauma or asphyxia. Aneurysms and arteriovenous malformations are less common causes of hemorrhage in children. Hypertension is rarely involved.

15. The answer is D. *(Gynecology; polycystic ovary disease)*
The major mechanism at work in polycystic ovary disease is an elevated luteinizing hormone (LH) level that is unresponsive to menstrual fluctuations. The body mass index is usually high. Although hirsutism is often seen, virilization is not. Menarche is usually normal.

16. The answer is D. *(General surgery; small bowel infarction)*
The patient has a small bowel infarction. These most commonly occur in elderly patients with atherosclerotic disease. In 50% of cases, the pathogenesis relates to sudden occlusion of the superior mesenteric artery by thrombosis over an atherosclerotic plaque (most common), embo-

lism from the left heart, vasculitis (uncommon), aortic aneurysm repair, or dissections of the aorta (uncommon). In 25% of cases, nonocclusive infarction can occur from vasospasm (e.g., from sympathomimetic drugs, digitalis), hypovolemia, and hypotension. Superior mesenteric vein occlusion also occurs in 25% of cases and is related to hypercoagulable states associated with polycythemia rubra vera, oral contraceptives, malignancy, and the hereditary hypercoagulable states (e.g., antithrombin III deficiency, protein C and S deficiencies).

Transmural, hemorrhagic infarctions damage the integrity of the mucosa, thus predisposing the bowel to secondary bacterial penetration and generalized peritonitis. The reestablishment of blood flow frequently results in further damage due to reavailability of oxygen to help form free radicals.

Small bowel infarction is often preceded by abdominal angina (mesenteric angina), with pain 30 minutes after eating. Because of the pain, patients have a fear of eating, and they lose weight. Findings associated with bowel infarction are the sudden onset of severe abdominal pain with vomiting and abdominal distention that is out of proportion with the physical findings. The bowel sounds are absent. Peritoneal signs (e.g., rebound tenderness) are generally late findings.

Laboratory findings include a striking neutrophilic leukocytosis with left shift. There is an increased serum amylase concentration of bowel origin that is often misinterpreted as representing acute hemorrhagic pancreatitis. Barium studies reveal "thumbprinting" of the mucosa due to submucosal hemorrhages and edema.

The treatment of the ischemic bowel must occur within 12 hours; otherwise a 100% mortality rate can be expected. Surgery is always indicated if a grossly obvious hemorrhagic infarction has already occurred. Visible peristalsis is the best way to determine if the bowel is viable or dead. Embolectomy and intra-arterial vasodilators are also used, depending on the cause of the ischemia.

The situation in this case is an unlikely clinical presentation for acute ulcerative colitis, which is most often seen in young adults. Although hemorrhagic pancreatitis involves an elevated concentration of serum amylase, it is not associated with diffuse abdominal pain and bloody diarrhea. An aortoenteric fistula is usually a late complication of repair of an abdominal aortic aneurysm.

17. The answer is B. *(Pediatrics; ataxia–telangiectasia)*
Ataxia–telangiectasia is an autosomal-recessive disorder and the most common of the degenerative ataxias. The ataxia usually begins at approximately 2 years of age. It is progressive until full loss of ambulation occurs by adolescence. Telangiectasia is seen in the eyes, bridge of the nose, ears, and exposed surfaces of the extremities. The skin also loses elasticity. Frequent sinopulmonary infections occur secondary to abnormal immune function. Low immunoglobulin A (IgA) and IgE levels are seen. The alphafetoprotein level is elevated. Children with ataxia–telangiectasia have a much higher risk of developing lymphoreticular and brain tumors.

18. The answer is A. *(Psychiatry; psychotherapy)*
Much literature suggests that cognitive psychotherapy approaches antidepressant medication in efficacy for a single episode of major depression without psychosis. The task in cognitive psychotherapy is to define and change the thoughts and beliefs that lead to the depressive mood. The effectiveness of this technique is not well documented for psychogenic amnesia, substance abuse and dependence, dementia caused by neurodegenerative disease, or borderline personality disorder.

19. The answer is E. *(Neurology; diabetes)*
The pure motor hemiparesis described would most likely be associated with a small lacunar infarct of the left internal capsule. The signs and symptoms are generally part of small-vessel disease, usually associated with diabetes, hypertension, or smoking. Large-vessel disease from the carotid artery is unlikely because a stroke in this area would also cause aphasia. Warfarin and aspirin have their place in medical management

of cardiac and large-vessel disease, respectively, but neither fits this scenario. Although this patient is also likely to be at risk for heart disease, cardiac medications would not necessarily confer protection to the central nervous system (CNS).

20. The answer is A. *(Gynecology; adenomyosis)*
Adenomyosis is a benign condition, usually developing in the later reproductive years, in which endometrial glands are found within the myometrium. Menstrual flow is frequently increased. Diagnosis is basically histologic, and the only effective treatment is surgical.

21. The answer is C. *(Health maintenance/promotion; stress)*
Dissociative symptoms are engendered by unbearable stress, and they are much more common during disasters. These symptoms include emotional numbing, amnesia, feelings of unreality, and peculiar personality changes. They are seen in such disorders as dissociative (psychogenic) amnesia, dissociative (psychogenic) fugue, depersonalization disorder, and acute and posttraumatic stress disorder.

22. The answer is D. *(Pediatrics; IgG_2 subclass deficiency)*
Patients with immunoglobulin G (IgG) subclass deficiencies present clinically like patients with panhypogammaglobulinemia; that is, they are susceptible to recurrent infections. However, laboratory studies show normal immunoglobulin levels. Only when subclasses of IgG are evaluated is an abnormality found. Patients with Chédiak-Higashi syndrome have a defect in the neutrophil granules. These patients have photophobia, nystagmus, and partial albinism. Their bleeding time is prolonged, but their platelet counts are normal. Chronic granulomatous disease (CGD) is another neutrophil disorder, characterized by recurrent infections with uncommon organisms. Wiskott-Aldrich syndrome shows elevated IgA and IgE levels, decreased IgM levels, and decreased platelets. Job syndrome is characterized by high levels of IgE.

23. The answer is B. *(Psychiatry; bipolar disorder)*
This patient's condition is highly suggestive of bipolar disorder. Although lithium is the drug of choice, approximately 25% of patients do not respond to it. It would be unwise to increase the dose in this patient, since his blood level is already at the top of the therapeutic range. Carbamazepine is the second drug of choice. Some patients who do not respond to lithium will respond to carbamazepine.

24. The answer is A. *(Endocrinology; congenital adrenal hyperplasia)*
The findings in the 8-month-old patient are compatible with 21-hydroxylase deficiency, an enzymatic defect in cortisol synthesis that characterizes congenital adrenal hyperplasia. The excess androgen causes external genital masculinization in the genetic female.

Cortisol production is reduced, with a subsequent increase in plasma levels of adrenocorticotropic hormone (ACTH). The decreased cortisol levels result in a loss of vigor and appetite, as well as hypoglycemia since cortisol is a gluconeogenic hormone.

In 21-hydroxylase deficiency, the urine concentration of 17-hydroxycorticosteroids is decreased (deoxycortisol and cortisol plus their metabolites comprise the 17-hydroxycorticosteroids). The weak mineralocorticoids (i.e., deoxycorticosterone and corticosterone) are decreased as well, which results in salt loss and volume depletion.

In 11-hydroxylase deficiency, the urine concentration of 17-hydroxycorticosteroids is increased since deoxycortisol is increased. Deoxycorticosterone is also increased, which produces salt retention and hypertension.

In 17-hydroxylase deficiency, both the 17-KS and 17-hydroxycorticosteroid concentrations are decreased. However, the mineralocorticoids are not inhibited; therefore, affected patients have hypertension. In addition, since 17-hydroxylase is also present in the ovaries and testes for the synthesis of 17-KS, testosterone, and estrogens, a deficiency of both male and female hormones results in both sexes having a female phenotype regardless of the genetic sex.

25. The answer is E. *(Gynecology; urinary stress incontinence)*
Genuine urinary stress incontinence is characterized by a loss of the urethral/vesicle angle when increases in intra-abdominal/intravesicle pressure fail to be transmitted to the urethra. No change occurs in voiding flow rate, residual urine, or bladder compliance.

26. The answer is C. *(General surgery; anal fissure)*
The patient has an anal fissure. Anal fissures produce severe rectal pain on defecation, bleeding, and anal tenderness. A sentinel pile is located below the fissure, and a hypertrophied papilla is above the fissure.

The mainstay for medical treatment is stool softeners. Increased water intake and topical hydrocortisone creams are also useful. If medical treatment is unsuccessful, internal sphincterotomy is indicated.

Hemorrhoids are dilated venous plexuses derived from the superior hemorrhoidal vein (internal hemorrhoids) or inferior hemorrhoidal veins (external hemorrhoids), or both. Predisposing conditions include pregnancy, straining at stool, and cirrhosis with portal hypertension.

Bleeding is the first symptom of internal hemorrhoids. Complications include thrombosis, strangulation, ulceration, infection, and anal fissures from passage of hard stools. The major modalities of therapy include patient education of proper dietary and bowel habits, banding, cryosurgery, sclerotherapy, laser surgery, and hemorrhoidectomy.

Thrombosed external hemorrhoids are treated with sitz baths, stool softeners, or by excision of the skin with evacuation of the thrombus if pain has not subsided in 48 hours.

Solitary rectal ulcers are uncommon. They produce pain on defecation and can be associated with massive lower gastrointestinal bleeding.

27. The answer is C. *(Pediatrics; chlamydial pneumonia)*
Chlamydial pneumonia in infants presents at 3 to 16 weeks of age. Typically the infants appear quite well, are afebrile, but have been ill with

tachypnea and a prominent cough. Rales, and sometimes wheezing, can be heard. Conjunctivitis is present in approximately 50% of patients. Hyperinflation and patchy infiltrates are seen on chest x-ray, and eosinophilia is apparent on complete blood count (CBC).

28. The answer is C. *(General medicine; treatment of hyperlipidemia)*
Dietary management [i.e., following a diet low in fat (less than 30% total fat)] is the most important initial step in lowering the cholesterol level. Following a low-fat diet can lower the cholesterol level by approximately 10%. Restricting carbohydrate intake decreases the synthesis of very-low-density lipoprotein (VLDL) by the liver, therefore decreasing the level of triglycerides. Increasing the intake of soluble fiber (e.g., psyllium) also lowers the cholesterol level.

Drugs are reserved for people who do not reach their ideal cholesterol level by diet and exercise after a minimum of 6 months. Reducing stress has no significant effect in lowering the cholesterol level.

29. The answer is B. *(Psychiatry; schizophrenia)*
This description suggests schizophrenia. Many studies indicate that readjustment to family life is improved if family stress and conflict, sometimes called expressed emotions, are kept as low as possible. Although it would be inadvisable to put too much pressure on the patient by insisting that he engage in stressful activities, gradual social involvement should be encouraged.

30. The answer is D. *(Neurology; lead toxicity)*
The patient likely has acute lead toxicity, which can present as wristdrop in an adult or as encephalopathy in a child. A nerve conduction velocity (NCV) study would only confirm the clinical diagnosis, not give the cause. X-rays and magnetic resonance imaging (MRI) scans would give uninformative structural information. Diabetes is the most common cause of neuropathy, but it would be very unlikely to present initially as a motor neuropathy, because it usually affects sensory fibers clinically first.

31. The answer is A. *(General surgery; Leriche syndrome)*
The patient has Leriche syndrome. This is due to aortoiliac atherosclerotic disease and is characterized by claudication on walking, atrophy of the calf muscles, diminished or absent femoral pulses, and impotence from involvement of the hypogastric arteries.

A herniated lumbar disc would not have a claudication history or problems with femoral pulses. Motor and sensory deficits would be present as well. Osteoarthritis in the hip produces pain that is relieved by the use of a cane. It is not associated with vascular findings. Phlegmasia alba dolens is a variant of femoral vein thrombosis in which there is femoral artery spasm, which produces a pale, cool leg with increased pulses.

32. The answer is C. *(Psychiatry; major depression)*
Maintenance therapy after response to antidepressants generally is recommended to continue for 6 months. Quick relapse is more likely if antidepressants are stopped earlier. Some studies now suggest much longer treatment after recovery from a depressive episode, but only if the patient has a history of multiple relapses.

33. The answer is D. *(Gynecology; male factor infertility)*
The normal values on semen analysis are as follows: sperm count is 20 to 250 million/ml; motility is greater than 50%; volume is 2 to 5 ml; morphology is greater than 50% normal forms; pH is 7.2 to 7.8. The parameters are normal in this man, except for the semen morphology.

34. The answer is B. *(Pharmacology; chemotherapy)*
HIV-positive patients with unexplained persistent fevers or oropharyngeal candidiasis are at risk for *Pneumocystis carinii* pneumonia and should receive prophylactic chemotherapy (e.g., trimethoprim–sulfamethoxazole). The physician has no reason to increase the zidovudine dose because the CD4 count has not dropped precipitously, but the count should be closely monitored. For mild oropharyngeal candidiasis, treatment

with clotrimazole in oral troche form is more appropriate than oral ketoconazole, which has the potential to cause adverse systemic effects.

35. The answer is C. *(Neurology; quadrantanopia)*
A lesion of the inferior chiasm would result in fibers crossing to the temporal areas, causing a bitemporal quadrantanopia, as may be seen in pituitary tumors. Choice A is incorrect because a parietal lesion would give an *inferior* quadrantanopia. Choice B violates the rule that lesions behind the chiasm give contralateral deficits. An enlarged blind spot (choice D) is associated with *high* intracranial pressure. Blindness in the left eye suggests a lesion anterior to the chiasm. A right occipital lesion would give a left homonymous hemianopsia.

36. The answer is D. *(Psychiatry; generalized anxiety disorder)*
This patient has generalized anxiety disorder. Buspirone is often considered the drug of second choice for this illness, and it is especially useful for patients who cannot tolerate the benzodiazepine-induced cognitive changes. Tapering the diazepam would be less likely to help, because the patient's residual anxiety would probably worsen. Alprazolam is less sedating, but its very short half-life and high potential for dependence make its use problematic for generalized anxiety disorder.

37. The answer is B. *(General surgery; subclavian steal syndrome)*
The patient has subclavian steal syndrome, which is characterized by the development of neurologic symptoms upon exercising. There is proximal subclavian stenosis or occlusion with reversal of flow through the vertebral artery (collateral for blood flow to the arm), which produces cerebral ischemia. Treatment consists of bypass grafting from the common carotid to the subclavian artery distal to the humerus.

Thoracic outlet syndrome refers to an abnormal compression of arteries, veins, or nerves in the neck. The compression can be secondary to a cervical rib, the anterior scalene muscle, or posi-tional changes. Patients present with pain, paresthesias, or numbness in the distribution of one or more trunks of the brachial plexus (commonly ulnar). Symptoms are associated with positional changes or downward traction of the shoulder or numbness during sleep. There is muscular atrophy in the hand, and the radial pulse is weakened by abduction of the arm with the head turned in the opposite direction (Adson's test). Percussion over the brachial plexus reproduces symptoms (Tinel's test). A bruit is frequently heard over the subclavian artery. The diagnosis is made with arteriography. Nerve conduction studies do not distinguish this disease from cervical disk disease. Treatment includes postural correction, physical therapy, first rib resection, or excision of the anterior scalene muscle.

Cervical disk disease produces compressive neuropathies with sensory and motor signs and symptoms. Computed tomography (CT) is useful in identifying nerve root encroachment in the vertebral foramens, while magnetic resonance imaging (MRI) is best for detecting spinal cord compression.

38. The answer is A. *(Gynecology; uterine leiomyomata)*
Submucosal myomata can distort the overlying endometrium altering its normal response to hormonal changes through the menstrual cycle. This change can lead to abnormal bleeding. Subserosal, intramural, intraligamentous, and pedunculated myomata, because of their anatomic locations, have no direct impact on uterine bleeding.

39. The answer is B. *(Biostatistics; positively skewed distribution)*
A positively skewed distribution has a few extreme values much greater than the other values. This aspect tends to drag the mean in the same direction as the skew. The median is much less affected, and the mode is the least affected. Therefore, the index of central tendency with the lowest magnitude would be the mode. The mean would have the highest magnitude, and the median would be midway.

40. The answer is D. *(Pediatrics; Wiskott-Aldrich syndrome)*
Wiskott-Aldrich syndrome is an X-linked recessive disorder. An eczematoid rash is often the first clinical manifestation. Recurrent and chronic infections (e.g., otitis and pneumonia) are common. Thrombocytopenia and lymphopenia are seen. Serum levels of immunoglobulin E (IgE) and IgA are elevated; the level of IgM is decreased. Patients are susceptible to malignant reticuloendotheliosis.

41. The answer is B. *(Gynecology; uterine leiomyomata)*
Carneous degeneration is associated with acute bleeding within the myoma. The irritation of the blood causes an inflammatory reaction and subsequent pain. Hyaline, calcareous, cystic, and myxomatous types of degeneration are gradual and are usually not associated with pain.

42. The answer is A. *(Psychiatry; opiate abuse)*
Methadone can be used to treat heroin addiction only in federally licensed programs that are mandated to provide a range of rehabilitative services. It can be administered only to patients who have a well-documented history of heroin addiction. Such programs have been demonstrated to be highly effective in improving psychosocial function in many patients. Unfortunately, concurrent use of methadone and heroin is quite common.

43. The answer is C. *(Pharmacology; chemotherapy)*
In addition to its activity against *Pneumocystis carinii,* trimethoprim–sulfamethoxazole is effective against *Nocardia* species and *Toxoplasma.* The drug combination has no significant activity against *Cryptococcus* or viral pathogens. Its role in prevention of bacterial infections due to Enterobacteriaceae in the acquired immune deficiency syndrome (AIDS) patient remains controversial, because resistant strains have emerged during prophylaxis and oral colonization with yeasts is increased.

44. The answer is C. *(Otolaryngology; otosclerosis)*
The patient has otosclerosis, which refers to sclerosis and fixation of the middle ear ossicles associated with a conductive type of hearing loss and possible deafness. It may be bilateral and has a strong autosomal-dominant inheritance pattern. It is the most common cause of conductive hearing loss in adults.

Presbycusis is the most common cause of nerve deafness in adults. It is associated with a progressive, predominantly symmetric, high-frequency hearing loss, and there is a loss of speech discrimination, particularly in noisy places. There is a genetic predisposition.

Chronic otitis media can be associated with the ingrowth of keratinizing squamous epithelium, which is called a cholesteatoma.

45. The answer is C. *(Behavioral science; cancer deaths in women)*
The leading causes of cancer death in the United States in women in descending order are lung, breast, and colorectal cancer. The increased rate of lung cancer is associated with the increased rate of smoking by American women.

46. The answer is E. *(Gynecology; cervical ectropion)*
Ectropion of the cervix is a condition in which columnar epithelium from the endocervical canal extends out to the ectocervix. This benign condition requires no treatment other than observation. Over time, under the influence of the normally acidic vaginal pH, the columnar epithelium will undergo squamous metaplasia to become stratified squamous epithelium.

47. The answer is D. *(Pediatrics; gray syndrome)*
Gray syndrome, a potentially fatal toxic reaction to chloramphenicol, is described in neonates. It probably occurs secondary to an immature liver, which cannot properly metabolize the drug, and high levels of unconjugated chloramphenicol are the result. Circulatory collapse occurs, and the infant develops an ashen or gray cyanosis.

48. The answer is A. *(Preventive medicine; drug abuse)*

Tertiary prevention refers to prevention of complications resulting from a given pathology. Disulfiram is used to prevent relapse into alcohol dependency by making it physically impossible to tolerate alcohol. Drug education would be a primary prevention measure since it is designed to prevent the onset of chemical dependence.

49. The answer is C. *(Psychiatry; cognitive disorder)*

Tacrine has been moderately effective in improving cognitive performance in patients with mild Alzheimer's dementia. Its therapeutic effectiveness is presumedly due to its inhibition of acetylcholinesterase and resultant higher levels of acetylcholine in the central nervous system (CNS). Because of potential hepatotoxicity, it is contraindicated in patients with liver disease.

50. The answer is A. *(Orthopedics; wrist bone fractures and avascular necrosis)*

The scaphoid is the most common bone that is fractured in the wrist and the bone most likely to be associated with avascular necrosis because of its poor blood supply. Approximately 2% to 5% of these fractures are not visible on radiograph, but they should be suspected if there is tenderness on the radial side of the wrist.

The hamate bone is infrequently fractured in golfers. The lunate bone is more commonly dislocated than fractured. It can be associated with avascular necrosis (Kienböck's disease). The triquetrum and capitate bones are protected and are very infrequently fractured.

51. The answer is E. *(Preventive medicine; drug abuse)*

A number of studies have demonstrated that teaching children and adolescents to resist peer pressure to use drugs is the most effective strategy for preventing substance abuse. Giving facts, issuing warnings, creating alternative activities, and improving general psychological health are good ends in themselves, but few data have suggested that these four approaches decrease substance abuse.

52–53. The answers are: 52-C, 53-B. *(Pharmacology; anesthesia and analgesia)*

The signs and symptoms described in this patient are consistent with a diagnosis of malignant hyperthermia. Although the occurrence rate of malignant hyperthermia during anesthesia is less than 1 in 10,000, the mortality rate is high (greater than 50%).

Malignant hyperthermia has generally been associated with halothane and succinylcholine administration, but it has occurred following the use of other halogenated gas anesthetics. In susceptible patients, abnormal excitation–contraction coupling occurs in muscle cells, resulting in prolongation of the myosin–actin interaction. Paradoxical contraction of jaw musculature (trismus) following succinylcholine administration is a possible premonitory sign.

Dantrolene interferes with muscle contraction by inhibiting calcium ion release from the sarcoplasmic reticulum. Dantrolene is a safe drug, although generalized muscle weakness may occur, resulting in respiratory insufficiency and sometimes aspiration pneumonitis.

Certain other diseases can present like malignant hyperthermic crisis, including sepsis, thyroid storm, and pheochromocytoma. A similar syndrome has also been described in patients early in treatment with antipsychotic drugs that block dopamine receptors in the nigrostriatal tracts of the brain.

54. The answer is B. *(Gynecology; endometriosis)*

Currently, surgery is the only definitive treatment for endometriosis. The condition typically occurs in the early reproductive years. The most common sites of occurrence, in order of frequency, are ovaries, cul-de-sac, uterosacral ligaments, broad ligaments, and oviducts. Endometriosis is not associated with endometrioid carcinoma of the ovary.

55. The answer is B. *(Behavioral science; informed consent)*

In order for a competent patient to make an informed decision, the physician is required to tell the patient the consequences of refusing treatment. The patient must understand the diagnosis, treatment, alternatives to treatment, and risks and benefits of agreeing to and of refusing a procedure.

56. The answer is B. *(Pediatrics; mycobacterial infection)*
Lymphadenitis is the most common presentation of atypical mycobacterial infection in children. The submandibular or anterior cervical nodes are most frequently involved. *Mycobacterium scrofulaceum* and *M. avium–intracellulare* infections are most common in the United States. Involvement is usually unilateral, and chest x-ray is normal. Many times there is no history of exposure to tuberculosis. Skin testing is usually negative or indeterminate. Differential diagnosis includes other mycobacterial infections as well as cat-scratch disease.

57. The answer is B. *(Infectious disease; herpes simplex keratoconjunctivitis)*
The patient has herpes simplex keratoconjunctivitis. A fluorescein stain exhibits the classic dendritic type of shallow ulcer with an irregular edge. Herpes labialis may or may not be present. Corneal involvement is frequently precipitated by topical corticosteroids or systemic corticosteroid therapy. Steroid therapy frequently results in deeper penetration of the ulcer.

Topical idoxuridine, vidarabine, or trifluridine can be used for treatment. Ophthalmologists frequently denude the infected corneal epithelium to enhance recovery.

Topical phenylephrine is a decongestant. Topical ketoconazole is used in fungal corneal ulcers, which are rare. Topical erythromycin and sulfacetamide are both useful for bacterial conjunctivitis.

58. The answer is A. *(Psychiatry; social phobia)*
Assertiveness training is the treatment of choice for social phobia. This technique involves education, role-reversal, desensitization, and role-playing. Some studies indicate that monoamine oxidase (MAO) inhibitors such as phenelzine are also useful. Buspirone is used occasionally.

59. The answer is C. *(Preventive medicine; geriatric health)*
Approximately half of medically hospitalized elderly patients have a diagnosable psychiatric illness. This percentage contrasts with a prevalence of 10% in the general elderly population. In nursing homes, the incidence of diagnosable mental disorders is well over 75%.

60. The answer is C. *(Gynecology; benign ovarian tumors)*
Endometrioid tumors, with characteristic psammoma bodies, have the highest malignant potential among the options listed. With respect to serous tumors, 70% are benign, 10% are borderline, and 20% are invasive malignancies. Serous histology appears to be derived from ciliated tubal epithelium. Of mucinous tumors, 85% are benign. Mucinous histology appears to be derived from columnar endocervical epithelium. Brenner's tumors, with histology that appears to be derived from transitional cell epithelium, are seldom malignant. Teratomas are rarely malignant.

61. The answer is A. *(Pharmacology; anesthesia and analgesia)*
Between 1% and 2% of all pregnant patients require surgery, with appendectomy being the most commonly performed abdominal surgery. Spinal anesthesia ("saddle block") would usually be preferred because it minimizes drug effects on the fetus. The risks of general anesthesia using inhalational agents (halothane or methoxyflurane) include failed intubation, pulmonary aspiration, and fetal drug exposure. Likewise, the highly lipid-soluble intravenous anesthetics rapidly equilibrate with fetal blood and would contribute to depressed Apgar scores if preterm labor and delivery occurred. The cardiac stimulant actions of ketamine would also increase blood loss. Epidural anesthesia requires high concentrations of local anesthetic, with attendant risks of unintentional intravascular or intrathecal injection.

62. The answer is A. *(Psychiatry; psychotherapy)*
Psychodynamic psychotherapy is often the most effective treatment for personality disorders and adjustment disorders. Although such therapy may be a useful adjunct for the other disorders listed, behavioral therapies are usually considered as treatments of first choice for substance abuse, obsessive–compulsive disorder, simple phobias, and social phobia. Antipsychotic medication combined with supportive and social psychotherapies is usually indicated in schizophrenia and schizophreniform disorder.

63. The answer is D. *(Sturge-Weber disease)*
Sturge-Weber disease is associated with a port-wine–stained nevus contralateral to the vascular malformation. The ash-leaf spot is associated with tuberous sclerosis. Mees lines are associated with arsenic poisoning. Pseudohypertrophy of the calves is associated with Duchenne and Becker muscular dystrophy; by contrast, patients with Charcot-Marie-Tooth disease have "stork legs."

64. The answer is C. *(Orthopedics; Legg-Calvé-Perthes disease)*
The patient has Legg-Calvé-Perthes disease. This disease is more common in boys than girls, primarily affecting children between the ages of 3 and 12 years. It presents as a slowly evolving, painless limp. Pain is most frequently referred to the groin area. The leg is shorter on the affected side. Radiographs reveal increased density in the femoral head. Magnetic resonance imaging (MRI), however, is preferred for making the diagnosis. Treatment varies from observation to surgery, in which the joint is braced so proper remodeling of bone can occur.

Osteoarthritis is a disease of the elderly and would not be expected in a 9-year-old patient.

Osteomyelitis is accompanied by other systemic signs and is most commonly located in the metaphysis of bone.

A slipped capital femoral epiphysis is most commonly seen in obese adolescent boys from 9 to 15 years of age. Pain is classically located on the medial aspect of the knee.

Osteogenic sarcoma is the most common primary malignant bone tumor. It is most often seen in adolescents and young adults and involves the distal femur or the proximal tibia.

65. The answer is C. *(Public health; hospital medical care)*
Most of the population receives medical care in voluntary hospitals, which are not-for-profit and are either owned privately or sponsored by churches, universities, or community governments. There are approximately 6000 voluntary hospitals in the United States. Investor-owned hospitals, which are for-profit facilities, number about 830; state mental hospitals about 300; and federal hospitals about 350.

66. The answer is B. *(Gynecology; amenorrhea)*
A positive progesterone challenge test indicates only that the patient has an adequate amount of estrogen to prepare her endometrium for ripening and shedding by progesterone. It is not helpful as a pregnancy test. It cannot rule out a pituitary adenoma. Even a spotting response is adequate to be a positive test. Primary and secondary amenorrhea can be differentiated from a good history.

67. The answer is A. *(Pediatrics; erythema infectiosum)*
Erythema infectiosum (fifth disease) is a mild exanthematous disease caused by a parvovirus. Usually there is no prodrome, and fever is low grade or absent. The rash usually starts on the cheeks, which appear to have been slapped. Following the bright-red and confluent rash, an erythematous maculopapular rash appears on the trunk, although it can precede the facial rash. The rash then fades, giving a lacy or reticular appearance. The rash is often pruritic, but does not desquamate, as seen with measles. Other symptoms include headache, rhinitis, arthralgia, and arthritis, but these symptoms are more common in adults.

68. The answer is E. *(Biostatistics; infant mortality rate)*
The infant mortality rate is calculated by dividing the number of deaths within the first year of life

by the total number of live births. In the scenario presented, there were 11 infant deaths and 2100 live births, so the correct answer is 11/2100.

69. The answer is A. *(Psychiatry; psychotherapy)*
Behavioral therapies are often effective for social phobia and drug abuse. In both disorders, the problematic behavior is well defined and measurable, and the disorders lend themselves to behavioral techniques. Behavioral therapy is also the treatment of choice for many psychiatric disorders of children.

70. The answer is B. *(Orthopedics; stress fractures)*
The patient has a stress fracture. These most commonly occur in the tibia and the second and third metatarsals. In the latter site, they are also called "march fractures," because they are associated with too much walking in ill-fitting shoes. Radiographs reveal new bone formation (callus) along the lines of microfracture in bone.

Greenstick fractures occur in children and refer to a break in the cortex on the convex side of the shaft but an intact concave side.

Osteochondritis refers to a localized area of avascular necrosis of bone, which, on a radiograph, appears as a lucency.

Sprains are a complete or partial tear of ligaments associated with swelling and tenderness. Physical examination confirms the diagnosis, because radiographs appear normal.

71. The answer is A. *(Gynecology; precocious puberty)*
Granulosa cell tumors, with Call-Exner bodies, have a low malignancy potential but can produce estrogens, resulting in precocious puberty. Fibrothecomas can produce estrogens from the theca cell line, but are less common than granulosa cell tumors. Sertoli-Leydig and hilar cell tumors, with characteristic crystals of Reinke, produce androgens and often cause virilization.

72. The answer is D. *(Pediatrics; rubeola)*
The lesions described in the mouth are known as Koplik's spots, which are pathognomonic of rubeola, or measles. They occur during the prodromal stage, which also presents with fever, cough, coryza, conjunctivitis, photophobia, and cervical lymphadenopathy. The temperature rises with the advent of the rash. Koplik's spots are transient, lasting approximately 12 to 18 hours. They are best seen opposite the lower molars.

73. The answer is D. *(Behavioral science; psychopathology in adoptees)*
Narcissistic injury, the hurt from knowing about being rejected as a child, often plays a significant role in the emotional life of adoptees. It sometimes manifests itself in an insecurity about acceptance by others. Over 80% of adoptions are considered successful, and IQ scores have been demonstrated to rise in some adoptive environments. However, the rate of psychopathology is higher among adoptees, as are parent–child problems.

74. The answer is C. *(Orthopedics; idiopathic scoliosis)*
The patient has idiopathic scoliosis. Forward bending is a school screening test for this disorder. This is usually accompanied by a prominent rib hump (paraspinus prominence) on the right caused by an abnormal lateral curvature of the spine. It is most commonly seen in adolescent girls from 10 to 16 years of age. Scoliosis refers to lateral displacement of the spine, while kyphosis refers to forward displacement of the spine.

Pott's disease of the spine refers to tuberculosis involving the vertebral column.

Ankylosing spondylitis is an HLA-B27 positive arthropathy that is more common in men. Sacroiliitis and fusion of the spine are prominent features of this disease. There is limited forward bending of the spinal column.

Osteomyelitis does not typically produce spinal abnormalities.

75. The answer is E. *(Behavioral science; child development)*
Attachment theory postulates that a healthy adult personality is in large part dependent on the formation of a secure attachment to caregivers in infancy and childhood. Conversely, early patho-

logic attachments, such as those that are threatening, inconstant, or absent, lead to developmental problems and personality disorders. Normal attachment is necessary for the development of basic trust and the ability to love others.

76. The answer is E. *(Obstetrics; dysmaturity syndrome)*
Dysmaturity syndrome is found in postmature pregnancies. It is characterized by dehydration of the fetoplacental unit. Therefore, excessive fundal height, placental thickening, and polyhydramnios are not found in this condition. Fetal subcutaneous tissue is decreased rather than being increased, as in macrosomatia. Decreased Wharton's jelly, which provides support to the umbilical blood vessels, is a classic finding in dysmaturity syndrome.

77. The answer is A. *(Biostatistics; sensitivity of test)*
Sensitivity is the ability to include persons with a specific disease in a study. Specificity is the ability to exclude those who are free of disease from a study.

78. The answer is B. *(General medicine; treatment of status epilepticus)*
Intravenous diazepam or lorazepam is the initial treatment of choice for status epilepticus. Both work well against tonic–clonic seizures, but are short-acting. Lorazepam has a slightly longer duration of action than diazepam and is associated with less respiratory depression and hypotension. Either drug can be given rectally if the intravenous route is not practical.

79. The answer is D. *(Pediatrics; Lyme disease)*
Lyme disease is caused by *Borrelia burgdorferi*. It is transmitted by the ticks of the *Ixodes* species, specifically the deer tick *Ixodes dammini* in the United States. It is endemic in the coastal areas of the Northeast, but has been described in 43 states, as well as Europe and Australia. Lyme disease is characterized by its rash, carditis, arthritis, and meningitis. The rash (erythema chronicum migrans) starts as an erythematous macule or papule at the site of the tick bite. The lesion continues to expand in a ring-like manner, with central clearing. Multiple secondary lesions may develop. Nonspecific symptoms of headache, fever, and chills accompany this stage, which resolves with or without treatment. Disseminated disease occurs in untreated patients after a latent period of weeks to months and can involve the central nervous system (CNS), heart, and musculoskeletal system. Persistent infection can occur. Treatment consists of tetracycline, penicillin, or erythromycin.

80. The answer is D. *(Behavioral science; child development)*
"Good-enough mothering" refers to Winnicott's widely accepted concept of mothering, which is sensitive and responsive enough to allow the child to develop a healthy relationship with the outside world. "Lock and key" and "goodness of fit" describe properties of the caregiver–child relationship. "Emerging competencies" usually refers to innate abilities that mature at given ages. "As if personality" refers to a particular type of pathologic relationship to the environment.

81. The answer is C. *(Otolaryngology; lingual thyroid)*
The patient has a lingual thyroid. This is a remnant of thyroid tissue in the foramen cecum, which is the initial site for thyroid tissue prior to migration into the neck. In 80% of the cases, this may be the only thyroid tissue, and excision would render the patient hypothyroid. Iodine-131 (^{131}I) uptake is useful diagnostically because it identifies the tissue as thyroid and determines whether there is any thyroid tissue in the neck. If thyroid hormone replacement therapy does not cause the mass to regress, it should be surgically excised and the patient should be kept on thyroid hormone. Needle biopsies and throat cultures serve no purpose in the workup of these lesions.

82. The answer is D. *(Gynecology; primary amenorrhea)*
Primary amenorrhea can be classified into four groups based on the presence or absence of normal breast development and a palpable uterus. This woman, with normal breast development but

without a uterus, has either testicular feminization syndrome or congenital uterine absence. In the former syndrome, a genetic male has a congenital lack of androgen receptors, and so the normal male levels of testosterone are unrecognized. Normal female hormonal status is associated with congenital uterine absence, including low levels of testosterone. Thus, measurement of serum testosterone would be the most useful test for this patient.

83. The answer is C. *(Pediatrics; German measles)*
Rubella (German or 3-day measles) in older children can present with joint manifestations, particularly in older girls and women. The joints of the hand and wrist are most commonly involved. Recently, most new cases have been in teenagers and young adults. The prodromal catarrhal stage is shorter than that of measles. Lymphadenopathy is the most characteristic sign, specifically of the posterior occipital, retroauricular, and posterior cervical lymph nodes. The rash begins on the face and spreads quickly, but also disappears quickly, usually within 3 days. Desquamation is minimal compared to that of rubeola.

84. The answer is C. *(Pulmonary medicine; lung abscess)*
The patient has a lung abscess that is due to aspiration of infected material from the oropharynx. This condition occurs in patients who are unconscious or obtunded from alcohol. Poor dental hygiene is invariably present. Gram's stain classically shows a mixture of aerobic and variable-staining anaerobic organisms, consisting of gram-positive cocci and a mixture of gram-positive and gram-negative rods with tapered ends. Common anaerobes include *Bacteroides melaninogenicus* (faint gram-negative rods), anaerobic streptococci (small gram-positive cocci), and *Fusobacterium nucleatum* (gram-negative rods with tapered ends). The basilar segments of the right lower lobe are the classic location for aspiration in the upright or sitting position. The posterior segment of the upper lobe is involved if aspiration occurs when the patient is lying on the right side. The superior segment of the lower lobe

is involved if the patient aspirates in the supine position. Penicillin plus vigorous bronchial toilet is usually effective in the treatment of anaerobic lung abscesses. Surgery is rarely indicated.

Gram-positive diplococci in the sputum are most commonly *Streptococcus pneumoniae,* the most common community-acquired pneumonia.

Fat gram-negative rods with capsules are usually *Klebsiella pneumoniae,* which is commonly associated with alcoholism. The abscesses are usually located within areas of lobar consolidation.

Gram-positive filamentous and branching bacteria in the sputum could be *Actinomyces* or *Nocardia. Actinomyces* is a strict anaerobe and is present within sulfur granules. It produces pleuropulmonary disease, with sinus tracts draining pus out to the skin. *Nocardia* is a strict aerobe and is partially acid-fast. Primary pulmonary disease with abscess formation is most commonly seen in immunocompromised hosts, particularly heart transplant patients.

Gram-positive rods (e.g., *Listeria, Clostridium* species, *Bacillus* species) are not common causes of lung abscesses.

85. The answer is B. *(Biostatistics; sensitivity versus specificity)*
Lowering the cutoff point on a screening test does increase the ability to include individuals with the disease (increases sensitivity) but at the same time it decreases the ability to exclude those free of disease (decreases specificity). This change would result in an increased false-positive rate and decreased false-negative rate.

86. The answer is E. *(Gynecology; vaginitis)*
The symptom history in this diabetic patient, combined with the gross description, is most consistent with a *Candida* vaginitis. Although a wet prep can show up the mycelia if they are profuse enough, the potassium hydroxide (KOH) prep that removes the epithelial debris would give the most prompt diagnosis in the simplest way. Gram's stain and culture are more expensive and time-consuming. A low pH would not be specific or sensitive.

87. The answer is B. *(Otolaryngology; nasopharyngeal carcinoma)*

Whenever a cervical lymph node contains a poorly differentiated carcinoma with no obvious primary site, a blind or direct visualization biopsy should be taken of the nasopharynx to rule out a nasopharyngeal carcinoma. These tumors have a putative relationship with Epstein-Barr virus, and are very common in China. Recent development of an Epstein-Barr virus vaccine in Britain may eradicate this disease.

Sputum cytology is not likely to be positive for malignancy with a normal chest radiograph from a nonsmoking woman nor are radiographic tomography studies of the lung.

Thyroid cancers are rarely poorly differentiated, so an iodine-131 (^{131}I) scan would not be indicated.

88. The answer is D. *(Pulmonary medicine;* Pneumocystis carinii *pneumonitis)*

The patient has a *Pneumocystis carinii* pneumonitis with the characteristic chest radiograph findings of "ground-glass" opacities in the lungs. Methenamine silver stains of lung tissue or bronchoalveolar lavage specimens frequently demonstrate densely clustered cysts that resemble crushed Ping-Pong balls. Because the patient is HIV positive and has an opportunistic infection, the patient qualifies as having AIDS.

Pneumocystis carinii is the most common initial manifestation and cause of death in patients with AIDS. Once considered a protozoan, DNA analysis now shows that the organism is more closely related to a fungus. The organism cannot be cultured. Patients are generally susceptible to infection when their CD4 helper T cell count approaches 200 cells/mm^3. It is contracted in immunosuppressed patients by inhalation and produces an interstitial pneumonitis with extreme hypoxemia. *Pneumocystis* predominantly affects the lungs, but it can also involve other head and neck organs, such as the thyroid, or the skin.

The treatment for *Pneumocystis carinii* is trimethoprim–sulfamethoxazole or pentamidine. Aerosolized pentamidine or low-dose sulfonamides are useful as prophylaxis against the infection. There is a 20% fatality rate with each

infection; therefore, lifetime prophylaxis is needed. The infection does not respond to amphotericin B or erythromycin.

Pneumocystis carinii is easily confused with *Histoplasma capsulatum,* but *Histoplasma* organisms are located in macrophages. Disseminated histoplasmosis could present with granulomas in the bone marrow. *Pneumocystis carinii* does not produce granulomatous inflammation. Amphotericin B is the treatment of choice for histoplasmosis.

89. The answer is B. *(Pediatrics; embryonal rhabdomyosarcoma)*

Rhabdomyosarcomas account for half the soft-tissue sarcomas. Those occurring before 5 years of age have a predilection for the neck, head, prostate, bladder, and vagina. A second peak occurs at 15 to 19 years of age, involving primarily the genitourinary tract. Embryonal rhabdomyosarcomas account for 60% of all rhabdomyosarcomas. Sarcoma botryoides is a form of embryonal rhabdomyosarcoma and accounts for 6% of the embryonal type. It occurs in the vagina, uterus, bladder, nasopharynx, and middle ear, and it looks like a bunch of grapes.

90. The answer is C. *(Gynecology; ectopic pregnancy)*

The most likely site for an ectopic pregnancy is the oviduct. Within the fallopian tube, the highest frequency is in the ampullae, followed by the infundibulum and then the isthmus.

91. The answer is E. *(Infectious disease; Rocky Mountain spotted fever)*

The boy has Rocky Mountain spotted fever, which is due to the bite of a hard tick (*Dermacentor andersoni*) carrying *Rickettsia rickettsii*. A diagnostic triad for the disease is a rash, fever, and history of exposure to a tick. The incubation period is approximately 2 to 12 days after exposure. Unlike the other rickettsial organisms, which cause a rash extending from the trunk to the extremities in centrifugal fashion, the rash of Rocky Mountain spotted fever begins on the palms and soles and spreads to the trunk. The rash is due to a vasculitis caused by the rickettsial organisms invading the endothelial cells of small vessels and producing petechial lesions. Oklahoma and North Carolina share the lead for the highest incidence of Rocky Mountain spotted fever.

The diagnosis is best made serologically using indirect immunofluorescent techniques rather than using the outdated Weil-Felix reaction, which has a positive *Proteus vulgaris* OX2 and OX19 reaction.

Chloramphenicol is the treatment of choice for children less than 8 years of age. Doxycycline is used for older children. The mortality rate is 20% without treatment and 5% with treatment.

92. The answer is B. *(Neurosurgery; basilar skull fracture with otorrhea)*
The patient has otorrhea with loss of cerebrospinal fluid (CSF) secondary to a basilar skull fracture. CSF, an ultrafiltrate of plasma, is primarily derived from the choroid plexus in the lateral ventricles and is resorbed by the arachnoid granulations. When compared with serum concentrations, CSF has a higher chloride (120–130 mEq/L versus 95–105 mEq/L), a lower protein (< 4 g/dl versus 6.0–7.8 g/dl), a lower glucose (60% of the plasma; 40–70 mg/dl versus 70–110 mg/dl), and fewer white blood cells (0–5 leukocytes/µl versus 4500–11,000 leukocytes/µl).

93. The answer is E. *(Obstetrics; isoimmunization)*
Isoimmunization occurs when the fetus has a paternally derived antigen for which the mother is negative. This situation allows the mother to make antibodies against the fetal antigen; these antibodies can then cross the placenta and hemolyze the fetal red blood cells (RBCs). The only options to consider are those in which the mother is negative, options A and E. The fetus is positive only in option E, so it is the correct answer.

94. The answer is C. *(Gastroenterology; antibiotic-induced pseudomembranous colitis)*
The association of this patient's complaints with antibiotic use and the appearance of the lesions argue against a parasitic cause of the diarrhea. The patient has antibiotic-associated pseudo-

membranous colitis. Colonoscopy in this disease shows whitish or yellowish plaques surrounded by hemorrhagic borders. It is due to an overgrowth of *Clostridium difficile*. Ampicillin and clindamycin are the most common antibiotics associated with pseudomembranous colitis.

The diagnosis is best made with a toxin assay of stool rather than culture or Gram's stain. Blood cultures are negative, because the damage to the mucosa and submucosa is toxin-induced and not invasive colitis.

Metronidazole and oral vancomycin are used for treatment.

95. The answer is B. *(Biostatistics; leading causes of death)*
The top ten causes of death in descending order of frequency are heart disease, cancer, cerebrovascular accident, accidents, chronic obstructive pulmonary disease (COPD), pneumonia and influenza, diabetes mellitus, suicide, chronic liver disease and cirrhosis, and human immunodeficiency virus (HIV). Tobacco and dietary factors are responsible for cancer being the second most common cause of death in this country. Tobacco is also a major risk factor for coronary artery disease.

96. The answer is A. *(Obstetrics; cytomegalovirus)*
Cytomegalovirus (CMV) is the most common congenital viral syndrome in the United States. Neither effective treatment nor prophylaxis exists, and the fetal risk with primary infection is equal in all trimesters. There is no advantage to be gained by cesarean delivery.

97. The answer is D. *(Laboratory medicine; effect of changing reference on sensitivity)*
Narrowing the reference interval of a test (0–7 mg/dl to 0–3 mg/dl) increases the test's sensitivity, because there will be fewer false-negatives in this range. However, increasing sensitivity automatically decreases specificity by increasing the number of false-positives. This relationship underscores the principle that there is always a trade-off when increasing either sensitivity or

specificity: Increasing one always decreases the other.

98. The answer is D. *(Clinical endocrinology; surreptitious insulin injection mimicking an insulinoma)*
Munchausen's syndrome occurs in those who purposefully make themselves sick in order to be admitted to a hospital. Injection of insulin to produce hypoglycemia that mimics an insulinoma is one example of this syndrome. Because C peptide is the internal marker of endogenous insulin release, a patient with an insulinoma (benign tumor of islet cells) would be expected to have a high C peptide, high serum insulin, and low serum glucose. If the C peptide is low, the patient must be taking insulin because exogenous insulin would lower the patient's own insulin production, therefore lowering the C peptide.

99. The answer is C. *(General surgery; metastatic papillary cancer of the thyroid)*
The patient has metastatic papillary adenocarcinoma of the thyroid to cervical lymph nodes. These are the most common thyroid cancers and are usually found in women between the ages of 20 and 60 years. They are papillary tumors that are often mixed with follicles. Psammoma bodies (calcium concretions) are an excellent marker for the cancer. Most patients initially present with palpable lymphadenopathy in the neck, which represents nodal metastasis via permeation of the lymphatics. They can produce a miliary pattern of metastasis to lung resembling miliary tuberculosis. Papillary carcinomas are treated with near-total thyroidectomy plus "node picking" of grossly involved nodes. Radioactive iodine ablates any follicular component of the tumor. The prognosis is worse with lymph node or distant metastases, age over 40 years, or the presence of direct extension into tissue. The overall 10-year survival rate is 80%.

Most vocal cord cancers are squamous carcinomas involving the true vocal cords.

The most common malignant parotid gland tumor is mucoepidermoid carcinoma.

The most common primary lung cancer is an adenocarcinoma with the formation of glandular structures.

The most common breast cancer is an infiltrating ductal carcinoma. Papillary cancers are very uncommon.

100. The answer is C. *(Gynecology; syphilis)*
The Venereal Disease Research Laboratories (VDRL) test is only for screening. It is not conclusive for syphilis. Among the many reasons for a false-positive is a recent immunization. In primary syphilis, the test may remain negative, but becomes positive by the time that condyloma lata are seen in secondary syphilis. The fluorescent treponemal antibody absorption (FTA-ABS) test is essential to confirm the diagnosis.

101. The answer is D. *(Biostatistics; cross-sectional study)*
The key element in this study design is the simultaneous determination of both exposure and disease outcome at a point in time and is characteristic of a cross-sectional study. A cohort study is incorrect because the case does not describe a cohort followed either historically or prospectively. A case-control study and a randomized controlled trial are incorrect because no control subjects were chosen. A crossover prospective study is erroneous because the design was not prospective nor was there a crossover strategy.

102–105. The answers are: 102-B, 103-A, 104-A, 105-A. *(Psychiatry; diagnosis of psychosis)*
Psychosis is indicated by the presence of bizarre delusions and thought disturbance. The patient's normal awareness and lack of memory impairment make delirium unlikely. Although the symptoms of dysphoria and anxiety are present, there is little evidence to suggest primary pathology, and they are readily explained by his psychosis.

Schizophrenia is the most likely diagnosis. A history of increasing pathology over the last year, a deterioration of function, the presence of psychosis, and social withdrawal are all suggestive. The lack of clear mood symptomatology makes bipolar disorder and major depression less likely. The patient has no history of cocaine use, and the girlfriend does not share his delusions.

A strong family history of psychiatric hospitalizations often indicates a genetic component to a patient's psychopathology. Of the heritable psychoses, schizophrenia would be the most likely condition in this patient. Although childhood conflicts, anxiety, and recent stressors can exacerbate psychopathology, they rarely cause psychosis.

Brief reactive psychosis cannot be diagnosed if a period of increasing pathology precedes a severe stressor. This characteristic distinguishes brief reactive psychosis from other disorders, which are simply exacerbated by stressors.

106–107. The answers are: 106-C, 107-D. *(Toxicology; mercury)*

Mercury is still widely used today in a variety of compounds (e.g., thimerosol is used in merthiolate and in contact-lens cleaning solutions). Acute poisoning causes predominantly gastrointestinal and renal symptoms. Oral intake of mercury can cause stomatitis, abdominal pain, nausea, vomiting, and explosive, bloody diarrhea. Kidney damage can lead to renal failure and death. Central nervous system (CNS) symptoms include ataxia, slurred speech, and visual and hearing impairment. Iron can cause a hemorrhagic gastroenteritis, but renal failure is not common; liver involvement manifests approximately 2 to 4 days after ingestion.

Treatment of mercury poisoning consists of correction of fluid and electrolyte imbalance and removal of mercury by gastric lavage. British antilewisite (BAL, dimercaprol) is the best therapy for mercury poisoning. Penicillamine may be used in patients who have adverse reactions to BAL, for example, nausea, vomiting, and fever. The combination of ethylenediaminetetraacetic acid (EDTA) and BAL is used for lead poisoning. Deferoxamine is recommended for iron poisoning.

108. The answer is E. *(Hematology; hemolytic anemia secondary to prosthetic valve)*

Prosthetic heart valves can sometimes damage red blood cells (RBCs) and produce a normocytic anemia secondary to intravascular hemolysis. As expected, the reticulocyte count is elevated in response to the loss of peripheral RBCs. Irregularly shaped RBCs secondary to the damage are called schistocytes. Haptoglobin is a "suicide protein" that is synthesized in the liver. Its main function is to bind free hemoglobin to form a haptoglobin–hemoglobin complex. This complex is removed by macrophages in the liver in order for amino acids and iron to be retrieved. Removal of the complex from the circulation results in a decreased concentration of serum haptoglobin as a marker of intravascular hemolysis. Unfortunately, in severe extravascular hemolytic anemias, some hemoglobin leaks out of macrophages, which destroys the RBCs, thus decreasing serum haptoglobin levels as well. Therefore, decreased serum haptoglobin cannot be used to clearly distinguish an intravascular from an extravascular hemolytic anemia.

109. The answer is B. *(Neurosurgery; subdural hematoma)*

The patient has a subdural hematoma, which is a collection of blood between the dura and the arachnoid membranes. It is most often the result of blunt trauma in an anteroposterior plane with or without an associated skull fracture (50% of cases). It is most commonly seen in elderly individuals and chronic alcoholics who have cerebral atrophy.

Bleeding in subdural hematomas is due to tearing of the bridging veins between the venous sinus and the cortex or from torn vessels in the underlying damaged brain. They may be acute or chronic and are frequently bilateral. Most subdural hematomas are located over the convexities of the cerebral hemisphere. The breakdown of blood clot material in the subdural space acts as an osmotic agent, which draws fluid from the adjacent subarachnoid space into the cavity, thus producing an expansile mass in the subdural space with compression of the underlying brain tissue.

The onset of symptoms in subdural hematomas is generally delayed. They become clinically manifested by fluctuating levels of consciousness. Ipsilateral headache is common. In 90% of cases, the pupil is dilated (mydriasis) on the side of the lesion.

Acute subdural hematomas have a mortality rate of 75% to 90% because of the frequent association with trauma to the brain. Chronic subdural hematomas are often undiagnosed, and patients frequently present with confusion, inattention, dementia, seizures, and coma (particularly in an elderly individual or chronic alcoholic). Subdural hematomas are easily detected by computed tomography (CT) or angiography. The clots must be surgically evacuated.

Subarachnoid hemorrhages are most commonly caused by a ruptured berry aneurysm rather than trauma.

Intracerebral hemorrhage is most commonly secondary to hypertension rather than trauma.

Hemorrhagic infarctions of the brain are most commonly secondary to embolism from the left side of the heart.

110. The answer is B. *(Gynecology; urinary stress incontinence)*

Genuine urinary stress incontinence is characterized by a loss of the urethral/vesicle angle when increases in intra-abdominal/intravesicle pressure fail to be transmitted to the urethra. Grand multiparity can be a cause. Multiple sclerosis, bladder tumor, interstitial cystitis, and detrusor instability all can be associated with types of incontinence other than stress.

111–112. The answers are: 111-C, 112-D. *(Rheumatology; osteoporosis)*

Osteoporosis is the most common metabolic abnormality of bone in the United States. Estrogen deficiency after menopause is the most common cause in women. Because most of the bone is lost in the first 3 to 6 years after menopause, early estrogen replacement is the key to prevention of osteoporosis. A partial list of other disorders that predispose to osteoporosis would include estrogen deficiency associated with exercise-induced amenorrhea or anorexia nervosa, primary hyperparathyroidism, Cushing's syndrome, chronic metabolic acidosis, heparin therapy, and the lack of gravity in space.

In osteoporosis, an imbalance occurs between the resorption of bone (osteoclastic activity) and the formation of bone (osteoblastic activity). The increased osteoclastic activity creates large holes that the osteoblasts are unable to fill. This imbalance is not related to increased secretion of osteoclast activating factor by macrophages or increased secretion of parathormone. Clinically, osteoporosis results in stress fractures of the vertebral bodies and femoral neck, a decrease in overall height, dowager's hump of the cervical spine, and pathological fractures. Serum calcium and phosphorus levels are usually normal in osteoporosis.

Progesterone alone is not used in either the prevention or treatment of osteoporosis. However, because the incidence of endometrial carcinoma increases 0.1% per year with unopposed estrogen, the addition of 2.5 mg of medroxyprogesterone is recommended.

If not contraindicated, estrogen is the gold standard for the prevention of osteoporosis and should be given to all postmenopausal women. An additional benefit is a 50% reduction in the incidence of ischemic heart disease. The usual dose is 0.625 mg/day of premarin. Contraindications for estrogen include pregnancy, breast cancer, undiagnosed vaginal bleeding, active thrombophlebitis, or thromboembolic disorders previously associated with estrogens. Additional pharmacologic agents are under study for their use in osteoporosis prevention or treatment, or both. Sodium fluoride increases bone formation in the spine, thus decreasing vertebral fractures, but it does so by reducing cortical bone mass. Bisphosphonates are potent inhibitors of bone resorption and have a place in the prevention and treatment of osteoporosis. Salmon calcitonin is primarily used in the treatment of osteoporosis, but is also useful in prevention if estrogens are contraindicated. Additional preventive measures include calcium and vitamin D supplementation and weight-bearing exercise.

113. The answer is E. *(Pediatrics; poststreptococcal glomerulonephritis)*
Poststreptococcal glomerulonephritis is characterized by hematuria, hypertension, and edema. Acute poststreptococcal glomerulonephritis typically occurs 1 to 2 weeks following a streptococcal infection by nephritogenic strains. Pharyngitis is associated with cold weather, whereas skin infections occur during warm weather. After uneventful recovery, the child develops symptoms of edema and hematuria. The hematuria may be microscopic. Renal involvement can progress to renal failure. Urinalysis shows red blood cells (RBCs) and RBC casts. The complement component C3 is low, and the antistreptolysin O titer is elevated, indicating a recent streptococcal infection.

114. The answer is A. *(General surgery; mammography)*
Mammography is most effective in detecting clinically occult, nonpalpable lesions in the breast. For women with palpable breast masses, however, it is less reliable as a diagnostic tool. In one study of patients with palpable breast cancer, the mammogram was negative (false negative) in approximately 9% of cases. This is true particularly when the mass is in a background of dense tissue, as often occurs with fibrocystic change. This underscores the fact that a "normal" mammogram does not necessarily indicate that a mass is not present or that the mass is benign. Typically, malignant breast tumors have irregular, spiculated margins with fine-stippled calcifications within a radius of 1 cm. These findings, however, can also be seen in traumatic fat necrosis and fibrocystic change. One current recommendation for screening is a baseline mammogram between 35 and 40 years of age, a mammogram every 1–2 years between the ages of 40 and 49, and a yearly mammogram after the age of 50.

115. The answer is D. *(Obstetrics; rubella infection)*
Rubella is a highly contagious viral syndrome with potentially disastrous pregnancy impact. However, gamma globulin is not helpful. Because the vaccine is a live virus, it is inappropriate to administer it to a pregnant woman. Breastfeeding is not contraindicated after maternal vaccination. Amniocentesis offers no benefit to offset the risk in a noninfected gravida. Avoiding pregnancy for 3 months after vaccination is essential.

116. The answer is C. *(Hematology; sickle cell disease presenting as dactylitis)*
Dactylitis is the most frequent initial manifestation of sickle cell disease, which is the most common hemoglobinopathy in the black population. The onset of symptoms usually occurs between the ages of 4 and 12 months, when the protective effect of fetal hemoglobin (Hgb F) against sickling is no longer present.

Dactylitis is characterized by soft tissue swelling of the hands, feet, or both, with associated heat and tenderness over the metacarpals, tarsals, and proximal phalanges. Radiographs at the onset of the disease reveal only soft tissue swelling. After 1 to 2 weeks, infarction and necrosis of the underlying bones are noted secondary to sickling of red blood cells in the sinusoids. This is followed by subperiosteal new bone formation. Absorption of the infarcted bone results in radiolucent areas. These areas of infarction are restored to normal within a few months, but recurrent disease is common.

Glucose-6-phosphate dehydrogenase (G6PD) deficiency is a sex-linked recessive hemolytic anemia that is initiated by oxidant stresses imposed on the patient from infection (most commonly) or drugs. The Mediterranean variant is the most severe form, since the enzyme is absent in both young and old red blood cells. It appears at birth as a brisk hemolytic anemia with subsequent indirect hyperbilirubinemia, which often requires an exchange transfusion in order to prevent kernicterus. This presentation does not occur in full-term black infants, since they have a weaker variant of the disease.

Salmonella osteomyelitis frequently occurs in sickle cell disease when functional hyposplenism is present from autoinfarction of the spleen. The highest risk of infection is between the ages of 1 and 10 years.

Coxsackieviruses in the A subgroup are associated with hand, foot, and mouth disease. This consists of ulcers on the tongue and oral mucosa and vesicles that do not ulcerate on the palms and soles.

Turner's syndrome, a sex chromosome abnormality with an XO pattern, is associated with nuchal edema as well as painless edema of the hands and feet in newborns.

117. The answer is A. *(Behavioral science; depression in the elderly)*
The prevalence of serious depressive illness in the geriatric population is estimated to be less than 10%. Including more loosely defined depression brings the prevalence to approximately 20%. While certain stresses are associated with old age, most studies show that rates of depressive illness are no higher than in the general population.

118. The answer is D. *(Infectious disease; enterobiasis)*
A cellophane-tape preparation from the perianal area is used to detect the eggs of *Enterobius vermicularis* (pinworm) in a patient with complaints of anal pruritus. Enterobiasis is the most common worm infection in the gastrointestinal tract. Patients acquire the infection by ingestion of the embryonated eggs. Larvae develop in the lumen of the small intestine. The adult worms have a superficial attachment to the cecum and appendix. Since the attachment is superficial, there is no peripheral blood eosinophilia. At night, the females lay eggs in the perianal area, which causes intense itching (pruritus ani) and a restless sleep. Pyrantel pamoate or mebendazole are the treatment options. All members of the family should be treated with the drug.

119. The answer is D. *(General surgery; esophageal carcinoma)*
The patient has an esophageal carcinoma. Squamous cell carcinoma accounts for 95% of esophageal cancers. Predisposing factors include smoking, alcohol, lye strictures, Plummer-Vinson syndrome, diverticular diseases, nitrosamines, and achalasia. Esophageal cancers are most commonly located in the mid-esophagus (50%). Dysphagia for solids, weakness, and weight loss are the usual presenting complaints. These cancers initially spread locally by lymphatics and drain into surrounding lymph nodes. Distant metastasis is to the liver (70%), lungs (60%), and adrenal glands (35%). Approximately 50% of esophageal carcinomas are resectable at the time of presentation. An esophagectomy is usually performed followed by radiation and chemotherapy. The 5-year survival rate is 5%.

Diffuse esophageal spasm, or "nutcracker esophagus," produces dysphagia and chest pain that is often relieved with nitroglycerin. A barium study reveals a "corkscrew" esophagus.

Zenker's diverticulum is the most common acquired diverticulum of the esophagus and is treated by surgery. Because of stagnant food collected in the pouch, the patient has halitosis.

Achalasia, a motor disorder of the distal esophagus due to failure of relaxation of the lower esophageal sphincter, is also associated with dysphagia for solids and liquids. The proximal esophagus is dilated and aperistaltic. It is treated with pneumatic dilatation, drugs that decrease lower esophageal sphincter tone (e.g., nifedipine), or surgery (esophagocardiomyotomy) in 20% to 25% of patients.

120. The answer is B. *(Pharmacology; anesthesia and analgesia)*
Intravenous morphine provides rapid relief of dyspnea from pulmonary edema and left ventricular failure. Central mechanisms proposed for this action include the relief of anxiety and a reduction in the perception of shortness of breath. Peripheral actions of morphine that are probably relevant include venous and arteriolar vasodilation, resulting in decreases in cardiac preload and afterload. Codeine or nonsteroidal anti-inflammatory drugs (NSAIDs) provide adequate analgesia for routine dental surgery. NSAIDs are also used for ductus arteriosus closure. Morphine and related drugs cause cerebral vasodilation [even analgesic doses increase the CO_2 tension (P_{CO_2})] which, in patients with elevated intracranial pressure, may cause lethal alterations in brain functions. Opioids have no anti-inflammatory actions.

121. The answer is A. *(Gynecology; vaginitis)*
The cause of the vaginitis is *Trichomonas vaginalis,* as evidenced by the pruritic discharge and the highly motile protozoan. The agent of choice is metronidazole. Clotrimazole and miconazole are antifungal agents. Acyclovir is used in genital herpes management. Spectinomycin is appropriate for treatment of gonorrhea.

122. The answer is B. *(Biostatistics; sensitivity of test)*
Sensitivity is the ability of a test to include those who have a diagnosis. In the table, 120 people who were screened have the disease. Only 40 of these 120 people were identified by a positive screening test; therefore, sensitivity is 33%.

123. The answer is E. *(Psychiatry; depression)*
"Masked depression" usually refers to depression that presents as physical complaints, without subjective complaints of mood disturbance by the patient. It is common in patients who are stoic, who are less introspective, and who come from backgrounds in which emotional pathology is less acceptable.

124. The answer is D. *(Dermatology; neurofibromatosis)*
The patient has two large café-au-lait macules on the right lower abdomen plus a family history that is consistent with neurofibromatosis. The disease is characterized by:

- An autosomal-dominant inheritance pattern with variable penetrance
- More than six café-au-lait macules on the skin or one café-au-lait patch greater than 5 cm
- Multiple neurofibromas dispersed on or in the body
- Pigmented iris hamartomas called Lisch nodules
- An increased incidence of meningiomas, optic nerve gliomas, acoustic neuromas of the eighth nerve, pheochromocytomas, and sarcomatous degeneration of neurofibromas involving large nerve trunks (i.e., neurofibrosarcomas)
- Massive distortion of the skin and soft tissue in some patients (e.g., "elephant man")

The dysplastic nevus syndrome is a variant type of nevus that predisposes the patient to malignant melanoma. The pigmented lesions measure 5 to 15 mm in size, have irregular borders, and have various shades of black, tan, and red. Patients with this syndrome frequently have over 100 nevi scattered over their body, one or more of which can be a precursor to malignant melanoma.

Sturge-Weber syndrome is a port-wine colored hemangioma that is located on the face in a characteristic trigeminal nerve distribution. It can be associated with ipsilateral arteriovenous malformation in the leptomeninges as well as mental retardation.

Tuberous sclerosis is an autosomal-dominant disease characterized by mental retardation, rhabdomyomas of the heart, angiomyolipomas of the kidney, periungual fibromas, intracranial calcifications, and skin nodules.

Tinea versicolor is a dermatophytosis that is characterized by many macular patches of various shapes and sizes.

125. The answer is C. *(Gynecology; contraception)*
The postcoital douche has the highest failure rate (40%). Reversible methods with the lowest failure rates include oral contraceptives (2% to 3%), intrauterine devices (IUDs; 5% to 6%), and spermicides and diaphragms (15% to 20%).

126. The answer is D. *(Behavioral science; mental retardation)*
The vast majority of mentally retarded adults (85%) have mild mental retardation. Such individuals can read at a sixth-grade level and manage simple jobs. They can be self-supporting and productive. While the incidence of substance abuse and the need for psychosocial services are higher in this population, these aspects do not characterize the majority of such individuals. The causes of mental retardation are varied and represent a wide variety of biologic and environmental factors. Only a minority of cases of mental retardation can be attributed to known biologic factors.

127. The answer is A. *(Pediatrics; scabies)*
Scabies is caused by the mite *Sarcoptes scabiei* and is transmitted by direct contact with other infected individuals. Burrows are usually absent in infants, but are demonstrable in 7% to 13% of adults. Although the face and scalp are spared in children and adults, they are common sites of infection in infants. Intertriginous areas are affected in infants, as well as the palms and soles. Red-brown nodules occasionally appear on the axillae, groin, and genitalia.

128. The answer is D. *(Emergency medicine; anaphylactic reaction to bee sting)*
Pain in the face followed by swelling of the face and respiratory difficulties while sunbathing on the grass is most likely due to an anaphylactic reaction caused by a bee sting. Bee stings are the most common cause of death from venomous animal bites in the United States. Most systemic reactions to insect stings are type I hypersensitivity reactions that occur in previously sensitized patients who have produced high titers of immunoglobulin E (IgE) antibodies against insect venom. These antibodies attach to mast cells and basophils and are distributed throughout the body. Reexposure to antigen with the bridging of two subjacent IgE antibodies by antigen on the surface of mast cells and basophils results in the release of histamine and other mediators that are vasodilators and bronchoconstrictors.

The predominant clinical findings involve the skin and the respiratory and cardiovascular systems. Clinical findings in mildly sensitized persons include a local wheal and flare reaction at the site of the bite, pain, hives, flushing, wheezing, rhinitis, conjunctivitis, and fever. A severely sensitized patient often presents with hypotension, diffuse urticaria, laryngeal edema, bronchospasm, diarrhea with abdominal cramping, and arrhythmias. Laryngeal obstruction is the most common cause of death in these patients, followed by cardiovascular collapse.

Initially, anaphylaxis is treated with subcutaneous or intramuscular administration of aqueous epinephrine 1:1000. The dose is 0.1 mg/kg with a maximal dose of 0.3 to 0.5 ml. This is repeated every 20 to 30 minutes if necessary. If there is no response to this therapy, or if the patient is in profound shock, a 1:10,000 dose of aqueous epinephrine is given intravenously. If orofacial swelling is present, the patient is intubated before laryngeal edema precludes this approach.

Other options in less severe envenomations include the use of diphenhydramine hydrochloride (1 mg/kg) either by mouth or parenterally. A nebulized β_2-agonist, such as albuterol, or intravenous aminophylline is useful in the treatment of bronchospasm. Intravenous administration of hydrocortisone is sometimes used in moderate-to-severe envenomations but does not appear to prevent recurrent waves of anaphylaxis.

The sting site should be examined and the stinger removed by scraping it out with a knife rather than using tweezers, which can introduce more venom into the wound.

Patients who have demonstrated exaggerated local cutaneous, respiratory, or cardiovascular reactions to insect stings should be prescribed an emergency epinephrine kit with syringe and should be taught how to use it. Venom immunotherapy is 95% effective in preventing anaphylaxis on subsequent exposures. Children with only localized cutaneous reactions are at low risk (< 10%) for developing systemic reactions; therefore, immunotherapy is not recommended in these patients.

129. The answer is B. *(Behavioral science; homelessness)*
Studies of the homeless population suggest that approximately one-third have chronic and severe mental illness. Common pathologies include schizophrenia and severe mood disorders. The prevalence of substance abuse in the homeless population is even higher, and includes a substantial percentage of the mentally ill homeless.

130. The answer is B. *(Gynecology; vulvar dystrophies)*
The lesion described is that of lichen sclerosis. The key finding is the atrophic skin description. The treatment of choice is testosterone cream. 5-Fluorouracil is used for neoplasias. Fluorinated corticosteroids are indicated for hyperplastic dys-

trophies of the vulva. Miconazole is an antifungal agent. Estrogen cream is not effective for lichen sclerosis.

131. The answer is A. *(Pediatrics; Friedreich's ataxia)*
Cardiac abnormalities are often associated with Friedreich's ataxia, and the heart condition may be the eventual cause of death. Diabetes, mental retardation, vision loss, and seizures are not particularly associated with Friedreich's ataxia, but both diabetes and retardation can be associated with myotonic dystrophy, and any number of conditions have associated seizures.

132. The answer is D. *(General surgery; pylephlebitis complicating acute appendicitis)*
The patient has pylephlebitis (inflammation of the portal vein) secondary to acute appendicitis, which is the most common cause. The presence of shaking chills and fever in a patient with appendicitis requires the prompt administration of antibiotics to prevent pylephlebitis. In addition to high fever and chills, there is jaundice and the potential for hepatic abscesses as infection spreads up into the portal tract, and also a potential for portal vein thrombosis. Computed tomography (CT) is considered the best test to detect gas and thrombosis in the portal vein.

Gallstone ileus is generally seen in elderly women with chronic cholecystitis. Adhesions occur between the gallbladder and bowel, resulting in the formation of a fistula. Gallstones can empty into the bowel and produce obstruction. Air is present in the biliary tree on an abdominal radiograph.

The Budd-Chiari syndrome involves hepatic vein thrombosis usually secondary to a hypercoagulable state [e.g., those with polycythemia rubra vera (most commonly) or those taking oral contraceptives]. There is painful hepatomegaly, jaundice, and ascites. Angiography is the best means of obtaining the diagnosis. Prompt surgical therapy is required due to a high mortality rate (50%–90%).

133. The answer is C. *(Pediatrics; infant mortality rate)*
In the United States, the mortality rate for black infants is 50% higher than the rate for white infants. The significantly higher mortality rate for black (and other nonwhite) infants can be partially attributed to social, economic, and cultural influences. Inadequate health education, limited access to health facilities and physicians, and lack of money to pay for health care (including prenatal and preventive medicine) contribute to the increased mortality rate.

134. The answer is E. *(Gynecology; vulvar lesions)*
Adequate assessment may require more than one biopsy. Colposcopy can be very helpful in identifying biopsy sites. Toluidine blue will not affect the histology and therefore should not be excluded. Large lesions should be biopsied on the margin of normal skin or at the worst-looking area. The definitive diagnosis is a histologic, not a clinical one.

135. The answer is D. *(Psychiatry; suicide)*
Schizophrenia is a significant risk factor for suicide. Other serious risk factors include divorce, widow- or widowerhood, or separation from a spouse; old age; and joblessness. Sexual orientation in and of itself does not seem to predispose to suicide, and, in general, suicide rates increase with age.

136. The answer is A. *(Pediatrics; recurrent otitis media)*
Hearing loss is the most common complication associated with recurrent otitis media. Temporary hearing loss can occur with acute infection, but this loss is reversible. Recurrent acute or chronic infection can cause permanent damage, leading to speech and learning problems. Cholesteatoma is a less common complication of otitis media. Abscess, thrombosis, and mastoiditis are even less frequent and occur via direct extension of the infection.

137. The answer is C. *(Neurosurgery; epidural hematoma)*
The patient had an epidural hematoma. Acute epidural hematomas generally result from trauma to the side of the head with fracture of the temporoparietal bone and severance of the middle meningeal artery, which lies between the dura and the inner table of frontal bone. Arterial bleeding in an epidural hematoma creates a potential space between the calvarium and dura, thus producing a true epidural compartment.

Typically, the patient is initially rendered unconscious and then regains consciousness (lucid interval). After 4 to 8 hours, when there is approximately 30 to 50 ml of blood in the space, the patient develops evidence of raised intracranial pressure (e.g., papilledema, convulsion) and may die of herniation unless the blood is surgically removed. There is a 20% mortality rate.

Subarachnoid and intracerebral hemorrhages are not associated with trauma. Subdural hematomas are most common in elderly individuals and chronic alcoholics who have cerebral atrophy.

138. The answer is C. *(Gynecology; dysmenorrhea)*
Primary dysmenorrhea is classically associated with normal pelvic examination findings. Onset is typically within 2 years of menarche and is probably due to excessive endometrial prostaglandin production. Symptoms end with the menses, and bleeding is usually normal. Treatment is pharmacologic, not surgical.

139. The answer is D. *(Biostatistics; specificity of test)*
Specificity is the ability of a test to exclude those who do not have the diagnosis. In the table, 60 people who were screened are disease free. Yet, only 40 of the 60 people had a negative screening test; therefore, specificity is 67%.

140. The answer is A. *(General surgery; ligation of right hepatic artery in gallbladder surgery)*
The right hepatic artery is the vessel that is most commonly injured during a cholecystectomy. If the origin of the cystic artery is distally placed on the right hepatic artery, there is a potential for ligating the right hepatic artery instead of the cystic artery, which could result in infarction of the liver. The liver is rarely infarcted because of a dual blood supply from the portal vein and hepatic artery. However, ligation of the main arterial branch can result in this fatal occurrence. The portal vein and inferior vena cava can also be injured in intra-abdominal operations. The right gastroepiploic artery is not usually injured.

141. The answer is E. *(Psychiatry; multiple personality disorder)*
A growing body of research suggests that multiple personality disorder is strongly associated with a history of childhood sexual abuse. The early necessity of dissociative defenses is postulated as the cause for the later development of a poorly integrated personality. Schizophrenia and autism are not correlated with any particular developmental pathology. Somatization disorder and antisocial personality disorder are associated with a higher incidence of childhood problems, including physical and sexual abuse. The causal link, however, is less established for these two disorders than it is for multiple personality disorder.

142. The answer is A. *(Ophthalmology; macular degeneration)*
Macular degeneration is the most common cause of permanent loss of visual acuity in the elderly. It is a strongly age-related phenomenon (prevalence of 22% by 75 years of age). Predisposing conditions include gender (in women more commonly than men), family history, occupational exposure to chemicals, blue eyes, cardiovascular disease, smoking, diastolic hypertension, and left ventricular hypertrophy.

Diabetic retinopathy is the most common cause of blindness in the United States but does not have a predilection only for the elderly population. Neovascularization of the retinal vessels portends a poor prognosis.

Optic neuritis is a cause of sudden, unilateral loss of vision.

Trauma and cataract surgery are not associated with a high rate of permanent loss of visual acuity.

143. The answer is A. *(Gynecology; pelvic relaxation)*
The patient in question has many risk factors for pelvic relaxation: She is white and postmenopausal, without estrogen replacement; she is multiparous and has delivered large infants; she has a long history of smoking. However, her symptoms are more referable to posterior vaginal relaxation with rectocele than anterior relaxation with cystocele.

144. The answer is E. *(Psychiatry; posttraumatic stress disorder)*
This veteran's symptoms suggest posttraumatic stress disorder. This illness is characterized by persistent reexperiencing of very traumatic events, coupled with anxiety and emotional numbing. The patient's wish for treatment appears well advised. Peer support groups to recall and discuss traumatic experiences seem to be an effective treatment.

145. The answer is A. *(Psychiatry; mechanisms of defense)*
Isolation describes the separation of a thought from its attached emotional tone, thereby making it tolerable. This mechanism is often used during highly stressful events. Depersonalization and derealization are other defenses that involve dissociation of mental functions, but both are more often accompanied by anxiety. Disorientation and intellectualization are not accompanied by odd calmness.

146. The answer is B. *(General medicine; treatment of cat bites)*
Pasteurella multocida is the organism that most commonly infects cat bites within 24 hours. Deep puncture wounds are characteristic of cat bites. (Wounds inflicted by cat claws are considered in the same category as bites.) *Pasteurella multocida* responds to penicillin VK. Wounds that develop after 24 hours are best treated by administration of cephradine or dicloxacillin.

Staphylococcus aureus and group A streptococci are not common pathogens in cat bites in the first 24 hours. *Afipia felis* is one of the causes of cat-scratch fever. In this disease, there are granulomatous microabscesses in lymph nodes draining the infection site.

In all bites (animal and human), the mainstay of therapy is proper cleansing of the wound with soap and water. All bites on the extremities should be treated aggressively because of the potential for septic arthritis and tenosynovitis. Antimicrobial ampicillin or penicillin prophylaxis is recommended for all human bites (the most serious bite) and most cat bites. High-risk dog bites requiring antibiotic prophylaxis (e.g., ampicillin) are those on the hand, those associated with puncture wounds, and wounds that are more than 6 to 12 hours old.

The risk of tetanus is always greater in contaminated wounds, puncture wounds, and wounds that come late to medical attention. In general, tetanus toxoid protects a person for 10 years. Tetanus immunoglobulin is reserved for dirty wounds in people who have never been immunized (never received the primary series of three doses of tetanus toxoid) or whose status is unknown.

The decision for rabies prophylaxis in animal bites depends on the circumstance of the bite and the local prevalence of rabies. In this country, rabies is most commonly contracted from the bites of bats, skunks, raccoons, and squirrels rather than dogs. In dogs or cats, a period of 10 days is sufficient to determine whether the animal is rabid. Strays or wild animals should be sacrificed and examined for rabies.

If postexposure prophylaxis is required, washing the wound with soap and water is the first step in management. Half the dose of rabies immune globulin should be administered in the wound site and the other half in the gluteal region. Rabies vaccine is administered the same day and given at varying time intervals. Without treatment, there is a 100% fatality rate.

147. The answer is C. *(Infectious disease; disseminated gonococcemia)*
The patient has disseminated gonococcemia and Gram-stain evidence of neutrophils with phago-

cytized gram-negative diplococci, representing *Neisseria gonorrhoeae.*

Approximately two-thirds of these cases occur in young, sexually active women. Patients present with either a septic arthritis involving the knees, wrists, or ankles or a tenosynovitis–dermatitis syndrome. *N. gonorrhoeae* is the most common cause of septic arthritis in the urban population.

The dermatitis is in the form of macules, papules, vesicles, or pustules, most commonly located on the distal extremities. Tenosynovitis often involves the fingers, wrists, knees, or ankles. There is an association with deficiencies of the terminal complement components C6 through C8. These patients are unable to mount a serum bactericidal response against gonococci or meningococci.

Hospitalization is recommended. Parenteral administration of ceftriaxone, ceftizoxime, or cefotaxime is the treatment option.

A deficiency of immunoglobulin G2 (IgG2) and IgG4 subclasses is seen in IgA deficiency. These patients are particularly prone to *Streptococcus pneumoniae* infections. Still's disease is juvenile rheumatoid arthritis. There is no relationship between this disease and disseminated gonococcemia. Reiter's syndrome is a seronegative spondyloarthropathy characterized by urethritis, conjunctivitis, and HLA B27–positive arthritis. It is associated with *Mycoplasma, Yersinia, Salmonella,* and *Shigella* infections.

148. The answer is E. *(Gynecology; androgen excess)*
Spironolactone, an aldosterone blocker, is used largely for its potassium-sparing diuretic properties. However, it also acts at the level of the hair follicle to block androgen stimulation. Prednisone and dexamethasone are both capable of suppressing adrenal androgen production but the danger of also suppressing cortisol production offsets their use in treating androgen excess. Progestogens and estrogens have no role in androgen excess treatment.

149. The answer is E. *(Hematology; chronic lymphocytic leukemia)*
This patient has chronic lymphocytic leukemia (CLL), which is the most common leukemia in patients more than 60 years of age. It is a malignancy of virgin B cells, which are long-lived, nonfunctioning lymphocytes. Clinical findings consist of generalized lymphadenopathy, hepatosplenomegaly, a predisposition for autoimmune hemolytic anemia (warm and cold types) and autoimmune thrombocytopenia, and an increased incidence of second malignancies (e.g., non-Hodgkin's lymphoma, carcinomas). Approximately 25% of patients are asymptomatic at the time of presentation.

The leukocyte count ranges from 15,000 to 200,000 cells/µl. The lymphocytes are mature in appearance and have a tendency to smudge when a peripheral smear is prepared. Approximately 50% of patients have a normocytic, normochromic anemia. Thrombocytopenia is due to either autoimmune destruction or destruction of megakaryocytes from diffuse infiltration of the bone marrow by leukemic cells. Bone marrow aspirates and biopsies reveal focal-to-diffuse infiltration by the neoplastic lymphocytes. Lymph node biopsies exhibit a diffuse, well-differentiated infiltrate that totally obscures normal nodal architecture. An immunoglobulin M (IgM) monoclonal gammopathy is frequently present. Hypogammaglobulinemia is the rule, since the virgin B cells are nonfunctional. This predisposes the patient to infections, which is the most common cause of death.

The survival of a patient with CLL depends on the stage of the disease at initial presentation. Nearly 50% of patients die of infection, most commonly pneumonia. Blast crises are extremely rare in CLL. Chemotherapy and radiation are the mainstays of therapy. Overall, the median survival of these patients is 4 to 6 years.

A positive tartrate-resistant acid phosphatase stain is present in hairy cell leukemia, which is a B-cell malignancy.

Chronic myelogenous leukemia most commonly terminates as an acute myelogenous leukemia.

Auer rods are splinter-to-rod–shaped cytoplasmic inclusions seen in myeloblasts in acute myelogenous leukemia.

150. The answer is A. *(Pediatrics; acute rheumatic fever)*

An increased anti–streptolysin O (ASO) titer is evidence of a preceding streptococcal infection but is not one of the major criteria. The major criteria are carditis, polyarthritis, chorea, subcutaneous nodule, and a rash (erythema marginatum). Minor criteria include fever, arthralgia, previous rheumatic fever, elevated acute phase reactants (erythrocyte sedimentation rate [ESR], C-reactive protein [CRP]), and prolonged P-R interval. Two major or one major and two minor criteria plus evidence of a recent streptococcal infection (e.g., elevated ASO titer) are required to consider the diagnosis of acute rheumatic fever.

151. The answer is A. *(Rheumatology; systemic lupus erythematosus)*

This patient has systemic lupus erythematosus (SLE) with a characteristic erythematous rash over both cheeks and the bridge of the nose ("butterfly" or malar rash), arthritis, and serositis manifested as pleuritis with a pleural effusion.

SLE is a connective tissue disorder resulting from an immunoregulatory disturbance of multifactorial etiology. It is thought to represent an interplay of genetic, hormonal, and environmental factors. The disturbance in the immune system results in polyclonal activation of B cells with the production of autoantibodies against DNA. Environmental factors that trigger attacks include sunlight and drugs (e.g., procainamide, hydralazine). In addition, there is increased conversion of estradiol to a metabolite with sustained estrogen activity.

Musculoskeletal disease is the most common symptom; 95% of patients present with it. Arthralgias and myalgias lead the list of musculoskeletal symptoms. Morning stiffness in the hands with symmetric fusiform swelling of the metacarpophalangeal joints and proximal interphalangeal joints occurs in 60% of patients. Unlike rheumatoid arthritis, the arthritis in SLE tends to be nonerosive and less disabling.

Cutaneous manifestations occur in 80% of cases. A butterfly rash on the face is present in up to 50% of patients. In SLE, a biopsy of uninvolved skin subjected to direct immunofluorescence (band test) reveals a band of fluorescence along the basement membrane against complement and IgG in 50% of cases. Immunofluorescence of a biopsied skin in an area of cutaneous involvement is positive in 80% to 100% of cases. In discoid lupus, which is lupus that is limited to the skin, only involved skin exhibits a positive band test.

Serositis, or inflammation of serosal surfaces, occurs in 30% to 50% of patients. Pericarditis is the most common manifestation of serositis, followed by pleuritis. The effusion is an exudate with predominantly monocytes and lymphocytes. In vivo lupus erythematosus (LE) cells are sometimes found in the inflammatory infiltrate. An LE cell is a neutrophil that has phagocytized altered DNA. Any unexplained pleural effusion in a young woman is diagnosed as SLE until proven otherwise.

Renal involvement occurs in 50% to 60% of patients. It is the most common cause of death. There is a high association of renal involvement if the patient has anti–double-stranded DNA. The majority of patients are nephritic (i.e., with hematuria, red blood cell casts, proteinuria) and have an immune complex etiology with a "lumpy-bumpy" immunofluorescent pattern.

Miscellaneous clinical findings include Libman-Sacks endocarditis, chronic interstitial lung disease, splenomegaly, generalized lymphadenopathy, central nervous system (CNS) involvement (e.g., loss of orientation, psychosis), autoimmune hematologic problems (e.g., hemolytic anemia, leukopenia, thrombocytopenia), and increased fetal wastage from anti-cardiolipin antibodies.

Corticosteroids are the mainstay of therapy. Long-term use results in osteoporosis, Cushing's syndrome, and aseptic necrosis of the femoral head.

152. The answer is A. *(Obstetrics; gestational trophoblastic disease)*

The outcome of gestational trophoblastic disease can be predicted by whether the findings fall into "good-prognosis" or "poor-prognosis" groups. Whereas 95%–100% of the former group of patients are cured, only 50%–70% of the latter are. Human chorionic gonadotropin (hCG), metastasis to the brain or liver, failure to respond to single-agent chemotherapy, and choriocarcinoma following a full-term delivery are all characteristics of the poor-prognosis group, but disease present less than 4 months from the antecedent pregnancy is not. Poor prognosis requires the disease to be present more than 4 months from the antecedent pregnancy.

153. The answer is E. *(Pediatrics; poststreptococcal glomerulonephritis)*

Edema is common to both acute poststreptococcal glomerulonephritis and minimal change disease (nephrotic syndrome). Serum albumin is decreased in minimal change disease. Red blood cell (RBC) casts are more common in glomerulonephritis. Hypertension is uncommon in minimal change disease.

154. The answer is D. *(Gynecology; cervical cancer)*

Cervical cancer is staged clinically, not surgically. Laparoscopy is a surgical procedure; therefore, it does not qualify for clinical staging.

155. The answer is B. *(Health maintenance/promotion; substance abuse)*

No studies demonstrate a strong association between therapeutic use of psychostimulants and later abuse. Although therapeutic use of opiates can lead to physical dependence, abuse rarely continues after detoxification. Peer drug use, social isolation, involvement in drug trafficking, and academic difficulties all have been identified as risk factors for substance abuse.

156. The answer is A. *(Pediatrics; complications of chickenpox)*

Secondary bacterial infection of skin lesions is the most common complication of varicella.

Thrombocytopenia can result in hemorrhages of skin and mucous membranes, but bloody diarrhea is not reported. Hemorrhagic vesicles can be seen. Encephalitis is the most common central nervous system (CNS) complication. Pneumonitis is more common in adolescents and adults than in children. Approximately 10% of cases of Reye's syndrome occur after a varicella infection.

157. The answer is E. *(Behavioral science; hospice care)*

Hospice care includes grief counseling, support groups, inpatient supportive care, and outpatient supportive care. Administration of pain medication as needed is an important concept in hospice care.

158. The answer is C. *(Gynecology; spouse abuse)*

In terms of findings in battered women, urinary tract infections are not related per se. Pelvic pain, insomnia, substance abuse, and gastrointestinal problems are signs or symptoms of battering in women.

159. The answer is B. *(Pediatrics; viral meningitis)*

Viral or aseptic meningitis usually presents with a normal to slightly elevated protein concentration. Glucose is normal as is the lactate concentration. No organisms are seen on Gram stain or routine cultures. White blood count (WBC) in the cerebrospinal fluid (CSF) is usually 100 to 700/μl, with polymorphonuclears early on, then lymphocyte predominance. Pressures are normal.

160. The answer is C. *(Hematology; iron deficiency secondary to colon cancer with metastasis to the liver)*

This 65-year-old man has iron deficiency anemia secondary to blood loss from a polypoid mass in the ascending colon, which on biopsy revealed an adenocarcinoma. In addition, there is laboratory evidence for metastasis to the liver.

Iron deficiency in a man more than 50 years of age is most likely due to colon cancer, which is the third most common cancer in men.

Carcinomas located in the right colon tend to bleed and produce iron deficiency, while those in the left tend to obstruct. A positive stood guaiac secondary to the blood loss should be expected in this patient. As the age of a patient increases, there is a higher predictive value for occult blood indicating cancer (i.e., 18% at 40–49 years versus 83% at 70+ years). Recent studies indicate a 33% reduction in the mortality rate from colorectal cancer in those patients who have a yearly stool guaiac test. Based on these studies, it is recommended that asymptomatic patients over the age of 50 years should have an annual stool guaiac and a flexible sigmoidoscopy examination every 3 to 5 years. Colonoscopy is considered the gold standard for the workup of positive stool guaiacs. Barium studies are not as sensitive in detecting colon cancer as is endoscopy performed by a skilled physician.

Serum enzyme studies in this patient reveal an increase in serum alkaline phosphatase, gamma glutamyltransferase, and lactate dehydrogenase, whereas the total bilirubin and transaminase concentrations are normal. This pattern is highly predictive for liver metastasis. Both serum alkaline phosphatase and gamma glutamyltransferase are excellent indicators of cholestasis in the presence of diffuse liver disease or focal disease in the liver due to granulomas or metastatic cancer. When tumor nodules in the liver compress the bile ducts, there is increased synthesis of alkaline phosphatase and gamma glutamyltransferase. Lactate dehydrogenase is a nonspecific enzyme marker of malignancy, since it is so widespread in tissue. The total bilirubin and transaminase levels are normal because there must be diffuse liver disease before they are increased. The increase in gamma glutamyltransferase is highly predictive of the alkaline phosphatase being of liver rather than bone origin, since gamma glutamyltransferase is not present in bone. This is a much easier way of distinguishing alkaline phosphatase of bone origin versus liver origin than is using isoenzyme analysis of alkaline phosphatase or heat stability tests.

Absolute monocytosis in this patient is due to malignancy. Monocytes are part of the immune surveillance system against tumors. Monocytosis is also a feature of chronic infections (e.g., tuberculosis) and chronic inflammation (e.g., autoimmune diseases).

161. The answer is D. *(Pediatrics; developmental defects)*

Valproic acid taken by a pregnant woman does not cause microcephaly; spina bifida and developmental delay are common effects, as are facial anomalies. Phenytoin does cause nail hypoplasia, growth retardation, and characteristic lip appearance (Cupid's bow). Isotretinoin is most teratogenic in the first trimester, and effects include brain malformations, microtia, thymic hypoplasia, and cardiac defects. Diethylstilbestrol (DES) is responsible for vaginal carcinoma and adenosis, as well as genitourinary anomalies in exposed males. Tobacco smoke is a common cause of small-for-gestational-age infants.

162. The answer is A. *(Cardiology; acute infective endocarditis)*

The patient has acute infective endocarditis due to *Staphylococcus aureus* involving the aortic valve. The high-pitched diastolic murmur between the right second and third intercostal space is aortic regurgitation. It is heard best with the patient exhaling while sitting up and leaning forward. The nail-bed finding is a splinter hemorrhage. Painful, erythematous, nodular lesions on the finger pad are called Osler's nodes. Both lesions are thought to be examples of immune complex vasculitis, although some cases of Osler's nodes are embolic in origin. Immune complexes are also operative in acute glomerulonephritis and Roth's spots in the retina, which are hemorrhages in the retinal vessels.

S. aureus is the most common organism to produce acute endocarditis. Due to its virulence, it can infect previously normal valves as well as damaged valves. There is a strong association with the presence of indwelling catheters and intravenous drug abuse. *Streptococcus viridans* is the most common pathogen in subacute bacterial endocarditis. Because it is a less virulent organism than *Staphylococcus,* it infects previously damaged valves (e.g., mitral valve in rheumatic fever). Bacterial adhesion factors, agglutinating antibodies, and the presence of platelet or fibrin deposits on these damaged valves favor infection by these organisms. Because the distinction between acute and subacute bacterial endocarditis is frequently arbitrary, the term infective endocarditis is most commonly used.

Overall, the mitral valve is most commonly involved in infective endocarditis. In intravenous drug abusers, the location is evenly split between the tricuspid and aortic valves.

Cardiac tamponade is not a feature of infective endocarditis.

Laboratory features of infective endocarditis include positive blood cultures in 95% of cases (if at least three cultures are taken 20 to 30 minutes apart) and the anemia of chronic disease.

Prophylactic antibiotics are usually administered to all patients with known valvular disease or known congenital heart disease, especially when they require dental procedures or manipulative procedures of the genitourinary tract.

The treatment of infective endocarditis is based on what organism is isolated from the blood. *S. viridans* responds to intravenous penicillin G plus gentamicin or streptomycin. Methicillin-susceptible *S. aureus* responds to intravenous nafcillin with or without gentamicin. Methicillin-resistant strains should be treated with intravenous vancomycin with or without gentamicin.

The mortality rate in subacute infective endocarditis is 10% to 20%, whereas in acute infective endocarditis it is 50%.

163. The answer is A. *(Pediatrics; fetal alcohol syndrome)*
Alcohol is the most common major teratogen to which the fetus may be exposed. Approximately one in six cases of cerebral palsy are the result of heavy alcohol exposure in utero. Full-blown fetal alcohol syndrome occurs after exposure to about 8 to 10 drinks per day, although more subtle features are seen with less intake. Findings include microcephaly, short palpebral fissures, maxillary hypoplasia, early tremors from hypoglycemia, smooth upper lip, smooth philtrum, and cardiac defects (ventricular septal defects, atrial septal defect). Average IQ is 63. The prognosis is pre-

dicted by the severity of maternal alcoholism and the pattern of malformation.

164. The answer is E. *(Gynecology; cervical conization)*
Stage IA$_2$ carcinoma is frankly invasive carcinoma. No change in treatment will be accomplished by a conization report. The other four options are appropriate indications for conization.

165. The answer is B. *(Oncology; role of tobacco in cancer)*
Tobacco has no direct or indirect effect in producing liver disease. Diseases associated with tobacco are oral, lung, laryngeal, esophageal, pancreatic, renal, cervical, and bladder cancers. Coronary artery disease, hypertension, and stroke have cardiovascular associations with smoking. Chronic obstructive pulmonary disease (COPD) and pneumonia are respiratory abnormalities associated with smoking. Sudden infant death syndrome (SIDS) and low–birth-weight infants are also associated with smoking.

166. The answer is D. *(Nutrition; role of diet in disease)*
Diet substantially contributes to the actual cause of death in coronary artery disease, strokes, hypertension, cancer (colon, breast, prostate), and diabetes mellitus. Half of all type II diabetes can be prevented by obesity control. Lack of insoluble fiber and high-fat diets have been implicated in cancer.

167. The answer is B. *(Pediatrics; pseudohypoparathyroidism)*
Patients with pseudohypoparathyroidism have normal or hyperplastic parathyroid glands that can synthesize and secrete parathormone. The disorder is associated with low calcium levels, and when calcium levels are low, parathormone levels are elevated. However, there seems to be unresponsiveness to parathormone at the receptor level, leading to hypoparathyroidism, and neither endogenous nor administered parathormone increases the calcium level. By contrast, patients

with hypoparathyroidism have a deficiency of parathormone.

168. The answer is D. *(Pharmacology; chemotherapy)*
Renal tubular injury is the dose-limiting toxicity of cisplatin, but it is largely avoided by hydration. Many effective drug-combination regimens include cisplatin, such as that with vinblastine and bleomycin (VBC) used in advanced testicular carcinoma. Sulfonamides displace methotrexate from the plasma protein binding site, causing pancytopenia. Etoposide acts mainly in late S–early G_2 phase of the cell cycle. Unfortunately, its major toxicities are to the hematopoietic and lymphoid systems.

169. The answer is B. *(Pediatrics; allergic diathesis)*
The Coombs' test is used to detect hemolytic anemia due to blood group incompatibility. The radioallergosorbent test (RAST) helps determine antigen-specific immunoglobulin E (IgE) concentrations in serum. The RAST is less sensitive than direct skin testing but brings no risk of allergic reactions. Nasal smears are an important tool because eosinophilia is common in allergic disorders. IgE levels are also increased in allergic disease.

170. The answer is B. *(Behavioral science; alcohol abuse)*
Women are less likely than men to abuse alcohol. However, alcohol use is increasing among women. Recently, the number of female smokers surpassed the number of male smokers. Women are more likely than men to visit doctors, be hospitalized, and suffer from unipolar depression.

171. The answer is D. *(Pediatrics; innocent heart murmur in children)*
Innocent murmurs are best heard in the supine position, not on the side. Innocent murmurs occur only in systole, never diastole. They are grade 1 to 2 out of a possible 6 and are commonly heard along the left sternal border in children 3 to 7 years of age. The murmur can intensify with fever or excitement or after exercise. Sitting up can make the murmur less intense. Innocent murmurs are just that—they have no cardiac significance, and treatment consists of reassurance of the parents.

172. The answer is D. *(Hematology; erythrocyte sedimentation rate)*
The erythrocyte sedimentation rate (ESR) is a measure of how fast red blood cells (RBCs) settle in a calibrated tube in millimeters/hour. If the density of RBCs is increased by an increase in gamma globulins, fibrinogen, or both, the RBCs settle faster and increase the ESR. A peripheral blood manifestation of this is rouleaux, which are RBCs stacked together like coins. Anemia enhances rouleaux formation, whereas polycythemia reduces rouleaux formation; therefore, the ESR is increased in the former and decreased in the latter. Sickle cell anemia is characterized by sickle cells in the peripheral blood that are unable to stack like coins. Therefore, the ESR is decreased. ESR is the screening test for temporal arteritis. If the ESR is elevated, and temporal arteritis is suspected, the patient should be started on prednisone to reduce the potential for blindness. A normal ESR effectively rules out the disease.

173. The answer is E. *(Rheumatology; Sjögren's syndrome with rheumatoid arthritis)*
The patient has severe rheumatoid arthritis (RA) involving both hands. An ulcer is present on the right fifth metacarpophalangeal (MCP; knuckle) joint. There is ulnar deviation of both hands and enlargement of the MCP and proximal interphalangeal (PIP) joints. Rheumatoid nodules extend in chain-like fashion down both forearms. The ulcer on the lower leg most likely represents rheumatoid vasculitis, which is commonly associated with high titer of rheumatoid factor.

RA is a chronic, systemic inflammatory disease that increases with age and is more prevalent in females. RA results in progressive destruction of the joint space accompanied by deformity and eventual disability in some patients.

The pathogenesis of RA is primarily immunologic. It involves an interplay of CD4 helper T cells, macrophages, and neutrophils and the release of inflammatory mediators as well as immune complex formation and deposition in synovial tissue. Neutrophils with phagocytized immune complexes in the cytoplasm are called ragocytes. Inflammation begins in the synovial tissue, which eventually proliferates and migrates over the articular surface with destruction of cartilage and bone. This is called a pannus. Reactive fibrosis eventually ankyloses the joint.

The disease begins with the insidious onset of morning stiffness lasting over 1 hour. This occurs most commonly in the hands, wrists, and foot joints. In the hands, it produces symmetric involvement of the MCP and PIP joints. In addition, there is ulnar deviation of the hands secondary to the laxity of the surrounding soft tissue. Radiologic findings in the hand include the presence of marginal bone erosions where pannus has destroyed bone, narrowing of the joint space from destruction of the articular cartilage, and fusion (ankylosis) of the joint in severe cases.

RA in the neck frequently involves the atlantoaxial joint, which can produce subluxation, which, in turn, could produce compression of the vertebral artery and vertebrobasilar insufficiency.

RA involving the knee is sometimes associated with formation of a synovial cyst in the popliteal fossa. This is called a Baker's cyst.

Nonsteroidal anti-inflammatory agents and salicylates are the first-line drugs. Methotrexate, gold salts, antimalarials (e.g., hydroxychloroquine), and penicillamine are used if the initial therapy is unsuccessful. Physical therapy is extremely important in order to prevent ankylosis of the involved joints.

174. The answer is B. (*Pediatrics; acquired immune deficiency syndrome*)
At least 75% of cases of pediatric acquired immune deficiency syndrome (AIDS) are perinatally acquired. Risk factors include maternal history of AIDS and intravenous drug abuse by the mother. Although all infants of mothers with AIDS test human immunodeficiency virus (HIV)-positive, this result usually represents passive transmission of maternal antibody and not actual infection. From 60% to 80% of antibody-

positive cases of HIV are just that—the test reverts to negative with time, and the children show no sign of infection. Neonatal AIDS infection presents as failure to thrive, with pneumonia and hepatosplenomegaly. Chronic candidiasis is common, as well as recurrent infections. Kaposi's sarcoma is unusual, occurring in fewer than 10% of cases.

175. The answer is A. (*Behavioral sciences; patient consent*)
Although informed consent must be obtained before any medical procedure, a formal document is not strictly required. For informed consent, a patient must understand the diagnosis, treatment, alternatives to treatment, and benefits as well as risks of a procedure. The patient must also understand that consent can be withdrawn at any time.

176. The answer is D. (*Pediatrics; generalized clonic–tonic seizures*)
The postictal phase of generalized tonic–clonic seizures lasts approximately 30 minutes to 2 hours. The actual seizure consists of loss of consciousness, followed by the eyes rolling back and tonic contractions. The clonic phase then ensues. Frequently, the patients bite their tongues. Urinary incontinence is common.

177. The answer is D. (*Gastroenterology; bile salt deficiency and malabsorption*)
Because cholesterol cannot be degraded by the liver, it is either solubilized in bile and excreted or converted into the primary bile acids, cholic acid and chenodeoxycholic acid. The primary bile acids are conjugated to glycine and taurine to form the bile salts, glycocholic acid and taurochenodeoxycholic acid. Bile salts are more effective than primary bile acids as detergents. They aggregate to form micelles in the small intestine, allowing fatty acids and 2-monoglycerides to enter these micelles for ease in absorption by the villi. Some of the bile salts in the intestine are deconjugated by bacteria into the secondary bile acids, deoxycholic acid and lithocholic acid. Approximately 95% of the primary (conjugated) bile salts and deoxycholic acid are

reabsorbed in the terminal ileum and recycled back to the liver.

Pancreatic insufficiency would not be expected to interfere with the bile salt pool. Deficiency of lipase results in maldigestion of long-chain saturated fatty acids; therefore, products such as fatty acids and 2-monoglycerides are not present in sufficient amounts to be taken up by the micelles formed by bile salts.

In cirrhosis of the liver, a decrease in the synthesis of primary bile salts accompanies an inability to recycle secondary bile acids and primary bile salts from the terminal ileum.

Crohn's disease is an inflammatory bowel disease that involves the terminal ileum in up to 80% of patients, either alone (30%) or in combination with colonic disease (50%). Recycling of primary bile salts and deoxycholic acid would be decreased owing to inflammation of the terminal ileum.

Diverticular disease of the small bowel predisposes to bacterial overgrowth, which causes a proportionately greater-than-normal deconjugation of the primary bile salts into secondary bile acids. This deconjugation interferes with micellarization and decreases the overall bile salt pool, because only conjugated primary bile salts and deoxycholic acid are normally reabsorbed. In addition, the increased secondary bile acids are thought to damage the mucosal surface of the bowel, and this damage also contributes to malabsorption.

Cholestyramine binds bile salts, an action that decreases the total bile salt pool. This decrease increases the uptake of cholesterol by the liver to replace the depleted bile salt pool, lowering the cholesterol level in the blood.

178. The answer is C. *(Pediatrics; Wilms' tumor)*
Wilms' tumor is the most common renal neoplasm in children. Prognosis depends on staging; the 4-year relapse-free survival rate ranges from 73% to 96.5%. Wilms' tumor is associated with congenital anomalies. Aniridia occurs in 1.1% of patients; a deletion in chromosome 11 was found in family members of children with aniridia and Wilms' tumor. Wilms' tumor usually presents as a unilateral abdominal mass, often discovered by the parent or during a routine physical examination. Diagnosis is usually made when the child is approximately 3 years of age. Hypertension is seen in approximately 60% of patients. Lung metastases are seen in 5% to 10% of patients at the time of diagnosis. Treatment is surgical removal, followed by chemotherapy, and occasionally radiotherapy.

179. The answer is C. *(Cardiology; treatment of left-heart failure)*
This patient has left-sided heart failure, based on the presence of dyspnea with exertion, the history of breathlessness at night, a third heart sound (the most common cardiac finding in heart failure), and rales in the lungs. The absence of jugular venous distention and peripheral edema excludes right-sided heart failure at this point. The marked breathlessness that the patient is experiencing is called paroxysmal nocturnal dyspnea. It occurs in left-sided heart failure when patients lie flat in bed at night. Excess venous return to the right side of the heart increases the load on the failed left side, resulting in the feeling of suffocation as blood builds up in the lungs. Patients frequently sleep using several pillows to elevate the head, which improves venous return to the heart and relieves the dyspnea. Dyspnea that occurs in the recumbent position and can be relieved by elevation of the head is called orthopnea.

Bed rest used to be a cornerstone of therapy in congestive heart failure, but is now thought to reduce exercise tolerance. Therefore, a carefully planned exercise program to increase exercise tolerance is an important part of therapy. Weight loss, cessation of smoking, and dietary restriction of salt are useful adjuncts to therapy. Diuretics are extremely useful in the setting of pulmonary congestion (as in this patient) and in peripheral edema from right-sided heart failure. Thiazide diuretics can be used in mild cases or loop diuretics, such as furosemide, in more advanced cases. Vasodilator therapy is a more recent advance in the treatment of congestive heart failure. Two regimens include the use of hydralazine and isosorbide dinitrate or captopril, an angiotensin converting enzyme (ACE) inhibitor. Vasodilatation decreases the afterload, which increases cardiac output. Because captopril blocks the renin–angiotensin–aldosterone circuit, angiotensin II levels are decreased, reducing vascular constriction and decreasing the afterload, and aldosterone levels are decreased, lowering volume overload (preload).

180. The answer is B. *(Pediatrics; viruses causing congenital abnormalities)*
Rubeola, or measles, is not associated with congenital abnormalities. Congenital varicella can be acquired early or late in pregnancy. If acquired in the first half of pregnancy, it may cause limb hypoplasia, microcephaly, seizures, and cataracts in the newborn. If transmitted in the last 3 weeks of pregnancy, varicella can be mild or involve fever and pneumonia. Congenital rubella syndrome occurs after German measles infection during pregnancy and causes a variety of congenital malformations. Cytomegalovirus (CMV) is associated with microcephaly, intracranial calcifications, seizures, and mental retardation in the newborn. Congenital herpes simplex virus infections can manifest as skin, central nervous system (CNS), or disseminated disease.

181. The answer is E. *(Behavioral science; involuntary treatment)*
In order to be committed for involuntary treatment, an individual must be both mentally ill and a danger to himself or others. The homeless schizophrenic man is not necessarily a danger. The depressed man who says he will commit suicide, the schizophrenic man who has threatened to kill his parents, the borderline patient who has threatened to kill his psychiatrist, and the Alzheimer's patient who regularly starts fires in his apartment are dangerous to themselves or others.

182. The answer is E. *(Pediatrics; febrile seizures)*
Febrile seizures rarely progress to epilepsy. They do, however, have a 50% chance of recurrence. Seizures are rare before 9 months or after 5 years of age, with a peak onset between 14 and 18 months. There is usually a strong family history of febrile seizures. Seizures are generalized, tonic–clonic, and usually last no longer than 15 minutes. The seizure is associated with a rapidly rising temperature, and often there is an associated viral infection or otitis media. Treatment consists of antipyretics.

183. The answer is C. *(Health maintenance/promotion; child abuse)*
Contrary to popular wisdom, only the minority of childhood sexual abuse is perpetrated by fathers and stepfathers. However, the abuser is often another relative or family friend.

184. The answer is C. *(Pediatrics; child abuse)*
Single parents are not any more likely to abuse their children then their married counterparts. Child abuse is any maltreatment of children or adolescents by their parents or caretakers. Approximately 4000 children die each year from abuse. Fatal abuse is more commonly associated with male than female caretakers. Poverty is one of the most important factors predisposing to abuse. Other factors include unwanted pregnancies, young parents, and socially and economically deprived parents. Many abusive parents were themselves abused as children. Spouse abuse doubles the chances of child abuse. Handicapped children are also more likely to be abused.

185. The answer is E. *(Gynecology; menopause)*
Menopause is the cessation of menses. Plasma levels of follicle-stimulating hormone (FSH) rise with advancing reproductive age. Vaginal epithelium atrophies, as do paravaginal tissues; therefore, some women develop a cystocele with loss of bladder support. Likewise, uterine leiomyomata usually atrophy with menopause, probably because of falling estrogen stimulation.

186. The answer is A. *(Pediatrics; Apgar score)*
Blood pressure is not a part of the Apgar score. The Apgar score is used as an immediate cardiorespiratory assessment of the newborn. A score of 0, 1, or 2 is given at 1 and 5 minutes after birth. Scores can also be given at succeeding 5-minute intervals to aid in evaluating efforts at resuscitation. Parameters observed are heart rate,

muscle tone, respiratory effort, response to catheter in the nose, and color.

187–190. The answers are: 187-F, 188-B, 189-H, 190-F. *(Neurology; stroke)*
Right–left disorientation is seen with damage to the dominant parietal lobe.

In Broca's (expressive) aphasia, caused by damage to the dominant frontal lobe, a patient can understand speech but is unable to speak himself.

This patient is probably suffering from transcortical aphasia because both speech and comprehension are impaired. This condition is caused by damage to the temporal–occipital–parietal junction.

Dyscalculia (i.e., problems doing mathematical calculations) is caused by damage to the dominant parietal lobe.

191–192. The answers are: 191-A, 192-E. *(Pharmacology; coagulation)*
Tissue plasminogen activator, produced by recombinant technology, preferentially activates plasminogen bound to fibrin, confining fibrinolysis to the formed thrombus and avoiding systemic activation. Aminocaproic acid competitively inhibits plasminogen activation. Anistreplase is an acylated plasminogen streptokinase-activated complex (APSAC) with strong thrombolytic activity, but is potentially antigenic due to the presence of bacterial protein.

Low doses of aspirin [acetylsalicylic acid (ASA)] inhibit platelet activation. The mechanism involves irreversible inhibition of platelet cyclooxygenase, which results in decreased formation of thromboxane (TX) A_2, an endogenous platelet activator. Basing its decision on results from a number of clinical studies, the Food and Drug Administration (FDA) approved the use of ASA at a dose of 325 mg/day for primary prophylaxis of myocardial infarction.

193–195. The answers are: 193-A, 194-G, 195-E. *(Psychiatry; psychological assessments)*
Because it is an objective paper and pencil test, the Minnesota Multiphasic Personality Inventory

(MMPI) can be used by a primary care physician to evaluate psychologic states in patients.

The Wide-Range Achievement Test (WRAT) is frequently used in medicine to evaluate achievement in areas in which a person has been instructed, for example, spelling, reading, and arithmetic.

The Halstead-Reitan Battery (HRB) is a neuropsychological test used to detect the presence of and to localize brain lesions.

196–198. The answers are: 196-E, 197-A, 198-C. *(Pharmacology; antihyperlipidemics)*
The primary action of gemfibrozil (and clofibrate) is to activate lipoprotein lipases in peripheral tissues. These drugs are most effective in hyperlipidemias characterized by elevated plasma very low-density lipoprotein (VLDL) levels, such as familial hypertriglyceridemia and dysbetalipoproteinemia. Gastrointestinal distress and myalgia occur with gemfibrozil and clofibrate, and both potentiate the actions of coumarin anticoagulants.

Several drugs that inhibit 3-hydroxy-3-methylglutaryl-coenzyme A (HMG-CoA) reductase, the first committed step in sterol biosynthesis, are now available for clinical use; the drugs include lovastatin and pravastin sodium. This action leads to increases in high-affinity low-density lipoprotein (LDL) receptors in hepatocytes, with increased clearance of LDL and VLDL from the plasma. Monitoring serum transaminases during lovastatin treatment is advised because the drug has hepatotoxic potential. In addition, lovastatin has caused muscle pain and myopathy, especially in patients taking cyclosporine, erythromycin, and other antihyperlipidemics.

The bile resins cholestyramine and colestipol block the jejunal reabsorption of bile acids, increasing their fecal excretion 10-fold. This increased bile acid excretion leads to increased catabolism of cholesterol (because of the necessity of synthesizing new bile acids) and to decreased plasma LDL because of the induction of tissue LDL receptors. These agents are useful only in hyperlipidemias involving elevated levels of LDL. Cholestyramine may interfere with gastrointestinal absorption of folic acid, vitamin K, and many drugs, including digitalis, thiazide diuretics, and warfarin.

199–200. The answers are: 199-C, 200-B.
(Psychiatry; mood disorder diagnosis)
Cyclothymia (graph B) is characterized by numerous periods of hypomanic symptoms followed by numerous periods of depressive symptoms. During none of these episodes do patients have full mania or depression. Cycling is often rapid.

The clinical course of bipolar II disorder (graph B) is characterized by depressive episodes and one or more periods of hypomania.

Bipolar I disorder (graph D) includes both manic and depressive episodes. Graph A represents major recurrent depression. Graph E represents dysthymia